Case Files™:
Family Medicine

NOTICE

Medicine is an ever-changing science. As new research and clinical experience broaden our knowledge, changes in treatment and drug therapy are required. The authors and the publisher of this work have checked with sources believed to be reliable in their efforts to provide information that is complete and generally in accord with the standard accepted at the time of publication. However, in view of the possibility of human error or changes in medical sciences, neither the editors nor the publisher nor any other party who has been involved in the preparation or publication of this work warrants that the information contained herein is in every respect accurate or complete, and they disclaim all responsibility for any errors or omissions or for the results obtained from use of the information contained in this work. Readers are encouraged to confirm the information contained herein with other sources. For example and in particular, readers are advised to check the product information sheet included in the package of each drug they plan to administer to be certain that the information contained in this work is accurate and that changes have not been made in the recommended dose or in the contraindications for administration. This recommendation is of particular importance in connection with new or infrequently used drugs.

Case Files™:
Family Medicine

EUGENE C. TOY, MD
The John S. Dunn, Senior Academic Chair
and Program Director
The Methodist Hospital-Houston OB/GYN
Residency Program, Houston, TX
Clerkship Director, Associate Clinical Professor
Department of Obstetrics and Gynecology
University of Texas
Medical School at Houston
Houston, Texas

DONALD BRISCOE, MD
Program Director
The Methodist Hospital–Houston Family Medicine
Residency Program
Houston, Texas

CARLOS A. DUMAS, MD
Assistant Professor
Department of Family Medicine
University of Texas
Medical School at Houston
Houston, Texas

JOE A. BEDFORD, MD
Associate Professor
Department of Family Medicine
University of Texas
Medical School at Houston
Houston, Texas

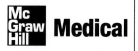

Mc
Graw
Hill **Medical**

New York   Chicago   San Francisco
Lisbon   London   Madrid   Mexico City
Milan   New Delhi   San Juan   Seoul
Singapore   Sydney   Toronto

Case Files™: Family Medicine

Copyright © 2007 by The McGraw-Hill Companies, Inc. All rights reserved. Printed in the United States of America. Except as permitted under the United States Copyright Act of 1976, no part of this publication may be reproduced or distributed in any form or by any means, or stored in a data base or retrieval system, without the prior written permission of the publisher.

Case Files™ is a trademark of The McGraw-Hill Companies, Inc.

3 4 5 6 7 8 9 0   FGR/FGR   0 9 8 7

ISBN 13: 978-0-07-147188-6
ISBN 10: 0-07-147188-X

This book was set in Times Roman by International Typesetting and Composition.
The editors were Marsha Loeb and Christie Naglieri.
The production supervisor was Catherine Saggese.
The cover designer was Aimee Nordin.
The index was prepared by Robert Swanson.
Quebecor World/Fairfield was printer and binder.

This book is printed on acid-free paper.

Cataloging-in-Publication Data is on file with the Library of Congress

International Edition ISBN 13: 978-0-07-110467-8; ISBN 10: 0-07-110467-4

Copyright © 2007. Exclusive rights by The McGraw-Hill Companies, Inc., for manufacture and export. This book cannot be re-exported from the country to which it is consigned by McGraw-Hill. The International Edition is not available in North America.

❖ DEDICATION

To my dearest brothers and sisters of the Partners of Faith class of Garden Oaks Baptist Church: who offer friendship and encouragement of the deepest nature.

—ECT

To Cal, Casey, and Heather.

—DB

This book is dedicated to past, current, and future residents. Their daily input and challenging questions certainly help to improve patient care.

—CD

❖ CONTENTS

❖ CONTRIBUTORS

Wael Aboughali, MD
Instructor
Department of Family and Community Medicine
The University of Texas–Houston Medical School
Houston, Texas
Approach to Asthma and Allergies
Approach to Respiratory Tract Infections
Approach to Depression

Olasunkanmi W. Adeyinka, MD
Assistant Professor
Department of Family and Community Medicine
The University of Texas–Houston Medical School
Houston, Texas
Approach to HIV/AIDS

Michael Altman, MD
Assistant Professor
Department of Family and Community Medicine
The University of Texas–Houston Medical School
Houston, Texas
Approach to Arrhythmia

Rolf Montalvo-Chen, MD
Chief Resident
Department of Family and Community Medicine
The University of Texas–Houston Medical School
Houston, Texas
Approach to Joint Pain
Approach to Abdominal Pain in Children

Ricca Dimalibot, MD
Resident
Department of Family Medicine
Methodist Hospital–Family Medicine Residency Program
Houston, Texas
Approach to Postoperative Fever
Approach to Wheezing in Children

Carrie L. Dodrill, PhD
Assistant Professor
Department of Family and Community Medicine
The University of Texas–Houston Medical School
Houston, Texas
Approach to Substance Abuse

Ajit Dwividi, MD
Resident Physician
Department of Family and Community Medicine
The University of Texas–Houston Medical School
Houston, Texas
Approach to Bowel Movement

Neeta Gautam, MD
Faculty
Department of Family Medicine
Methodist Hospital–Family Medicine Residency Program
Houston, Texas
Approach to Tobacco Use
Adult Female Health Maintenance

Orlando D. Gutierrez, MD
Chief Resident
Department of Family and Community Medicine
The University of Texas–Houston Medical School
Houston, Texas
Approach to GI Bleeding
Approach to Congestive Heart Failure

Jaime Hurtado, MD
Resident
Department of Family and Community Medicine
The University of Texas–Houston Medical School
Houston, Texas
Approach to TIA and Stroke

Vijaya L. Mallela, MD
Assistant Professor
Department of Family and Community Medicine
The University of Texas–Health Science Center
Houston, Texas
Approach to Pneumonia

David Michalak, MD
Resident
Department of Family Medicine
Methodist Hospital–Family Medicine Residency Program
Houston, Texas
Approach to Skin Lesions
Approach to Calcium Disorders

Jana Miller, MD
Assistant Professor
Department of Family and Community Medicine
The University of Texas–Houston Medical School
Houston, Texas
Approach to Chest Pain

Phuc Duc Nguyen, MD
Assistant Clinical Professor
Department of Family and Community Medicine
The University of Texas–Houston Medical School
Houston, Texas
Approach to Geriatric Health Maintenance
Approach to Family Planning

Anush Pillai, MD
Faculty
Department of Family Medicine
Methodist Hospital FMRP
Approach to Prenatal Care
Approach to Hematuria

Bal Reddy, MD
Assistant Professor
Department of Family and Community Medicine
The University of Texas–Houston Medical School
Houston, Texas
Approach to Thyroid Disease
Approach to Vaginitis
Approach to Headache

Yogesh Reddy, MD
Resident
Department of Family and Community Medicine
The University of Texas–Houston Medical School
Houston, Texas
Approach to Bites

Julia Reyser, MD
Assistant Professorr
Department of Family and Community Medicine
The University of Texas–Houston Medical School
Houston, Texas
Approach to Dementia

Nahid Rianon, MD
Chief Resident
Department of Family and Community Medicine
The University of Texas–Houston Health Science Center
Houston, Texas
Approach to Anemia

Angela Stotts, PhD
Assistant Professor
Department of Family and Community Medicine
The University of Texas–Houston Medical School
Houston, Texas
Approach to Substance Abuse

Terah Tower, MD
Instructor
Department of Family and Community Medicine
The University of Texas–Houston Medical School
Houston, Texas
Approach to Chronic Kidney Disease

Deepa Vasudevan, MD
Assistant Professor
Department of Family and Community Medicine
The University of Texas–Houston Medical School
Houston, Texas
Approach to Obesity

Carman Hall Whiting, MD
Assistant Professor
Department of Family and Community Medicine
The University of Texas–Houston Health Science Center
Houston, Texas
Approach to Ethics

❖ ACKNOWLEDGMENTS

The curriculum that evolved into the ideas for this series was inspired by two talented and forthright students, Philbert Yau and Chuck Rosipal, who have since graduated from medical school. It has been a pleasure to work with Dr. Don Briscoe, a brilliant, compassionate and dedicated teacher and leader, and Dr. Carlos A. Dumas, who is eloquent and well spoken. Likewise, it has been a pleasure to work with my good friend, Dr. Joseph Bedford, who has trained countless medical students in family medicine. I am greatly indebted to my editor, Catherine Johnson, who is now twice a mother, and whose exuberance, experience, and vision helped to shape this series. I appreciate McGraw-Hill's believing in the concept of teaching through clinical cases, and I would like to especially acknowledge Marsha Loeb and Christie Naglieri for the excellent editing and Catherine Saggese and Gita Raman for their fantastic production skills. I appreciate Dottie Mersinger and Jo McMains for their sage advice and support. At the Methodist Hospital, I thank Dr. Marc Boom, Dr. Dirk Sostman, Dr. Judy Paukert, Dr. Alan Kaplan, and Mr. John N. Lyle VII for their phenomenal encouragement. I appreciate Hospital Partners of America, especially Todd Johnson, Stephen Puckett, Terry Linn, Phil Robinson, Laura Fortin, Pat Mathews, and Janet Matthews who have provided a bright future for our hospital and residency. Most of all, I appreciate my ever-loving wife Terri, and four wonderful children, Andy, Michael, Allison, and Christina for their patience, encouragement, and understanding.

Eugene C. Toy, MD

❖ INTRODUCTION

Mastering the cognitive knowledge within a field such as family medicine is a formidable task. It is even more difficult to draw on that knowledge, procure and filter through the clinical and laboratory data, develop a differential diagnosis, and, finally, to form a rational treatment plan. To gain these skills, the student often learns best at the bedside, guided and instructed by experienced teachers, and inspired toward self-directed, diligent reading. Clearly, there is no replacement for education at the bedside. Unfortunately, clinical situations usually do not encompass the breadth of the specialty. Perhaps the best alternative is a carefully crafted patient case designed to stimulate the clinical approach and decision making. In an attempt to achieve that goal, we have constructed a collection of clinical vignettes to teach diagnostic or therapeutic approaches that are relevant to family medicine. Most importantly, the explanations for the cases emphasize the mechanisms and underlying principles, rather than merely rote questions and answers.

This book is organized for versatility: to allow the student "in a rush" to go quickly through the scenarios and check the corresponding answers, as well as enable the student who wants thought-provoking explanations to take a slower path. The answers are arranged from simple to complex: a summary of the pertinent points, the bare answers, an analysis of the case, an approach to the topic, a comprehension test at the end for reinforcement and emphasis, and a list of resources for further reading. The clinical vignettes are purposely placed in random order to simulate the way that real patients present to the practitioner. Section III includes a listing of cases to aid the student who desires to test his/her knowledge of a certain area, or to review a topic including basic definitions. Finally, we intentionally did not primarily use a multiple choice question (MCQ) format because clues (or distractions) are not available in the real world. Nevertheless, several MCQs are included at the end of each scenario to reinforce concepts or introduce related topics.

HOW TO GET THE MOST OUT OF THIS BOOK

Each case is designed to simulate a patient encounter with open-ended questions. At times, the patient's complaint is different from the most concerning issue, and sometimes extraneous information is given. The answers are organized with four different parts.

PART I

1. The **Summary** identifies the salient aspects of the case, filtering out the extraneous information. The student should formulate his/her summary from the case before looking at the answers. A comparison to the summation in the answer will help to improve one's ability to focus on the important data, while appropriately discarding the irrelevant information, a fundamental skill in clinical problem solving.

2. A **straightforward answer** is given to each open-ended question.

3. The **Analysis of the Case**, which is comprised of two parts:
   a. **Objectives** of the Case—a listing of the two or three main principles that are crucial for a practitioner in managing the patient. Again, the student is challenged to make educated "guesses" about the objectives of the case upon initial review of the case scenario, which help to sharpen his/her clinical and analytical skills.
   b. **Considerations**—a discussion of the relevant points and a brief approach to the specific patient.

PART II

The **Approach to the Disease Process** has two distinct parts:

1. **Definitions or pathophysiology**—terminology or basic science correlates that are pertinent to the disease process; and

2. **Clinical Approach**—a discussion of the approach to the clinical problem in general, including tables, figures, and algorithms.

PART III

The **Comprehension Questions** for each case is composed of several multiple-choice questions that either reinforce the material or introduce new and related concepts. Questions about material not found in the text have explanations in the answers.

PART IV

Clinical Pearls are a listing of several clinically important points that summarize the text, and allow for easy review of the material, such as before an examination.

SECTION I

How to Approach Clinical Problems

PART 1. APPROACH TO THE PATIENT

Applying "book learning" to a specific clinical situation is one the most challenging tasks in medicine. To do so, the clinician must not only retain information, organize facts, and recall large amounts of data but also apply all of
this to the patient. The purpose of this text is to facilitate this process.

The first step involves gathering information, also known as establishing
the database. This includes taking the history, performing the physical examination, and obtaining selective laboratory examinations, special studies, and/or
imaging tests. Sensitivity and respect should always be exercised during the
interview of patients. A good clinician also knows how to ask the same question
in several different ways, using different terminology. For example, patients may
deny having "congestive heart failure" but will answer affirmatively to being
treated for "fluid on the lungs."

> ## CLINICAL PEARL
>
> ❖ The history is usually the single most important tool in obtaining a
>   diagnosis. The art of seeking this information in a nonjudgmental,
>   sensitive, and thorough manner cannot be overemphasized.

History

1. Basic Information:
   a. Age: Some conditions are more common at certain ages; for instance,
      chest pain in an elderly patient is more worrisome for coronary
      artery disease than the same complaint in a teenager.
   b. Gender: Some disorders are more common in men, such as abdominal
      aortic aneurysms. In contrast, women more commonly have autoim-
      mune problems, such as chronic idiopathic thrombocytopenic purpura
      or systemic lupus erythematosus. Also, the possibility of pregnancy
      must be considered in any woman of child-bearing age.
   c. Ethnicity: Some disease processes are more common in certain
      ethnic groups (such as type II diabetes mellitus in the Hispanic
      population).

> ## CLINICAL PEARL
>
> ❖ Family Medicine illustrates the importance of longitudinal care;
>   that is, seeing the patient in various phases and stages of life.

2. Chief Complaint: What is it that brought the patient into the hospital? Has there been a change in a chronic or recurring condition or is this a completely new problem? The duration and character of the complaint, associated symptoms, and exacerbating/relieving factors should be recorded. The chief complaint engenders a differential diagnosis, and the possible etiologies should be explored by further inquiry.

CLINICAL PEARL

❖ The first line of any presentation should include *Age, Ethnicity, Gender, Marital Status, and Chief Complaint.* Example: A 32-year-old married White male complains of lower abdominal pain of 8 hours' duration.

---

3. Past Medical History:
   a. Major illnesses such as hypertension, diabetes, reactive airway disease, congestive heart failure, angina, or stroke should be detailed.
      i. Age of onset, severity, end-organ involvement
      ii. Medications taken for the particular illness, including any recent changes to medications and reason for the change(s).
      iii. Last evaluation of the condition (for example: When was the last stress test or cardiac catheterization performed in the patient with angina?)
      iv. Which physician or clinic is following the patient for the disorder?
   b. Minor illnesses such as recent upper respiratory infections.
   c. Hospitalizations no matter how trivial should be queried.

4. Past Surgical History: Date and type of procedure performed, indication, and outcome. Laparoscopy versus laparotomy should be distinguished. Surgeon and hospital name/location should be listed. This information should be correlated with the surgical scars on the patient's body. Any complications should be delineated including anesthetic complications, difficult intubations, etc.

5. Allergies: Reactions to medications should be recorded, including severity and temporal relationship to medication. Immediate hypersensitivity should be distinguished from an adverse reaction.

6. Medications: A list of medications, dosage, route of administration and frequency, and duration of use should be developed. Prescription, over-the-counter, and herbal remedies are all relevant. If the patient is currently taking antibiotics, it is important to note what type of infection is being treated.

7. Immunization History: Vaccination and prevention of disease is a principal goal of the family physician; hence, recording the immunizations received including dates, age, route, and adverse reactions, if any, is critical.

8. Screening History: Cost-effective surveillance for common diseases or malignancy is another cornerstone responsibility of the family physician. An organized record-keeping is important to a time-efficient approach to this area.

9. Social History: Occupation, marital status, family support, and tendencies toward depression or anxiety are important. Use or abuse of illicit drugs, tobacco, or alcohol should also be recorded.

10. Family History: Many major medical problems are genetically transmitted (e.g., hemophilia, sickle cell disease). In addition, a family history of conditions such as breast cancer and ischemic heart disease can be a risk factor for the development of these diseases. Social history, including marital stressors, sexual dysfunction, and sexual preference, are of importance.

11. Review of Systems: A systematic review should be performed but focused on the life-threatening and the more common diseases. For example, in a young man with a testicular mass, trauma to the area, weight loss, and infectious symptoms are important to note. In an elderly woman with generalized weakness, symptoms suggestive of cardiac disease should be elicited, such as chest pain, shortness of breath, fatigue, or palpitations.

Physical Examination

1. General Appearance: mental status, alert versus obtunded, anxious, in pain, in distress, interaction with other family members and with examiner.

2. Vital Signs: Record the temperature, blood pressure, heart rate and respiratory rate. An oxygen saturation is useful in patients with respiratory symptoms. Height and weight are often placed here with a body mass index calculated (weight in kg/height in m squared = kg/m^2).

3. Head and Neck Examination: Evidence of trauma, tumors, facial edema, goiter and thyroid nodules, and carotid bruits should be sought. In patients with altered mental status or a head injury, pupillary size, symmetry, and reactivity are important. Mucous membranes should be inspected for pallor, jaundice, and evidence of dehydration. Cervical and supraclavicular nodes should be palpated.

4. Breast Examination: Inspection for symmetry and skin or nipple retraction, as well as palpation for masses. The nipple should be assessed for discharge, and the axillary and supraclavicular regions should be examined.

5. Cardiac Examination: The point of maximal impulse (PMI) should be ascertained, and the heart auscultated at the apex and base. It is important to note whether the auscultated rhythm is regular or irregular. Heart sounds (including S_3 and S_4), murmurs, clicks, and rubs should be characterized. Systolic flow murmurs are fairly common as a result of the increased cardiac output, but significant diastolic murmurs are unusual.

6. Pulmonary Examination: The lung fields should be examined systematically and thoroughly. Stridor, wheezes, rales, and rhonchi should be recorded. The clinician should also search for evidence of consolidation (bronchial breath sounds, egophony) and increased work of breathing (retractions, abdominal breathing, accessory muscle use).

7. Abdominal Examination: The abdomen should be inspected for scars, distension, masses, and discoloration. For instance, the Grey-Turner sign of bruising at the flank areas may indicate intraabdominal or retroperitoneal hemorrhage. Auscultation should identify normal versus high-pitched and hyperactive versus hypoactive bowel sounds. The abdomen should be percussed for the presence of shifting dullness (indicating ascites). Then careful palpation should begin away from the area of pain and progress to include the whole abdomen to assess for tenderness, masses, organomegaly (i.e., spleen or liver), and peritoneal signs. Guarding and whether it is voluntary or involuntary should be noted.

8. Back and Spine Examination: The back should be assessed for symmetry, tenderness, and masses. The flank regions particularly are important to assess for pain on percussion that may indicate renal disease.

9. Genital Examination
   a. Female: The external genitalia should be inspected, then the speculum used to visualize the cervix and vagina. A bimanual examination should attempt to elicit cervical motion tenderness, uterine size, and ovarian masses or tenderness.
   b. Male: The penis should be examined for hypospadias, lesions, and discharge. The scrotum should be palpated for tenderness and masses. If a mass is present, it can be transilluminated to distinguish

between solid and cystic masses. The groin region should be carefully palpated for bulging (hernias) upon rest and provocation (coughing, standing).

c. Rectal examination: A rectal examination will reveal masses in the posterior pelvis and may identify gross or occult blood in the stool. In females, nodularity and tenderness in the uterosacral ligament may be signs of endometriosis. The posterior uterus and palpable masses in the cul-de-sac may be identified by rectal examination. In the male, the prostate gland should be palpated for tenderness, nodularity, and enlargement.

10. Extremities/Skin: The presence of joint effusions, tenderness, rashes, edema, and cyanosis should be recorded. It is also important to note capillary refill and peripheral pulses.

11. Neurologic Examination: Patients who present with neurologic complaints require a thorough assessment including mental status, cranial nerves, strength, sensation, reflexes, and cerebellar function.

CLINICAL PEARL

A thorough understanding of functional anatomy is important to optimally interpret the physical examination findings.

12. Laboratory Assessment Depends on the Circumstances.
    a. CBC, or complete blood count, can assess for anemia, leukocytosis (infection), and thrombocytopenia.
    b. Basic metabolic panel: electrolytes, glucose, BUN (blood urea nitrogen), and creatinine (renal function).
    c. Urinalysis and/or urine culture to assess for hematuria, pyuria, or bacteriuria. A pregnancy test is important in women of child-bearing age.
    d. Aspartate aminotransferase (AST), alanine aminotransferase (ALT), bilirubin, alkaline phosphatase for liver function; amylase and lipase to evaluate the pancreas.
    e. Cardiac markers (creatine kinase myocardial band [CK-MB], troponin, myoglobin) if coronary artery disease or other cardiac dysfunction is suspected.
    f. Drug levels such as acetaminophen level **in possible overdoses.**
    g. Arterial blood gas measurements give information about oxygenation, but also carbon dioxide and pH readings.

13. Diagnostic Adjuncts
    a. Electrocardiogram if cardiac ischemia, dysrhythmia, or other car-
        diac dysfunction is suspected.
    b. Ultrasound examination is useful in evaluating pelvic processes in
        female patients (e.g., pelvic inflammatory disease, tuboovarian
        abscess) and in diagnosing gall stones and other gallbladder dis-
        ease. With the addition of color-flow Doppler, deep venous throm-
        bosis and ovarian or testicular torsion can be detected.
    c. Computed tomography (CT) is useful in assessing the brain for
        masses, bleeding, strokes, skull fractures. CTs of the chest can eval-
        uate for masses, fluid collections, aortic dissections, and pulmonary
        emboli. Abdominal CTs can detect infection (abscess, appendicitis,
        diverticulitis), masses, aortic aneurysms, and ureteral stones.
    d. Magnetic resonance imaging (MRI) helps to identifies soft tissue
        planes very well. In the emergency department setting, this is most
        commonly used to rule out spinal cord compression, cauda equina
        syndrome, and epidural abscess or hematoma.
    e. Screening tests: Fasting lipid panel can demonstrate the choles-
        terol level, including the low-density lipoprotein (LDL) levels,
        which have prognostic significance in coronary heart disease; fast-
        ing glucose and thyroid tests may be important; in many centers,
        dual-energy x-ray absorptiometry (DEXA) is the test of choice to
        monitor bone mineral density; the mammogram is the examination
        of choice to assess for subclinical breast cancer; the double-contrast
        barium enema and colonoscopy are used to detect colonic polyps or
        malignancy.

PART 2. APPROACH TO CLINICAL PROBLEM-SOLVING

Classic Clinical Problem-Solving

There are typically four distinct steps that the family physician undertakes to
systematically solve most clinical problems:

1. Making the diagnosis
2. Assessing the severity of the disease
3. Treating based on the stage of the disease
4. Following the patient's response to the treatment

MAKING THE DIAGNOSIS

This is achieved by carefully evaluating the patient, analyzing the information,
assessing risk factors, and developing a list of possible diagnoses (the differential). Usually a long list of possible diagnoses can be pared down to a few
of the most likely or most serious ones, based on the clinician's knowledge,

experience, and selective testing. For example, a patient who complains of upper abdominal pain and has a history of nonsteroidal antiinflammatory drug (NSAID) use may have peptic ulcer disease; another patient who has abdominal pain, fatty food intolerance, and abdominal bloating may have cholelithiasis. Yet another individual with a 1-day history of periumbilical pain that now localizes to the right lower quadrant may have acute appendicitis.

CLINICAL PEARL

The first step in clinical problem solving is making the diagnosis.

ASSESSING THE SEVERITY OF THE DISEASE

After establishing the diagnosis, the next step is to characterize the severity of the disease process; in other words, to describe "how bad" the disease is. This may be as simple as determining whether a patient is "sick" or "not sick." Is the patient with a urinary tract infection septic or stable for outpatient therapy? In other cases, a more formal staging may be used. For example, cancer staging is used for the strict assessment of extent of malignancy.

CLINICAL PEARL

The second step is to establish the severity or stage of disease. This usually impacts the treatment and/or prognosis.

TREATING BASED ON STAGE

Many illnesses are characterized by stage or severity because this affects prognosis and treatment. As an example, a formerly healthy young man with pneumonia and no respiratory distress may be treated with oral antibiotics at home. An older person with emphysema and pneumonia would probably be admitted to the hospital for IV antibiotics. A patient with pneumonia and respiratory failure would likely be intubated and admitted to the intensive care unit for further treatment.

CLINICAL PEARL

The third step is tailoring the treatment to fit the severity or "stage" of the disease.

FOLLOWING THE RESPONSE TO TREATMENT

The final step in the approach to disease is to follow the patient's response to the therapy. Some responses are clinical, such as improvement (or lack of improvement) in a patient's pain. Other responses may be followed by testing (e.g., monitoring the anion gap in a patient with diabetic ketoacidosis). The clinician must be prepared to know what to do if the patient does not respond as expected. Is the next step to treat again, to reassess the diagnosis, or to follow-up with another more specific test?

CLINICAL PEARL

❖   The fourth step is to monitor treatment response or efficacy. This may be measured in different ways—symptomatically or based on physical examination or other testing. For the emergency physician, the vital signs, oxygenation, urine output, and mental status are the key parameters.

PART 3. APPROACH TO READING

The clinical problem-oriented approach to reading is different from the classic "systematic" research of a disease. Patients rarely present with a clear diagnosis; hence, the student must become skilled in applying textbook information to the clinical scenario. Because reading with a purpose improves the retention of information, the student should read with the goal of answering specific questions. There are several fundamental questions that facilitate clinical thinking. These are:

1. What is the most likely diagnosis?
2. How would you confirm the diagnosis?
3. What should be your next step?
4. What is the best screening strategy in this situation?
5. What are the risk factors for this condition?
6. What are the complications associated with the disease process?
7. What is the best therapy?

CLINICAL PEARL

❖   Reading with the purpose of answering the seven fundamental clinical questions improves retention of information and facilitates the application of "book knowledge" to "clinical knowledge."

What Is the Most Likely Diagnosis?

The method of establishing the diagnosis was discussed in the previous section. One way of determining the most likely diagnosis is to develop standard "approaches" to common clinical problems. It is helpful to understand the most common causes of various presentations, such as "the worst headache of the patient's life is worrisome for a subarachnoid hemorrhage" (see the Clinical Pearls at end of each case).

The clinical scenario would be something such as:

A 38-year-old woman is noted to have a 2-day history of a unilateral, throbbing headache with photophobia. What is the most likely diagnosis?

With no other information to go on, the student would note that this woman has a unilateral headache with photophobia. Using the "most common cause" information, the student would make an educated guess that the patient has a migraine headache. If instead the patient is noted to have "the worst headache of her life," the student would use the Clinical Pearl

The worst headache of the patient's life is worrisome for a subarachnoid hemorrhage.

CLINICAL PEARL

❖ The more common cause of a unilateral, throbbing headache with photophobia is a migraine, but the main concern is subarachnoid hemorrhage. If the patient describes this as "the worst headache of her life," the concern for a subarachnoid bleed is increased.

How Would You Confirm the Diagnosis?

In the scenario above, the woman with "the worst headache" is suspected of having a subarachnoid hemorrhage. This diagnosis could be confirmed by a CT scan of the head and/or lumbar puncture. The student should learn the limitations of various diagnostic tests, especially when used early in a disease process. The lumbar puncture (LP) **showing xanthochromia (red blood cells) is the "gold standard" test for diagnosing subarachnoid hemorrhage, but it may be negative early in the disease course.**

What should be your next step? This question is difficult because the next step has many possibilities; the answer may be to obtain more diagnostic information, stage the illness, or introduce therapy. It is often a more challenging question than "What is the most likely diagnosis?" because there may be insufficient information to make a diagnosis and the next step may be to pursue more diagnostic information. Another possibility is that there is enough information for a probable diagnosis, and the next step is the stage the disease. Finally, the most appropriate answer may be to treat. Hence, from clinical data, a judgment needs to be rendered regarding how far along one is on the road of:

**1. Make a diagnosis → 2. Stage the disease →
3. Treat based on stage → 4. Follow response**

Frequently, the student is taught "to regurgitate" the same information that someone has written about a particular disease, but is not skilled at identifying the next step. This talent is learned optimally at the bedside, in a supportive environment, with freedom to take educated guesses and with constructive feedback. A sample scenario might describe a student's thought process as follows:

1. MAKE THE DIAGNOSIS: "Based on the information I have, I believe that Mr. Smith has a small bowel obstruction from adhesive disease *because* he presents with nausea and vomiting, abdominal distension, and high-pitched hyperactive bowel sounds, and has dilated loops of small bowel on x-ray."
2. STAGE THE DISEASE: "I don't believe that this is severe disease as he does not have fever, evidence of sepsis, intractable pain, peritoneal signs, or leukocytosis."
3. TREAT BASED ON STAGE: "Therefore, my next step is to treat with nothing per mouth, nasogastric (NG) tube drainage, IV fluids, and observation."
4. FOLLOW RESPONSE: "I want to follow the treatment by assessing his pain (I will ask him to rate the pain on a scale of 1 to 10 every day), his bowel function (I will ask whether he has had nausea, or vomiting, or passed flatus), his temperature, abdominal exam, serum bicarbonate (for metabolic acidemia), and white blood cell count, and then reassess him in 48 hours."

In a similar patient, when the clinical presentation is unclear, perhaps the best "next step" may be diagnostic such as an oral contrast radiologic study to assess for bowel obstruction.

CLINICAL PEARL

❖   Usually, the vague query, "What is your next step?" is the most difficult question because the answer may be diagnostic, staging, or therapeutic.

What Is the Best Screening Strategy in This Situation?

A major role of the family physician is screening for common and/or dangerous conditions where there may be interventions to alleviate disease. Cost-effectiveness, ease of the screening modality, wide availability, and presence of intervention are some of the important issues. The age, gender, and risk factors for the disease process in question play roles. In general, age is one of the most important risk factors for cancer. For instance, with breast cancer, an annual mammography is recommended in women older than age 50 years. This imaging technique is widely available, inexpensive, safe, decreases mortality, and is cost-effective.

What Are the Risk Factors for This Process?

Understanding the risk factors helps the practitioner to establish a diagnosis and to determine how to interpret tests. For example, understanding risk-factor analysis may help in the management of a 55-year-old woman with anemia. If the patient has risk factors for endometrial cancer (such as diabetes, hypertension, anovulation) and complains of postmenopausal bleeding, she likely has endometrial carcinoma and should have an endometrial biopsy. Otherwise, occult colonic bleeding is a common etiology. If she takes NSAIDs or aspirin, then peptic ulcer disease is the most likely cause.

CLINICAL PEARL

❖ Being able to assess risk factors helps to guide testing and develop the differential diagnosis.

What Are the Complications to This Process?

Clinicians must be cognizant of the complications of a disease, so that they will understand how to follow and monitor the patient. Sometimes the student has to make the diagnosis from clinical clues and then apply his/her knowledge of the consequences of the pathologic process. For example, "A 26-year-old male complains of right lower-extremity swelling and pain after a trans-Atlantic flight" and his Doppler ultrasound reveals a deep vein thrombosis. Complications of this process include pulmonary embolism (PE). Understanding the types of consequences also helps the clinician to be aware of the dangers to a patient. If the patient has any symptoms consistent with a PE, a ventilation–perfusion scan or CT scan angiographic imaging of the chest may be necessary.

What Is the Best Therapy?

To answer this question, not only does the clinician need to reach the correct diagnosis and assess the severity of the condition, but (s)he must also weigh the situation to determine the appropriate intervention. For the student, knowing exact dosages is not as important as understanding the best medication, route of delivery, mechanism of action, and possible complications. It is important for the student to be able to verbalize the diagnosis and the rationale for the therapy.

CLINICAL PEARL

❖   Therapy should be logical and based on the severity of disease and
     the specific diagnosis. An exception to this rule is in an emergent
     situation, such as respiratory failure or shock, when the patient
     needs treatment even as the etiology is being investigated.

SUMMARY

1. There is no replacement for a meticulous history and physical examination.
2. There are four steps in the clinical approach to the family medicine patient: making the diagnosis; assessing severity; treating based on severity; and following response.
3. There are seven questions that help to bridge the gap between the textbook and the clinical arena.

REFERENCES

Taylor RB, David AK, Fields SA, Phillips DM, Scherger JE. Family medicine, principle and practice. 6th ed. New York: Springer-Verlag, 2002.

SECTION II
Clinical Cases

A 52-year-old man comes to your office for a routine physical examination. He is a new patient to your practice. He has no significant medical history and takes no medications regularly. His father died at the age of 74 of a heart attack. His mother is alive at the age of 80. She has hypertension. He has 2 younger siblings with no known chronic medical conditions. He does not smoke cigarettes, drink alcohol, use any recreational drugs, and does not exercise. On examination, his blood pressure is 127/82 mm Hg, pulse is 80 beats/min, respiratory rate is 18 breaths/min, height is 67 inches, and weight is 190 lb. On careful physical examination, no abnormalities are noted.

◆ **What screening test(s) for cardiovascular disease should be recommended for this patient?**

◆ **What screening test(s) for cancer should be recommended?**

◆ **What immunization(s) should be recommended?**

ANSWERS TO CASE 1: Adult Male Health Maintenance

Summary: A 52-year-old man with no active medical problems is being evaluated during an "annual physical." He has no complaints on history and a normal physical examination.

◆ **Recommended screening tests for cardiovascular conditions:** Blood pressure measurement (screening for hypertension) and lipid measurement (screening for dyslipidemia)

◆ **Recommended screening tests for cancer:** Fecal occult blood testing, flexible sigmoidoscopy (with or without occult blood testing), colonoscopy or double-contrast barium enema to screen for colorectal cancer; there is insufficient evidence to recommend for or against universal prostate cancer screening by prostate-specific antigen (PSA) testing

◆ **Recommended immunizations:** Tetanus-diphtheria (Td), if he has not had one within 10 years; influenza vaccine annually, in the fall or winter months

Analysis

Objectives

1. Know the components of an adult health-maintenance visit.
2. Learn the screening tests and immunizations that are routinely recommended for adult men.

Considerations

For years, one of the cornerstones of primary care was the "annual physical," which often consisted of a complete physical examination, blood tests, including complete blood counts (CBCs) and multichemistry panels, and, frequently, annual chest x-rays and electrocardiograms (EKGs). The concept of the "annual physical," or "health-maintenance examination" is still important; however, the components of the examination have changed over time.

The purposes of the health-maintenance visit are to identify the individual patient's health concerns, manage the patient's current medical conditions, identify the patient's risks for future health problems, perform rational and cost-effective health screening tests, and promote a healthy lifestyle. Prevention is divided into primary prevention and secondary prevention. **Primary prevention** is an intervention designed to prevent a disease before it occurs. It usually involves the identification and management of risk factors for a disease. Examples of this would be the use of a statin medication to reduce low-density lipoprotein (LDL) cholesterol in order to lower the risk of coronary artery disease or the removal of colon polyps to prevent the development of colon cancer. **Secondary prevention** is an intervention intended to reduce the recurrence or exacerbation of a disease. An example of secondary prevention is the use of a statin medication after a person has had a myocardial infarction so as to reduce the risk of a second heart attack.

Effective screening for diseases or health conditions should meet several established criteria. First, the disease should be of **high enough prevalence** in the population to make the screening effort worthwhile. There should be a time frame during which the person is asymptomatic, but during which the disease or risk factor can be identified. There needs to be a test available for the disease that has **sufficient sensitivity and specificity, is cost-effective,** and is **acceptable** to patients. Finally, there must be an intervention that can be made during the asymptomatic period that will prevent the development of the disease or reduce the morbidity/mortality of the disease process.

The United States Preventive Services Task Force (USPSTF) is an independent panel of experts in primary care and preventive medicine that reviews evidence and makes recommendations on the effectiveness of clinical preventive services, specifically in the areas of screening, immunization, preventive medications, and counseling. USPSTF recommendations are "gold standards" for clinical preventive medicine. The recommendations of the USPSTF are available online for free at www.preventiveservices.ahrq.gov. USPSTF grades its recommendations in 5 categories:

A—There is strong evidence that the intervention improves health outcomes and its benefits substantially outweigh its potential harms. These services are strongly recommended.

B—There is at least fair evidence that the intervention improves health outcomes and its benefits outweigh its potential harms. These services are recommended.

C—The balance of the benefits and potential harms is too close to justify making a general recommendation.

D—There is at least fair evidence that the service is ineffective or the potential harms outweigh the benefits. These services are not recommended.

I—There is insufficient evidence, or the available evidence is of such poor quality, that the balance of benefits and harms cannot be weighed and recommendations for or against the service cannot be made.

CLINICAL APPROACH

Screening Tests

Cardiovascular Diseases

Diseases of the cardiovascular system are the leading cause of death in adult men and the management of risk factors for these diseases reduces both morbidity and mortality from these diseases. The USPSTF strongly recommends (Level A) screening of adults for **hypertension** by measurement of blood pressure, as screening causes little harm and management of hypertension is effective at reducing the risk of cardiovascular diseases. USPSTF also strongly recommends (Level A) screening middle age and older adults for **lipid disorders** and recommends (Level B) screening adults older than age 20 years who are at increased risk for cardiovascular diseases. The screening can take the form of nonfasting total cholesterol and high-density lipoprotein (HDL)-cholesterol levels or fasting lipid panels that include the low-density lipoprotein (LDL)-cholesterol. Ultrasonography to assess for **abdominal aortic aneurysm** is recommended (Level B) for men ages 65–75 years who have ever smoked. There is no recommendation (Level C) for abdominal aortic aneurysm screening for men who have never smoked and it is recommended against (Level D) for women, regardless of smoking status.

The routine use of electrocardiogram (EKG), exercise stress testing, or computed tomography (CT) scanning for coronary calcium is not recommended (Level D) for screening for **coronary artery disease** in adults at low risk for coronary events. There is insufficient evidence to recommend for or against these modalities (Level I) in adults at higher risk of coronary events. Screening for **peripheral arterial disease** in asymptomatic adults is not recommended (Level D) because of the low prevalence of the problem in asymptomatic adults and the lack of evidence for improved outcomes from treatment in the asymptomatic stage.

Cancer

Adults (men and women) older than 50 years are strongly advised (Level A) to have screening for **colorectal cancer.** This screening can take the form of fecal occult blood testing (FOBT) using guaiac cards on three consecutive bowel movements collected at home, flexible sigmoidoscopy with or without occult blood testing, double-contrast barium enema, or colonoscopy. The optimal intervals for testing are not clear, but FOBT is generally recommended annually, sigmoidoscopy and barium enema every 3–5 years, and colonoscopy every 10 years. An abnormal test result of FOBT, sigmoidoscopy, or barium enema leads to the performance of a colonoscopy.

The USPSTF currently finds insufficient evidence to recommend for or against routine screening (Level I) for **prostate cancer** using digital examination or prostate-specific antigen (PSA). Although testing improves detection of prostate cancer, the evidence for improved outcomes is inconsistent. Level I ratings are also given to screening for **lung cancer** using CT scanning, chest x-rays, sputum cytology, or combinations of these, and to screening for skin cancer or oral cancer.

Screening for **bladder, testicular, pancreatic, or thyroid cancer** in asymptomatic adults is not recommended (Level D).

Other Health Conditions

Screening for **obesity** by measuring body mass index (BMI) and providing intensive counseling and behavioral interventions to promote weight loss are recommended for all adults (Level B). There is insufficient evidence to recommend screening of asymptomatic adults for **type 2 diabetes mellitus** (Level I), although screening is recommended (Level B) for adults with hypertension or hyperlipidemia. **Depression** screening is recommended (Level B) if there are mechanisms in place for assuring accurate diagnosis, treatment, and follow up. Screening and counseling to identify and promote cessation of **tobacco use** is strongly recommended (Level A) and to identify and prevent the **misuse of alcohol** is recommended (Level B).

Immunizations

As is the case for well child care, the provision of age- and condition-appropriate immunizations is an important component of well-adult care. Recommendations for immunizations change from time to time and the most up-to-date source of vaccine recommendations is the Advisory Committee on Immunization Practices. Its immunization schedules are widely published and are available at the Centers for Disease Control website (among other places) at www.cdc.gov.

A booster vaccination for **tetanus and diphtheria** (Td) is recommended every 10 years for all adults who previously have had a primary series of immunizations. If there is no history of having received a primary series for Td, the following schedule should be used: 2 injections of Td vaccine should be given at least 4 weeks apart, followed by a third injection 6–12 months later. This is followed by routine boosters every 10 years.

Influenza vaccination is recommended every year for adults older than age 50 years. It is also recommended annually for those younger than age 50 years with certain medical conditions and for persons who may transmit the infection to others who are at high risk (healthcare or nursing home workers, household contacts of high risk individuals, etc.). High-risk conditions include chronic diseases of the cardiovascular, pulmonary, and renal systems, metabolic diseases such as diabetes, hemoglobinopathies, and immunodeficiencies.

Pneumococcal polysaccharide vaccination is recommended as a single dose for all adults age 65 years or older. It is also recommended for adults younger than age 65 years who have chronic cardiovascular, pulmonary, renal, or hepatic diseases, diabetes, or an immunodeficiency, or who are functionally asplenic. One-time revaccination after 5 years is recommended for those with chronic kidney or hepatic disease, immunodeficiency, or asplenia. One-time revaccination is also recommended for those older than age 65 years if they were vaccinated longer than 5 years previously and were younger than age 65 years at the time of initial vaccination.

Other vaccinations may be recommended for specific populations, although not for all adults. **Hepatitis B** vaccination should be recommended for those at high risk of exposure, including healthcare workers, those exposed to blood or blood products, dialysis patients, intravenous drug users, persons with multiple sexual partners or recent sexually transmitted diseases, and men who engage in sexual relations with other men. **Hepatitis A** vaccine is recommended for persons with chronic liver disease, who use clotting factors, who have occupational exposure to the hepatitis A virus, who use IV drugs, men who have sex with men, or who travel to countries where hepatitis A is endemic. **Varicella** vaccination is recommended for those with no reliable history of immunization or disease, who are seronegative on testing for varicella immunity, and who are at risk for exposure to varicella virus. **Meningococcal** vaccine is recommended for persons with certain complement deficiencies, functional or anatomic asplenia, or who travel to countries where the disease is endemic.

Healthy Lifestyle

Along with the discussion of screening and promotion of tobacco cessation and prevention of alcohol misuse, other aspects of healthy living should be promoted by physicians. **Exercise** has been consistently shown to reduce the risk of cardiovascular disease, diabetes, obesity, and overall mortality. Even exercise of moderate amounts, such as walking for 30 minutes a day, has a positive effect on health. The benefits increase with increasing the amount of exercise performed. Studies performed on counseling physically inactive persons to exercise have shown inconsistent results. However, the benefits of exercise are clear and should be promoted. Counseling to promote a healthy **diet** in persons with hyperlipidemia, other risk factors for cardiovascular disease, or other conditions related to diet is beneficial. Intensive counseling by physicians or, when appropriate, referral to dietary counselors or nutritionists, can improve health outcomes. In selected patients, recommendations regarding **safer sexual practices,** including the use of condoms, may be appropriate to reduce the risk or recurrence of sexually transmitted diseases. Finally, all patients should be encouraged to use **seat belts** and avoid driving while under the influence of alcohol or drugs, as motor vehicle accidents remain a leading cause of morbidity and mortality in adults.

Comprehension Questions

[1.1] For which of the following conditions is screening recommended for all men older than 50 years?

    A. Prostate cancer
    B. Lung cancer
    C. Abdominal aortic aneurysm
    D. Colon cancer

[1.2]   A 62-year-old man with recently diagnosed emphysema presents to
your office in November for a routine examination. He has not had any
immunizations in more than 10 years. Which of the following immunizations would you recommend?

A. Tetanus–diphtheria (Td) only
B. Td, pneumococcal, and influenza
C. Pneumococcal and influenza
D. Td, pneumococcal, influenza, and meningococcal

[1.3]   Which of the following statements regarding exercise is correct?

A. To be beneficial, exercise must be performed everyday.
B. Walking for exercise has not been shown to improve meaningful
clinical outcomes.
C. Counseling patients to exercise has not been shown consistently to
increase the number of patients who exercise.
D. Intense exercise offers no health benefit over mild to moderate
amounts of exercise.

Answers

[1.1]   **D.** Colon cancer screening is given a Level A recommendation by the
USPSTF and is routinely recommended for all adults older than 50 years.
There is insufficient evidence to recommend for or against routine lung
or prostate cancer screening. Abdominal aortic aneurysm screening is
recommended in men age 65–75 years who have smoked.

[1.2]   **B.** In an adult with a chronic lung disease, one-time vaccination with
pneumococcal vaccine and annual vaccination with influenza vaccine
are recommended. A Td booster should be recommended to all adults
who have had a primary series of Td but who have not had a booster
within 10 years.

[1.3]   **C.** Although the benefits of exercise are clear, the benefit of counseling patients to exercise is not. Counseling has not been consistently
shown to increase the number of patients who exercise.

CLINICAL PEARLS

❖   There is no such thing as "routine blood tests" or a "routine chest
x-ray." All tests that are ordered should have evidence to support
their benefit.

❖   High-quality, evidence-based recommendations for preventive health
services are available at www.preventiveservices.ahrq.gov.

REFERENCES

United States Preventive Services Task Force website: www.preventiveservices.ahrq.gov.

Centers for Disease Control website: www.cdc.gov.

A 52-year-old man presents to your office for an acute visit because of coughing and shortness of breath. He is well known to you because of multiple office visits in the past few years for similar reasons. He has a chronic "smoker's cough," but reports that in the past 2 days his cough has increased, his sputum has changed from white to green in color, and he has had to increase the frequency with which he uses his albuterol inhaler. He denies having a fever, chest pain, peripheral edema, or other symptoms. His medical history is significant for hypertension, peripheral vascular disease, and 2 hospitalizations for pneumonia in the past 5 years. He has a 60-pack-year history of smoking and continues to smoke 2 packs of cigarettes a day.

On examination, he is in moderate respiratory distress. His temperature is 98.4°F, his blood pressure is 152/95 mm Hg, his pulse is 98 beats/min, his respiratory rate is 24 breaths/min, and he has an oxygen saturation of 94% on room air. His lung examination is significant for diffuse expiratory wheezing and a prolonged expiratory phase of respiration. There are no signs of cyanosis. The remainder of his examination is normal. A chest x-ray done in your office shows an increased anteroposterior (AP) diameter and flattened diaphragms, but otherwise clear lung fields.

◆ **What is the most likely cause of this patient's dyspnea?**

◆ **What acute treatment(s) are most appropriate at this time?**

◆ **What interventions would be most helpful to reduce the risk of future exacerbations of this condition?**

ANSWERS TO CASE 2: Dyspnea (Chronic Obstructive Pulmonary Disease [COPD])

Summary: A 52-year-old male with a long smoking history presents with dyspnea, increased sputum production, coughing, and wheezing.

◆ **Most likely cause of current symptoms:** Acute exacerbation of chronic obstructive pulmonary disease (COPD)

◆ **Appropriate treatment of exacerbation:** Antibiotic, bronchodilators, systemic corticosteroids

◆ **Interventions to reduce exacerbations:** Smoking cessation, long-acting bronchodilator, inhaled corticosteroid, influenza vaccination

Objectives

1. Be able to diagnose and determine the stage of COPD in adults
2. Know the management of stable COPD and COPD exacerbations

Considerations

Two of the most common causes of dyspnea and wheezing in adults are asthma and COPD. There can be substantial overlap between the two diseases, as patients with chronic asthma can develop chronic obstructive disease over time. As in most medical situations, the patient's history will usually provide the key information to the appropriate diagnosis. Asthma often presents earlier in life, may or may not be associated with cigarette smoking and is characterized by episodic exacerbations with return to relatively normal baseline lung functioning. COPD, on the other hand, tends to present in midlife or later, is usually the result of a long-term history of smoking, and is a slowly progressive disorder in which measured pulmonary functioning never returns to normal.

In the setting of an acute exacerbation, the differentiation between an exacerbation of asthma and an exacerbation of COPD is not necessary for determination of the immediate management. The assessment of the patient presenting with dyspnea should always start with the ABCs—Airway, Breathing, and Circulation. Intubation with mechanical ventilation should be performed when the patient is unable to protect his own airway (for example, when he has a reduced level of consciousness), when he is tiring because of the amount of work required to overcome his airway obstruction or when adequate oxygenation can not be maintained.

For both asthma and COPD exacerbations, the mainstays of medical therapy are oxygen, bronchodilators, and steroids. All dyspneic patients should have an assessment of their level of oxygenation. Clinical signs of hypoxemia, such as cyanosis of the perioral region or digits, should be noted on examination. Objective levels of oxygenation using pulse oximetry or arterial blood gas measurements should also be performed. Hypoxemia must be addressed by providing supplemental oxygen. Inhaled β_2-agonists, most commonly albuterol, can rapidly result in bronchodilation and reduction in airway obstruction. The addition of an inhaled anticholinergic agent, such as ipratropium, may work synergistically with the β-agonist. Corticosteroids, given systemically (orally, intramuscularly, or intravenously), act to reduce the airway inflammation that underlies the acute exacerbation. Clinically significant effects of steroids take hours to occur; consequently, steroids should be used with bronchodilators because bronchodilators act rapidly. Steroids used in combination with bronchodilators significantly improve short-term outcomes in the management of acute exacerbations of asthma and COPD.

APPROACH TO COPD

Definitions

> **Chronic Bronchitis:** Cough and sputum production on most days for at least 3 months during at least 2 consecutive years.
> **Emphysema:** Shortness of breath caused by the enlargement of respiratory bronchioles and alveoli caused by destruction of lung tissue.

Evaluation

COPD is defined as airway obstruction that is not fully reversible, is usually progressive, and is associated with chronic bronchitis, emphysema, or both. The most common etiology is **cigarette smoking,** which is **associated with approximately 90% of cases of COPD.** Other etiologies of COPD include passive exposure to cigarette smoke ("second-hand smoke") and occupational exposures to dusts or chemicals. A rare cause of COPD is a genetic deficiency in α_1-**antitrypsin,** which should be considered when emphysema develops at younger ages, especially in non-smokers.

COPD is a disease of inflammation of the airways, lung tissue, and vasculature. Pathologic changes include mucous gland hypertrophy with hypersecretion, ciliary dysfunction, destruction of lung parenchyma, and airway remodeling. The results of these changes are narrowing of the airways, causing a fixed airway obstruction, poor mucous clearance, cough, wheezing, and dyspnea.

The most common initial symptom of COPD is cough, which is at first intermittent and then frequently becomes a daily occurrence. The cough is often productive of white, thick mucus. Patients will present with intermittent episodes of worsening cough, with change in mucus from clear to yellow/green, and often with wheezing. These exacerbations are usually caused by viral or bacterial infections.

As lung function continues to deteriorate, dyspnea develops. Dyspnea is the primary presenting symptom of COPD. Dyspnea also tends to worsen over time—initially the dyspnea will occur only with significant effort, then with any exertion, and finally at rest. **By the time dyspnea develops, lung function (as measured by forced expiratory volume at 1 second [FEV_1]) has been reduced by about half and the COPD has been present for years.**

Examination of a patient with mild or moderate COPD, who is not having an exacerbation, is usually normal. As the disease progresses, patients are often noted to have "barrel chests" (increased anteroposterior chest diameter) and distant heart sounds, as a result of hyperinflation of the lungs. Breath sounds may also be distant and expiratory wheezes with a prolonged expiratory phase of respiration may be noted. During an acute exacerbation, patients often appear anxious and tachypneic; they may be using accessory muscles of respiration, usually have wheezes or rales, and may have signs of cyanosis.

Chest x-rays in patients with COPD are typically normal until the disease is advanced. In more severe cases, hyperinflation of the lungs with an increased posteroanterior (PA) diameter and flattening of diaphragms may be seen. Bullae—areas of pulmonary parenchymal destruction—can also be seen in x-rays in more severe disease.

The primary diagnostic test of lung function is spirometry. In normal aging, both the forced vital capacity (FVC) (a measure of the total amount of air that can be expired after a maximal inspiration) and forced expiratory volume in 1 second (FEV_1) reduce gradually over time. In normal-functioning lungs, the ratio of the FEV_1 to FVC is greater than 0.7. **In COPD, both the FVC and FEV_1 are reduced and the ratio of FEV_1 to FVC is less than 0.7,** indicating an airway obstruction. Using a bronchodilator may result in some improvement of both FVC and FEV_1, but neither will return to normal, making the diagnosis of a fixed obstruction. The severity of COPD, which can help to determine treatment, can be assessed using these measurements (Table 2–1).

Management of Stable COPD

The goals of COPD management are to relieve symptoms, slow disease progression, reduce/prevent/treat exacerbations, and reduce/prevent/treat complications. Several components of treatment are common to all stages of COPD, whereas pharmacologic treatment is guided by the stage of disease.

All patients with COPD should be encouraged to quit smoking. The pulmonary function of smokers declines more rapidly than that of nonsmokers. **Although smoking cessation does not result in significant improvement in pulmonary function, smoking cessation does reduce the rate of further deterioration to that of a nonsmoker.** Cessation also reduces the risks of other comorbidities, including cardiovascular diseases and cancers. Chapter 7 more thoroughly discusses smoking cessation. All patients with COPD should receive a pneumococcal and annual influenza vaccination. Influenza vaccination reduces the frequency and complications of exacerbations. Regular exercise and efforts to maintain normal body weight should be encouraged.

Short-acting bronchodilators used as needed are the recommended treatment in stage I COPD. These include β_2-agonists (albuterol) and anticholinergics

Table 2–1

CLASSIFICATION OF COPD SEVERITY

STAGE	CLASSIFICATION	FINDINGS
0	At risk	Cough, sputum production Normal Spirometry
I	Mild COPD	$FEV_1/FVC <0.7$ $FEV_1 \geq 80\%$ predicted With or without symptoms
II	Moderate COPD	$FEV_1/FVC <0.7$ FEV_1 50–80% predicted With or without symptoms
III	Severe COPD	$FEV_1/FVC <0.7$ FEV_1 30–50% predicted With or without symptoms
IV	Very Severe COPD	$FEV_1/FVC <0.7$ $FEV_1 <30\%$ predicted or $FEV_1 <50\%$ predicted with chronic hypoxemia

Adapted from: NHLBI/WHO. Global initiative for chronic obstructive lung disease, executive summary, 2005.

(ipratropium). **Inhaled medications are preferred over oral,** as they tend to have fewer side effects. The choice of specific agent is based on availability, individual response to therapy, and side effects.

In stage II COPD, a long-acting bronchodilator should be added. Commonly used agents in the United States are salmeterol (an inhaled β_2 agonist) and tiotropium (an inhaled anticholinergic). Oral methylxanthines (aminophylline, theophylline) are also options, but have narrow therapeutic windows (high toxicity) and multiple drug–drug interactions, making their use less common. The use of long-acting bronchodilators is more convenient and more effective than using short-acting agents, but is much more expensive and does not replace the need for short-acting agents for rescue therapy in exacerbations.

Inhaled steroids do not affect the rate of decline of lung function in COPD but do reduce the frequency of exacerbations. For that reason, **inhaled steroids are recommended for stages III and IV COPD with frequent exacerbations.** Long-term treatment with oral steroids is not recommended, as there is no evidence of benefit, but there can be multiple complications (myopathy, osteoporosis, glucose intolerance, etc).

Oxygen therapy is recommended in stage IV COPD if there is evidence of hypoxemia ($PaO_2 \leq 55$ mm Hg or $SaO_2 \leq 88\%$ at rest) or where the PaO_2 is

≤ 60 mm Hg and there is polycythemia, pulmonary hypertension or peripheral edema suggesting heart failure.

Management of Exacerbations of COPD

Acute exacerbations of COPD are common and typically present with change in sputum color or amount, cough, wheezing, and increased dyspnea. Viral and bacterial infections are a common precipitant of acute exacerbations of COPD. Diagnoses that can cause similar symptoms (e.g., pulmonary embolism, congestive heart failure, myocardial infarction) must be excluded so that appropriate therapy can occur.

The severity of the exacerbation should be evaluated by history, examination, assessment of oxygenation, and focused testing. Oxygen should be given to keep saturation greater than 90% or PaO_2 levels at about 60 mm Hg. Patients with more severe symptoms, comorbidities, altered mental status, an inability to care for themselves at home, or whose symptoms fail to respond promptly to office or emergency room treatments should be hospitalized.

All acute exacerbations should be treated with short-acting bronchodilators. Combinations of short-acting agents with different mechanisms of action (i.e., β-agonist and anticholinergic) can be used until symptoms improve. **Systemic steroids shorten the course of the exacerbation and may reduce the risk of relapse.** A steroid dose of 40 mg prednisone (or equivalent) for 10–14 days is recommended.

Exacerbations associated with increased amounts of sputum or with purulent sputum should be treated with antibiotics. *Pneumococcus, Haemophilus influenzae,* and *Moraxella catarrhalis* are the most common bacteria implicated. In milder exacerbations, treatment with oral agents directed against these pathogens is appropriate. In severe exacerbations, Gram-negative bacteria (*Klebsiella, Pseudomonas*) can also play a role, so antibiotic coverage needs to be broader.

Comprehension Questions

[2.1]   A 38-year-old woman presents with progressively worsening dyspnea and cough. She has never smoked cigarettes, has no known passive smoke exposure, and does not have any occupational exposure to chemicals. Pulmonary function testing shows obstructive lung disease that does not respond to bronchodilators. Which of the following is the most likely etiology?

   A. Radon exposure at home
   B. Cigarette use that the patient is not telling you about
   C. α_1-Antitrypsin deficiency
   D. Asthma

[2.2]   A 60-year-old male is diagnosed with stage II COPD. Which of the following reasons would justify smoking cessation at this point?

A. By quitting, his pulmonary function will significantly improve.
B. His rate of pulmonary decline will slow.
C. Smoking cessation at this point will not alter the course of his disease.
D. Smoking cessation will not alter the course of his COPD but will reduce his risk of developing lung cancer.

[2.3]   A 68-year-old patient of your practice with known COPD has pulmonary function testing showing an FEV_1 of 40% predicted and has been having frequent exacerbations of his COPD. Which of the following medication regimens is the most appropriate?

A. As-needed inhaled albuterol only
B. Salmeterol BID and albuterol as needed
C. Oral albuterol daily and an inhaled steroid
D. An inhaled steroid, tiotropium BID, and inhaled albuterol as needed

Answers

[2.1]   **C.** α_1-Antitrypsin deficiency should be considered in a patient who develops COPD at a young age, especially if there is no other identifiable risk factor.

[2.2]   **B.** Smoking cessation will not result in reversal of the lung damage that has already occurred, but can result in a slowing in the rate of decline of pulmonary function. In fact, cessation can result in the rate of decline returning to that of a nonsmoker.

[2.3]   **D.** This patient has stage III COPD with frequent exacerbations. He is best treated by a long-acting bronchodilator and an inhaled steroid used regularly, along with an inhaled, short-acting agent on an as-needed basis.

CLINICAL PEARLS

❖ All smokers should be counseled on the benefits of smoking cessation before they develop symptomatic COPD; by the time symptoms develop, the patient's FEV_1 will have reduced by approximately 50%.

❖ Always remember to evaluate the ABCs—Airway, Breathing, Circulation—when evaluating a dyspneic patient.

REFERENCES

Anthonisen N. Chronic bronchitis, obstructive pulmonary disease. In: Goldman L. and Ausiello D (eds). Cecil Textbook of Medicine. WB Saunders, 2004.

Hunter MH, King DE. COPD: management of acute exacerbations and chronic stable disease. Am Fam Physician 2001;64:603–12, 621–2.

National Heart, Lung and Blood Institute/World Health Organization. Global initiative for chronic obstructive lung disease. Executive summary. Updated 2005 (based on an April 1998 NHLBI/WHO workshop). Available at: http://www.goldcopd. com/Guidelineitem.asp?l1=2&l2=1&intId=996

A 45-year-old white male presents to your office complaining of left knee pain that started last night. He says that the pain started suddenly after dinner and was severe within a span of 3 hours. He denies any trauma, fever, systemic symptoms, or prior similar episodes. He has a history of hypertension for which he takes hydrochlorothiazide (HCTZ). He admits to consuming a great amount of wine last night with dinner.

On exam, his temperature is 98°F, his pulse is 90 beats/min, his respirations are 22 breaths/min, and his blood pressure is 129/88 mm Hg. Heart and lung examinations are unremarkable. The patient is reluctant to flex the left knee, wincing in pain at touch, and passive range of motion. The knee is edematous, hot to touch, and has erythema of the overlying skin. No crepitation or deformity is apparent. No other joints are involved. Inguinal lymph nodes are not enlarged. Complete blood count reveals a white blood cell count of 10,900 cells/mm^3 and is otherwise normal.

◆ **What is the next diagnostic step?**

◆ **What is the most likely diagnosis?**

◆ **What is the next step in therapy?**

ANSWERS TO CASE 3: Joint Pain

Summary: This is a 45-year-old male who presents with the sudden onset of monoarticular, nontraumatic joint pain. Evolution from onset to severe pain was rapid. The patient denies any trauma, systemic signs of illness, or any prior episodes. That he takes hydrochlorothiazide and drank a lot of alcohol the night that his symptoms started are important. His vital signs are stable, and he does not appear to be systemically ill. There is pain to movement and touch of the left knee, with evident edema, erythema, and warmth of the joint. No other joints are involved. His white blood cell count is not indicative of an acute infectious process.

◆ **Next diagnostic step:** Joint aspiration for examination of joint fluid to identify crystals and exclude infection.

◆ **Most likely diagnosis:** Crystal-induced gout of the left knee.

◆ **Next step in therapy:** Nonsteroidal antiinflammatory drug and provide analgesia; may consider using colchicine.

Analysis

Objectives

1. Have a differential diagnosis for nontraumatic joint pain, based on clinical presentation.
2. Become familiar with the most common diagnostic tests for the above conditions, and have a rationale when ordering these tests.
3. Know the most common treatment options in the acute onset of gout and infectious arthritis, as well as the chronic management of rheumatoid arthritis and osteoarthritis.

Considerations

This 45-year-old male presents with the sudden onset of monoarticular joint pain. **The first diagnosis that needs to be excluded is an infected joint.** A joint becomes septic by blood inoculation, by contiguous infection (such as from bone or soft tissue), or from direct inoculation from trauma or surgery. Exclusion of an infectious etiology is paramount as cartilage can be destroyed within the first 24 hours of infection. In this case, the patient's history and clinical scenario do not favor an infectious cause, although it cannot be excluded by history and physical examination alone.

There are several additional pieces of information that guide the diagnosis in this case. Most gout attacks occur between the ages of 30 and 50 years in men, with a later onset in postmenopausal women (50 to 70 years of age). The patient's recent increase in alcohol consumption can be considered an exacerbating factor. Other factors that may also increase the risk of a gout attack include trauma, surgery, or a large meal that induces hyperuricemia. Finally, the patient's history of taking a **thiazide diuretic** is also important, as these drugs **may induce hyperuricemia.**

The examination of a joint aspirate is essential for the diagnosis. The **gross appearance of fluid is not very specific,** as both a septic aspirate and a heavily condensed crystal-induced arthritis may have a thick, yellowish/chalky appearance. To diagnose crystal-induced arthritis, polarizing microscopy has to reveal monosodium urate (MSU) crystals, which will look like needles and have a strong negative birefringence. Other crystals that may be seen are:

- **Calcium pyrophosphate dihydrate**—rod shaped, rhomboid, weakly positive birefringence
- **Calcium hydroxyapatite**—seen by electron microscopy, cytoplasmic inclusions that are nonbirefringent.
- **Calcium oxalate**—bipyramidal appearance, strongly positive birefringence; seen mostly in end-stage renal disease patients

In crystal-induced arthritis, the white blood cell count of the joint aspirate is on average 2,000 to 60,000/µL, with less than 90% neutrophils, while a septic joint will have an average of 100,000 white blood cells/µL (25,000–250,000 cells) with a >90% neutrophil count. Aspirate that has been determined to be crystal-induced must also be cultured so as to rule out a coexisting infection.

APPROACH TO NONTRAUMATIC JOINT PAIN/SWELLING

Depending on the etiology, pain may be present in 1, 2, or more joints. Considering the patient's age, medical history, and medication profile is important. The patient's lifestyle and social history should also be considered, as certain activities may predispose a patient to specific infections. Among **the major diagnoses that have to be considered in a nontraumatic swollen joint are gout (or any crystal-induced arthritis), infectious arthritis, osteoarthritis, and rheumatoid arthritis.** A short discussion on low back pain is included.

Clinical Presentation

Gout's first episode can often be confused with cellulitis. It presents with swelling and pain, usually of 1 joint, accompanied by erythema and warmth. **Classically, a gout attack involves the metatarsophalangeal joint of the first toe,** called **podagra,** but it may involve any joint in the body. Some cases left untreated resolve spontaneously within 3 to 10 days, with no residual signs or symptoms. **During an acute attack, the serum uric acid level may be normal or even low,** likely as a result of the existing deposition of the urate crystals. Uric acid levels are, however, useful in monitoring hypouricemic therapy between attacks. Radiographs may show cystic changes in the joint surface, with punched-out lesions and soft-tissue calcifications. These findings are nonspecific and are also seen in osteoarthritis and rheumatoid arthritis.

An infection usually involves only 1 joint if it is of bacterial origin (>90% of cases). The knee, hip, and shoulder are the 3 most commonly involved joints. A *chronic* monoarticular arthritis or involvement of 2–3 joints may be caused by fungi or mycobacteria. In the case of acute polyarticular (>3 joints) arthritis, the etiology may be from endocarditis or a disseminated gonococcal infection.

Bacterial infections of a joint occur most commonly in persons with rheumatoid arthritis. The chronic inflammation of joints coupled with the use of steroids predisposes this group to *Staphylococcus aureus* infections. HIV-positive patients may develop pneumococcal, salmonella, or even *Haemophilus influenzae* joint infections. Intravenous drug users are most likely to get a streptococcal, staphylococcal, Gram-negative, or *Pseudomonas* infection.

Range of motion (ROM) of the joint is an important maneuver of the physical examination. **A septic joint will have a very limited ROM,** coupled with effusion and fever. However, a nearby cellulitis, bursitis, or osteomyelitis will usually maintain the ROM of a joint. The aspirate of a septic joint will have a positive culture in >90% of cases.

Osteoarthritis (OA) is most commonly found in people older than 65 years of age (68% of patients) and is associated with trauma, history of repetitive joint use, and obesity (specifically for knee OA). It primarily affects the cartilage, but ends up damaging the bone surface, synovium, meniscus, and ligaments. The clinical presentation is usually that of a dull, deep, ache-type pain. The onset is usually gradual, with activity exacerbating the pain, and rest decreasing it. In the latter stages, pain is usually constant. On physical examination, a bony crepitus may be felt on passive ROM. There may be a small joint effusion and periarticular muscle atrophy. In the advanced stage, joint deformity with decreased ROM will be seen. **X-rays are usually normal at first,** with the gradual development of bone sclerosis, subchondral cysts, and osteophytes.

Rheumatoid arthritis (RA) is another common disorder that may affect people from any age group, but will usually present initially in those 30–55 years old. The presentation of RA can be varied, ranging from a monoarticular arthritis that is intermittent, to a polyarthritis that progresses gradually in intensity, leading to disability. It affects more women than men (3:1), and the treatment will usually depend on the stage at which the disease is diagnosed. The American Rheumatism Association has delineated **specific diagnostic criteria to aid in the diagnosis of RA,** among which are these:

1.   Morning stiffness
2.   Involvement of 3 or more joints

3. Involvement of hand joints
4. Symmetric arthritis
5. Presence of rheumatoid nodules
6. Positive rheumatoid factor
7. Radiographic changes which include erosions or decalcifications

Of all these diagnostic criteria, the **first 4 must be present for at least 6 weeks,** and the **fulfillment of any 4 of these criteria is sufficient to diagnose RA.** Among the laboratory tests that may be abnormal in patients with RA are an elevated erythrocyte sedimentation rate, an elevated C-reactive protein, anemia, thrombocytosis, and low albumin. The level of hypoalbuminemia usually correlates with the severity of the disease.

Treatment

Analgesia is a common factor to consider in therapy for all the conditions described above. In the case of an acute gout attack, colchicines, nonsteroidal antiinflammatory drugs (NSAIDs), and glucocorticoids are the drugs mainly used. In the elderly population, one must take into account the possibility of GI complications from the above medications. To reduce these risks, intraarticular steroids, ice packs, and low-dose colchicine are more often used. In patients with recurrent gout attacks, chronic medication therapy can be used to maintain serum uric acid levels below 5 mg/dL. The maintenance therapy is usually with either probenecid, which increases the urinary excretion of uric acid, or allopurinol, which reduces the production of uric acid.

A **septic joint requires surgery** for drainage of infectious material followed by IV antibiotics. Methicillin-resistant *Staphylococcus aureus* (MRSA) will usually require vancomycin, but coverage with antibiotics is dependent on the specific organisms isolated.

Degenerative joint disease treatment involves mobility exercises, maintenance of adequate range of motion, and weight loss, if appropriate. Intraarticular corticosteroid injections may provide relief for varying amounts of time, but should only be done every 4–6 months so as to avoid cartilage destruction. Surgery, such as joint replacement, is usually reserved for people with severe disease that affects their daily functions.

Therapy for rheumatoid arthritis involves multiple modalities. Education and counseling of the patient regarding disease progression, treatment options, and implications to lifestyle is essential. Exercises, such as those that maintain joint mobility and muscle strength, are very important, as the natural course of RA is to develop a stiff joint that becomes disabling. Physical therapy and occupational therapy are important to address specific areas in which the patient may need additional devices to perform activities of daily living.

Many different categories of medications are used in RA. These include NSAIDs, glucocorticoids, **disease-modifying antirheumatic drugs (DMARDs), anticytokines, and topical analgesics.** Among the DMARDs are sulfasalazine and methotrexate. Infliximab and etanercept are examples of anticytokine agents. Treatment regimens are individualized, and will often include a combination of two or three of these agents. Although effective, monitoring for hepatotoxicity must be performed.

Low Back Pain

Low back pain (LBP) is a very common complaint that will require a different work-up, depending on the patient's age, history, and clinical findings. Approximately 93% of patients will present with LBP only. If the patient is younger than 50 years old and has no "red flag symptoms or signs" (Table 3–1), conservative treatment is recommended (NSAIDs, local heat, exercises) for 6 weeks. If the patient is older than 50 years of age, the likelihood pain being from a musculoskeletal source is still approximately 95%, but a lumbar spine x-ray is indicated. If this is abnormal, then imaging with magnetic resonance imaging (MRI) should be considered. A different picture is seen with patients who complain of sciatic nerve pain or symptoms consistent with a radiculopathy. If the involvement is unilateral and there is no bladder or bowel incontinence, then conservative treatment for 4 weeks is recommended followed by an MRI if no improvement. An urgent MRI or computed tomography (CT) scan should be obtained if symptoms are in saddle distribution or if there is involvement of bladder/bowel sphincters, as this may signal the "cauda equina syndrome," which is a surgical emergency.

Table 3–1
"RED FLAG" SYMPTOMS AND SIGNS IN PATIENTS
WITH BACK PAIN

Unrelenting night pain
Unrelenting pain at rest
Neuromotor deficit
Fever
Loss of bowel or bladder control
Suspicion of ankylosing spondylitis
Trauma
History or suspicion of cancer
Osteoporosis
Chronic corticosteroid use
Immunosuppression
Drug or alcohol abuse

Comprehension Questions

Match the most likely diagnosis with the clinical vignette:

    A. Rheumatoid arthritis
    B. Crystal induced arthritis
    C. Infectious arthritis
    D. Degenerative joint disease

[3.1]   A 26-year-old male with fever and left knee pain and swelling 2 weeks after his bachelor party.

[3.2]   A 44-year-old female with a 5-month history of malaise and stiff hands in the morning that improve as the day goes by.

[3.3]   A 52-year-old morbidly obese patient with bilateral knee pain for 1 year.

[3.4]   A 35-year-old male with hypertension and right big toe pain that resolved spontaneously at home after 1 week of taking ibuprofen.

Answers

[3.1]   **C.** Infectious arthritis would need to be high on the differential diagnosis for two reasons in this scenario. Both the possibility of trauma that may lead to direct infection and the possibility of gonococcal arthritis from sexual activity must be considered.

[3.2]   **A.** Morning stiffness, involvement of the hands and symmetric arthritis are three of the criteria necessary for the diagnosis of rheumatoid arthritis.

[3.3]   **D.** Obesity is a risk factor for osteoarthritis, which is common in the knees and typically presents with a gradual onset and worsening of symptoms.

[3.4]   **B.** Gouty arthritis often initially presents in the big toe ("podagra") and the use of HCTZ, a common treatment for hypertension, also can increase the risk.

CLINICAL PEARLS

❖ A red, swollen joint **must** be aspirated to rule out a joint infection.
❖ Most low back pain can be treated conservatively. The presence of "red flag" symptoms or signs should prompt a more aggressive work-up.

REFERENCES

Atlas, SJ, Deyo, RA. Evaluating and managing acute low back pain in the primary care setting. J Gen Intern Med 2001;16:120.

Canoso J. Rheumatoid arthritis. In: Canoso JJ (ed.). Rheumatology in primary care. 1st ed. Philadelphia, PA: Saunders WB, 1997:59–63.

Canoso J. Crystal-induced arthritis. In: Canoso JJ (ed.). Rheumatology in primary care. 1st ed. Philadelphia, PA: Saunders WB, 1997: 150–8.

Helfgott SM. Evaluation of the adult with monoarticular pain. Up to Date, version 13.3, updated November 8, 2004.

Institute for Clinical Systems Improvement (ICSI). Adult low back pain. Bloomington, MN: Institute for Clinical Systems Improvement (ICSI), September 2005.

Van Tulder MW, Koes BW, Bouter LM. Conservative treatment of acute and chronic nonspecific low back pain. A systematic review of randomized controlled trials of the most common interventions. Spine 1997;22:2128.

A 22-year-old woman who has never been pregnant before presents to you after having a positive home pregnancy test. She has no significant medical history. Upon further questioning, she states that she is unsure of the date of her last menstrual period. She denies any symptoms and is worried as she has not felt the baby move thus far. She is also concerned as she recently had dental x-rays taken prior to discovering that she was pregnant. Patient denies the use of any drugs, alcohol, or tobacco. She inquires about when she can get an ultrasound and a genetic test to rule out Down syndrome.

◆ **When is an ultrasound indicated in prenatal care?**

◆ **What laboratory studies are routinely indicated at an initial prenatal visit?**

◆ **What is the risk to the pregnancy based on the radiation exposure that the patient has encountered?**

◆ **When is the optimal time for screening with a trisomy screen test?**

ANSWERS TO CASE 4: Prenatal Care

Summary: A 22-year-old primigravida female with no significant past medical history presents for initial prenatal care visit. She has numerous questions regarding her care and recently has had dental x-rays taken.

◆ **Indications for an ultrasound in pregnancy:** According to the American College of Obstetricians and Gynecologists (ACOG), an ultrasound is not mandatory in routine, low-risk prenatal care. An ultrasound is indicated for the evaluation of uncertain gestational age, size/date discrepancies, vaginal bleeding, multiple gestations, or other high-risk situations.

◆ **Laboratory studies recommended at the initial prenatal visit:** Complete blood count (CBC), hepatitis B surface antigen (HBsAg), HIV testing, syphilis screening with a rapid plasma reagin (RPR), urinalysis and urine culture, rubella antibody, blood type and Rh status with antibody screen, Papanicolaou (Pap) smear, and cervical swab for gonorrhea and Chlamydia.

◆ **Risk to the pregnancy based on the radiation exposure from dental x-rays:** Risk for the baby is increased once the radiation exposure is greater than 5 rads; the radiation exposure from routine dental x-rays is 0.00017 rads.

◆ **The optimal time for the trisomy screen:** The optimal time is 16–18 weeks' gestation; however, it may be performed between 15 and 20 weeks' gestation, if necessary. Emerging evidence shows first trimester screening may be as effective in some centers.

Analysis

Objectives

1. Learn the components of the preconception counseling and the initial prenatal visit.
2. Know the recommended screening tests and visit intervals in routine prenatal care.
3. Learn the relevant psychosocial aspects of providing prenatal care, including important counseling issues.

Considerations

Prenatal, or antenatal, care affords the opportunity to both perform appropriate medical testing and provide counseling and anticipatory guidance. Pregnancy can be a time of anxiety and patients frequently have many questions. One of the goals of prenatal care is to provide appropriate education in order to help reduce anxiety and help women to be active participants in their own care.

Preconception

In the United States, the first visit for prenatal care frequently is at 8 weeks of gestation or later, and yet it is the time preceding this that poses the greatest risk to fetal development. **A preconception visit is an ideal opportunity for the patient to discuss with her physician any issue related to possible pregnancy or contraception occurring within 1 year of pregnancy.** The preconception visit can be included during visits for many reasons, including fertility problems, contraception, periodic health assessment, recent amenorrhea or specifically for preconception counseling. Roughly one-half of patients with a negative pregnancy test may have some risk that could adversely affect a future pregnancy. Because roughly 50% of pregnancies are unplanned or unintended, physicians should consider the potential of pregnancy when writing each prescription.

Women who intend to become pregnant should be advised to avoid, whenever possible, potentially harmful agents such as radiation, drugs, alcohol, over-the-counter (OTC) medications, herbs, and other environmental agents. **Radiation exposure greater than 5 rads is associated with fetal harm. Most commonly performed x-ray procedures, including dental, chest, and extremity x-rays, expose a fetus to only very small fractions of this amount of radiation.** Whenever possible, the abdomen and pelvis should be shielded and x-rays performed only when the benefit outweighs the potential risk. Magnetic resonance imaging studies have not been proven to cause harm, but are not recommended in pregnancy, if avoidable. Ultrasound has not been shown to be harmful.

Women should refrain from OTC medicines, herbs, vitamins, minerals, and nutritional products until cleared by their obstetric provider. They should also be instructed to start a folic acid supplement at least 1 month prior to attempting to conceive. **For low-risk women, 400 µg of folic acid daily is recommended to reduce the risk of neural tube defects.** Higher doses are recommended in the presence of certain risk factors. For women with diabetes mellitus or epilepsy, 1 mg of folic acid a day is recommended. **A woman who has had a child with a neural tube defect should take 4 mg of folic acid daily.**

Women from certain ethnic backgrounds may be offered specific genetic screening. African and African-American women may be offered sickle cell trait screening. A French-Canadian or Ashkenazi Jewish background is an indication to consider screening for a Tay-Sachs carrier state. Southeast Asian and Middle Eastern women may be offered screening for thalassemia.

Women who will be 35 years old or older at the anticipated time of delivery should be educated about age-related risk, particularly the increased risk of Down syndrome. They should be counseled about the available screening and diagnostic testing available, along with the appropriate time frame in which each test may be performed.

Women with medical conditions such as diabetes, asthma, thyroid disease, hypertension, lupus, thromboembolism, seizures should be referred to providers with experience in managing high risk pregnancies. Women with psychiatric disorders should be comanaged with a psychiatrist and counselor/therapist so that the patient can benefit from pharmacologic and behavioral therapy. These patients may require more frequent visits. Patients who have drug, tobacco, or alcohol dependence should be educated about the risks and referred to rehab/treatment centers to quit the drug prior to conception. Women should also be educated about proper nutrition and exercise during pregnancy. Preconception counseling may also address issues such as financial readiness, social support during pregnancy and the postpartum period, and issues of domestic violence.

Initial Prenatal Visit

The initial visit should address all the concepts in the preconception visit, if no preconception counseling was done. Ideally, the initial visit should be in the first trimester. A detailed history and physical examination, initial obstetric labs, and counseling regarding the logistics for prenatal care should be done at this visit. The history should begin with an assessment of the last menstrual period (LMP) and its reliability. **One of the most crucial pieces of information is the accuracy of the dating.** The first day of the LMP is used to obtain the estimated delivery date using Naegele's rule (from the first day of the LMP subtract 3 months and add 7 days). The LMP is considered reliable if the following criteria are met: the date is certain, the last menstrual period was normal, there has been no contraceptive use in the past 1 year, the patient has had no bleeding since the LMP, and her menses are regular. If these criteria are not met, an ultrasound should be performed. ACOG has established further criteria that can be used to ensure that a fetus is mature at the time of delivery (Table 4–1).

Table 4–1
ACOG CRITERIA FOR ASSUMPTION OF FETAL MATURITY

Fetal heart tones have been documented for 20 weeks by nonelectronic fetoscope or for 30 weeks by Doppler.

It has been 36 weeks since a positive serum or urine human chorionic gonadotropin pregnancy test was performed by a reliable method.

An ultrasound measurement of the crown-rump length, obtained at 6–11 weeks, supports a gestational age of 39 weeks or more.

An ultrasound scan obtained at 12–20 weeks confirms the gestational age of 39 weeks or more as determined by clinical history and physical examination.

Information from American College of Obstetricians and Gynecologists. Fetal maturity assessment prior to elective repeat cesarean delivery. ACOG Committee Opinion 98. Washington, DC: ACOG, 1999.

History should also be obtained with particular attention to medical history, prior pregnancies, delivery outcomes, pregnancy complications, neonatal complications, and birth weights. Gynecologic history should focus on the menstrual history, contraceptive use, and history of sexually transmitted diseases (STDs). Allergies, current medications—both prescription and OTC—and substance use should also be investigated. Social history should consider whether the pregnancy was planned, unplanned, or unintentional. A discussion of social supports for the patient during the prenatal and postpartum period is also warranted. Genetic history should be obtained for the patient and partner's family, if known.

The initial examination should be thorough and should assess height, weight, blood pressure, thyroid, breast, and general physical and pelvic examinations. Pregnancy-specific examinations, including an estimation of gestational age by uterine size or fundal height measurement and an attempt to hear fetal heart tones by Doppler fetoscope should be performed. Heart tones should be obtainable by 10 weeks' gestation using a handheld Doppler fetoscope. Pelvimetry has been removed as a recommended required intervention, but it may be useful to have a subjective assessment for risks of problems during delivery.

The initial laboratory screen should include blood type and Rh status antibody screen, rubella status, HIV, hepatitis B surface antigen, rapid plasma reagin (RPR), urinalysis, urine culture, Pap smear, cervical swab for gonorrhea and *Chlamydia*, and a CBC.

The logistics of the prenatal visits should be addressed. A typical protocol includes follow-up visits every 4 weeks until 28 weeks' gestation, every 2 weeks from 28–36 weeks' gestation, and every week from 36 weeks' gestation until delivery. More frequent visits should be performed if any problems arise or if all issues are not addressed in the scheduled visits.

The **ACOG does not require ultrasonography in patients without complications.** Nevertheless, ultrasonography should be performed in patients without reliable dating criteria, with a discrepancy between the measured and expected uterine growth, in a postdates pregnancy, suspicion for twin gestation, suspicion for placental issues, chromosomal abnormalities, or with other problems. For gestational age estimations, ultrasonography is accurate for within 1 week if performed in the first trimester, 2 weeks in the second trimester, 3 weeks in the third trimester. If the ultrasound dates and LMP are off by more than the aforementioned intervals, the due date should be recalculated based on the ultrasound findings.

The visit should end with an adequate explanation of all patient/partner concerns. Women should be counseled that sexual activity is not associated with any harm during an uncomplicated pregnancy, although there may be conditions that arise during the course of a pregnancy that would make sexual activity inadvisable. A follow-up visit should be scheduled prior to her leaving the office. She should also be educated about preterm labor precautions, signs of ectopic pregnancy, and situations in which to call the physician or go to the obstetrics triage unit for evaluation.

Subsequent Visits

At follow-up prenatal visits, concerns or questions brought up by the patient should be addressed. The examiner should ask questions specifically targeted at symptoms suggestive of complications that include pregnancy-induced hypertension (PIH), preeclampsia, infections (urinary tract, vaginal, etc.), fetal compromise, placenta previa/abruption, and preterm labor or premature rupture of membranes. At each visit, the patient should be asked about vaginal bleeding, loss of fluid, headaches, visual changes, abdominal pain, dysuria, facial or upper-extremity edema, vaginal discharge, and subjective sensation of fetal movements.

The examination on each subsequent visit should include weight, blood pressure, fundal height measurement, and fetal heart tones by hand-held Doppler. In addition, a urinalysis should be performed at every visit to assess for protein and glucose.

Subsequent Testing and Laboratory Studies

At 15–20 weeks' gestation (preferably between 16 and 18 weeks' gestation) a trisomy screen should be offered to patients. The most common test in use now is the triple screen, which tests serum human chorionic gonadotropin (hCG), unconjugated estriol, and α-fetoprotein. This test screens for trisomy 21, trisomy 18, and neural tube defects. **The triple screen is approximately 65% sensitive and 95% specific for detecting aneuploidy.** More recently, adding inhibin as a fourth analyte for the so-called quad screen increases the sensitivity to approximately 80% without increasing the false-positive rate. The most common cause for a false-positive serum screen is incorrect gestational age dating. In some centers, fetal nuchal translucency can be measured by ultrasonography combined with maternal serum analyte levels (i.e., free hCG and pregnancy-associated plasma protein A [PAPP-A]). This testing can be performed at 10–14 weeks' gestation. Sensitivity and specificity of these tests is determined by the risk cutoff used (e.g., for trisomy 21, sensitivity is 85.2% when specificity is 90.6%; at 95% specificity, the sensitivity is 78.7%). Women should be counseled about the limited sensitivity and specificity of the tests, the psychological implications of a positive test, the potential impact of delivering a child with Down syndrome, the risks associated with prenatal diagnosis and second-trimester abortion, and delays inherent in the process.

Women at increased risk of aneuploidy should be offered prenatal diagnosis by amniocentesis or chorionic villus sampling (CVS). Persons at increased risk include women who will be older than age 35 years at delivery and who have a singleton pregnancy (older than age 32 years at delivery for women pregnant with twins); women carrying a fetus with a major structural anomaly identified by ultrasonography; women with ultrasound markers of aneuploidy (including increased nuchal thickness); women with a previously affected pregnancy; couples with a known translocation, chromosome inversion, or aneuploidy; and women with a positive maternal serum screen. Amniocentesis may be performed after 15 weeks' gestation and is associated with a 0.5% risk of spontaneous abortion. CVS is performed at 10–12 weeks' gestation and has a 1.0–1.5% risk of spontaneous abortion. CVS may be associated with transverse limb defects (1 per 3000 to 1 per 1000 fetuses). Women undergoing CVS also should be offered maternal serum α-fetoprotein testing for neural tube defects. Women older than age 35 years at time of delivery may opt for serum screening and ultrasonography before deciding whether to proceed with amniocentesis. **Although the risk for trisomy 21 increases with maternal age, an estimated 75% of affected fetuses are born to mothers younger than age 35 years at time of delivery.**

The American College of Obstetricians and Gynecologists and the American Diabetes Association recommend that all pregnant women be screened for gestational diabetes at 24–28 weeks' gestation, except women who are at low risk (e.g., younger than age 25 years, belonging to a low-risk ethnic group, normal prepregnancy weight, no history of abnormal glucose metabolism, no previous poor obstetric outcomes, and no first-degree relatives with diabetes). Screening is standard in the United States, with 94% of physicians reporting universal screening.

At 24–28 weeks' gestation, patients should be screened for gestational diabetes with a 1-hour glucose challenge test. This is done by giving the patient a 50-g glucose load and obtaining a blood sugar 1 hour later. The patient does not need to fast prior to this test. Most guidelines consider a value above 140 mg/dL as abnormal, whereas new studies advocate using a value of 135 mg/dL. If the test is positive, a 3-hour glucose tolerance test (GTT) should be performed (after an overnight fast) by giving the patient a 100-g glucose load and obtaining fasting, 1-hour, 2-hour, and 3-hour postload serum glucose samples; 2 out of 4 positive values generally constitute a positive 3-hour GTT.

At 28 weeks' gestation, a repeat RPR and hemoglobin/hematocrit should be obtained in those at risk for syphilis and anemia, respectively. In addition, a patient who is Rh-negative should receive $Rh_O(D)$ immune globulin (RhoGAM) at this time. An Rh-negative patient should also receive $Rh_O(D)$ immune globulin at delivery and in any instance of trauma. Nonsensitized, Rh-negative women also should be offered a dose of $Rh_O(D)$ immune globulin after spontaneous or induced abortion, ectopic pregnancy termination, CVS, amniocentesis, cordocentesis, external cephalic version, abdominal trauma, and second- or third-trimester bleeding. Administration of $Rh_O(D)$ immune globulin can be considered before 12 weeks' gestation in women with a threatened abortion and live embryo, but Rh alloimmunization is rare.

The Centers for Disease Control and Prevention and ACOG recommend that **all women be offered group B streptococcus (GBS) screening by vaginorectal culture at 35–37 weeks' gestation** and that colonized women be treated with intravenous antibiotics at the time of labor or rupture of membranes in order to reduce the risk of neonatal GBS infection. The **proper method of collection is to swab the lower vagina, perineal area, and rectum.** Of tested women, 10–30% will test positive for GBS colonization. Because GBS bacteriuria indicates heavy maternal colonization, women with GBS bacteriuria at any time during their pregnancy should be offered intrapartum antibiotics and do not require a vaginorectal culture. Similarly, women with a previous infant who was diagnosed with a GBS infection should be offered intrapartum antibiotics.

If a patient does not go into labor spontaneously by 42 weeks' gestation, induction of labor should be considered to reduce the risk of neonatal mortality and morbidity. Several studies have shown reduced risks with induction at 41 weeks' gestation. ACOG recommends testing for fetal well-being in prolonged pregnancies, starting in the 42nd week of gestation.

Vaccinations During Pregnancy

Women who will be in their third trimester during flu season should be offered the influenza vaccine. Influenza vaccine is safe in any stage of pregnancy provided there is no allergy to any of its components. Tetanus toxoid vaccination can also be given safely during pregnancy. Varicella and rubella vaccinations are not advised during pregnancy.

Comprehension Questions

[4.1]   A 24-year-old woman presents for an initial prenatal visit. She is at 9 weeks' gestation based on her LMP but, on further questioning, she isn't certain of the first day of her LMP. The most accurate estimate of her gestational age at this time would come from:

   A. Using her LMP if her uterine size is consistent
   B. A first trimester ultrasound
   C. A second trimester ultrasound
   D. A quantitative serum hCG level

[4.2]   A 38-year-old pregnant female presents for initial visit at 22 weeks' gestation. She requests a "genetic screen" but doesn't want amniocentesis performed. How would you advise the patient?

   A. If no prior personal or family history of genetic defects, no screen is needed
   B. Draw and send blood for the triple screen, as patient has advanced maternal age
   C. Discuss with patient that optimal time for the triple screen is over and the test may be inaccurate outside of this time period
   D. Offer the patient chorionic villus sampling

[4.3]   A 28-year-old female with a history of epilepsy presents for a preconception consultation visit. What is the recommended dose of folic acid supplementation that you would advise her to take?

   A. 100 mg/d
   B. 1 mg/d
   C. 400 µg/d
   D. 4 mg/d
   E. 400 mg/d

Answers

[4.1] **B.** A first trimester ultrasound is accurate to within ±1 week for gestational dating.

[4.2] **C.** A triple screen should be offered at 16–18 weeks, but can be done between 15 and 20 weeks. Outside of this time frame, the results are considered inaccurate. CVS is generally performed between 10 and 12 weeks' gestation.

[4.3] **B.** Women with a history of epilepsy should receive 1 mg of folic acid supplementation daily.

CLINICAL PEARLS

❖ The initial prenatal visit often is scheduled after fetal organogenesis has occurred. For this reason, a preconception visit can be very beneficial. Furthermore, when prescribing medications, physicians must consider the possibility that any woman of reproductive age may become pregnant.

❖ Genetic counseling should be offered to any woman who *will be* 35 years old or older at her estimated date of confinement (EDC).

REFERENCES

Briscoe D, Nguyen H, Mencer M, et al. Management of pregnancy beyond 40 weeks' gestation. Am Fam Physician 2005;71(10):1935–41.

Brundage SC. Preconception health care. Am Fam Physician 2002;65(12):2507–14.

Cline MK, Baxley EG, Noller KL. Prenatal care. Available at: www.familypractice. com/references/referencesframe.htm?main=/references/ABFPGuides/Pregnancy/ pregnancy.htm.

Graves JC, Miller KE, Sellers AD. Maternal serum triple analytic screening in pregnancy. Am Fam Physician 2002;65(5):915–20.

Institute for Clinical Systems Improvement (ICSI). Routine prenatal care. Bloomington, MN: Institute for Clinical Systems Improvement (ICSI), August 2005.

Kirkham C, Harris S, Grzybowski S. Evidence-based prenatal care: part I. General prenatal care and counseling issues. Am Fam Physician 2005;71(7): 1307–16.

Kirkham C, Harris S, Grzybowski S. Evidence-based prenatal care: part II. Third-trimester care and prevention of infectious diseases. Am Fam Physician 2005; 71(8):1555–60.

National Collaborating Centre for Women's and Children's Health. Antenatal care: routine care for the healthy pregnant woman. London: RCOG Press, 2003.

Veterans Health Administration, Department of Defense. DoD/VA clinical practice guideline for the management of uncomplicated pregnancy. Washington, DC: Department of Veteran Affairs, 2002.

A 6-month-old male is brought to your office by his mother for a routine well child visit. His mother is concerned that he is not yet saying "mama," because her best friend's baby said mama by age 6 months. Your patient was born to a full-term, uncomplicated pregnancy to a 23-year-old gravida$_1$, para$_1$ mother. He was delivered by a spontaneous vaginal delivery and there were no complications in the neonatal period. You have been following him since his birth. He has had appropriate growth and development up to this age and is up-to-date on his routine immunizations. He had one upper respiratory infection at age 5 months that was treated symptomatically. There is no family history of any developmental, hearing, or speech disorders. He has been fed since birth with an iron-fortified infant formula. Cereals and other baby foods were added starting at age 4 months. He lives with both parents, neither of whom smokes cigarettes.

On examination, he is a vigorous infant who is at the 50th percentile for length and weight and 75th percentile for head circumference. His physical examination is normal. On developmental examination, he is seen to sit for a short period of time without support, reach out with one hand for your examining light, pick up a Cheerio with a raking grasp and put it in his mouth, and he is noted to babble frequently.

◆ **What immunizations would be recommended at this visit?**

◆ **By what age should an infant say "mama" and "dada"?**

◆ **The child's mother asks when she can place him in front-facing car seat. What is your recommendation?**

ANSWERS TO CASE 5: Well Child Care

Summary: A 6-month-old healthy child is brought in for a routine well child examination.

◆ **Recommended immunizations for a 6-month well child visit (in a child who is up-to-date on routine immunizations):** *Diphtheria, tetanus,* and acellular *pertussis* (DTaP) no. 3, hepatitis B no. 3, and *Haemophilus influenzae* type b (HIB) no. 3; inactivated polio vaccine no. 3 can be given between 6 and 15 months of age.

◆ **Age by which a child should say "mama" and "dada":** Most children will start to say "dada" or "mama" nonspecifically between ages 6 and 9 months. It usually becomes specific between ages 8 and 12 months.

◆ **Recommendations for continuing in a rear-facing car seat:** A child should stay in a rear-facing car seat until the child weighs at least 20 lb and is at least 1 year old.

Analysis

Objectives

1. Learn the basic components of a well child examination.
2. Know the routine immunization schedule for children.
3. Know common developmental milestones for young children.

Considerations

The pediatric well child examination serves many valuable purposes. It provides an opportunity for parents, especially first-time parents, to ask questions about, and for the physician to address specific concerns regarding, their child. It allows the physician to assess the child's growth and development in a systematic fashion and to perform an appropriate physical examination. It also allows for a review of both acute and chronic medical conditions. When performed at recommended time intervals, it gives the opportunity to provide age-appropriate immunizations, screening tests, and anticipatory guidance. Finally, it supports the development of a good doctor–patient–family relationship, which can promote health and serve as an effective tool in the management of illness.

CLINICAL APPROACH

Definitions

Amblyopia: Reduction in loss of vision in one eye from lack of use. Strabismus is the most common cause of amblyopia.
Strabismus: Ocular misalignment.

Pediatric History

For the purposes of routine well child visits, a comprehensive history should be obtained at the initial visit with more focused, interval histories obtained at subsequent encounters. The initial history should include an opportunity for the parent to raise any questions or concerns that the parent may have. New parents, especially first-time parents and young parents, often have many questions or anxieties about their child. The ability to discuss them with the physician will help to engender a positive physician–patient–family relationship and improve the parent's satisfaction with their child's care.

A complete past medical history should be obtained. This should start with a detailed prenatal and pregnancy history, including the duration of the pregnancy, any complications of pregnancy, any medications taken, the type of delivery performed, the child's birth weight, and any neonatal problems. Any significant chronic or acute illnesses should be recorded. The use of any medications, both prescription and over-the-counter, should be reviewed.

A detailed family history, including information (when available) on both maternal and paternal relatives should be obtained. A thorough social history is critical in pediatric care. Information, including the parents' education levels, relationships, religious beliefs, use of substances (tobacco, alcohol, drugs) and socioeconomic factors can provide significant insight into the health and development of the child.

Efforts should be made to obtain old medical records, if any are available. Growth charts, immunization records, results of screening tests and other valuable information that can assist with the child's assessment and reduce the unnecessary duplication of previously performed interventions can often be found.

Growth

At each well child visit, the child's height and weight should be recorded and plotted on a standard growth chart. Head circumference is measured and plotted in children 3 years of age and younger. Children older than age 3 years should have their blood pressure recorded using an appropriate-size pediatric cuff. Significant variances from accepted, age-adjusted, population norms, or growth that deviates from predicted growth curves, may warrant further evaluation. **Failure to thrive** is defined by some as weight below the third or fifth percentile for age, and by others as decelerations of growth that have crossed two major growth percentiles in a short period of time. Either significant loss or gain of weight may prompt an in-depth discussion of nutrition and caloric intake.

Development

An assessment of the child's development in the areas of **gross motor, fine motor/adaptive, language, and social/personal** skills is an important aspect of each well child visit. Numerous screening tools, such as the Denver II developmental screening test, the Parents' Evaluations of Developmental Status (PEDS), and others, are available to assist with these assessments. These assessments typically involve both responses from the parents regarding the child's behavior at home and observations of the child in the office setting. Persistent delays in development, either globally or in individual skill areas, should prompt a more in-depth developmental assessment, as early intervention may effectively aid in the management of some developmental abnormalities. Table 5–1 summarizes many of the important motor, language and social developmental milestones of early childhood.

Screening Tests

Each state requires screening of all newborns for specified congenital diseases; however, the specific diseases for which screening is done vary from state to state. **All states require testing for phenylketonuria (PKU) and congenital hypothyroidism,** as early treatment can prevent the development of profound mental retardation. Diseases for which testing commonly occurs include hemoglobinopathies (including sickle cell disease), galactosemia, and other inborn errors of metabolism. This screening is done by collecting blood from newborns prior to discharge from the hospital. In some states, newborn screening is repeated at the first routine well visit, usually at about 2 weeks of age.

Nationwide, the prevalence of childhood lead poisoning has declined, primarily because of the use of unleaded gasoline and lead-free paints. However, in some communities, the risk of lead exposure is higher. Universal screening for lead poisoning is recommended by the Centers for Disease Control and Prevention and the American Academy of Pediatrics for children ages 9–12 months and again at age 2 years in communities where ≥27% of homes were built before 1950 or where ≥12% of children have a venous lead concentration >10 µg/dL. In other communities, screening should be targeted to high-risk children (Table 5–2).

Iron deficiency is the most common cause of anemia in children. Iron-containing formula and cereals have helped to reduce the occurrence of iron deficiency. Children who drink more than 24 ounces of cow's milk, have iron-restricted diets, or were low birth weight or preterm, or whose mother was iron deficient, are at higher risk. Iron deficiency can be evaluated by a hemoglobin or hematocrit measurement, usually taken between 6 and 12 months of age. Repeat testing can be considered annually, especially in high-risk children, up

Table 5–1
DEVELOPMENTAL MILESTONES

AGE	MOTOR	LANGUAGE	SOCIAL	OTHER
1 month	• Reacts to pain	• Responds to noise	• Regards human face • Establishes eye contact	
2 months	• Eyes follow object to midline • Head up prone	• Vocalizes	• Social smile • Recognizes parent	
4 months	• Eyes follow object past midline • Rolls over	• Laughs and squeals	• Regards hand	
6 months	• Sits well unsupported • Transfers objects hand to hand (switches hands) • Rolls prone to supine	• Babbles	• Recognizes strangers	• Babbles • Six strangers switch sitting at 6 months
9 months	• Pincer grasp (10 months) • Crawls • Cruises (walks holding furniture)	• Mama/dada • Bye-bye	• Starts to explore	• Can crawl, therefore can explore • It takes 9 months to be a "mama" • Pinches furniture to walk
12 months	• Walks • Throws object	• 1–3 words • Follows 1-step commands	• Stranger and separation anxiety	• Walking away from mom cause anxiety • Know 1 word at 1 year
2 years	• Walks up and down stairs • Copies a line • Runs • Kicks ball	• 2–3-word phrases • One half of speech is understood by strangers • Refers to self by name • Pronouns	• Parallel play	• Puts 2 words together at 2 • At age 2, $2/4$ ($1/2$) of speech understood by strangers

(Continued)

Table 5–1

DEVELOPMENTAL MILESTONES (*CONTINUED*)

AGE	MOTOR	LANGUAGE	SOCIAL	OTHER
3 years	• Copies a circle • Pedals a tricycle • Can build a bridge of 3 cubes • Repeats 3 numbers	• Speaks in sentences • Three-fourth of speech is understood by strangers • Recognize 3 colors	• Group play • Plays simple games • Knows gender • Knows first and last name	• Tricycle, 3 cubes, 3 numbers, 3 colors, 3 kids make a group • At age 3, $1/4$ of speech understood by strangers
4 years	• Identifies body parts • Copies a cross • Copies a square (4.5 years) • Hops on one foot • Throws overhand	• Speech is completely understood by strangers • Uses past tense • Tells a story	• Plays with kids, social interaction	• Song "head, shoulder, knees, and toes," 4 parts reminds you that at age 4 can identify body parts • At age 4, $4/4$ of speech is understood by strangers • When using past tense, speaks of thins that happened before • If a 2-year-old can copy 1 line, a 4-year-old can copy 2 lines to draw a cross and a square, which has 4 sides
5 years	• Copies a triangle • Catches a ball • Partially dresses self	• Writes name • Counts 10 objects		
6 years	• Draws a person with 6 parts • Ties shoes • Skips with alternating feet	• Identifies left and right		• At 6 years: skips, shoes, person with 6 parts.

Reproduced, with permission, from Hay: Current pediatric diagnosis and treatment. 17th ed. New York: McGraw-Hills, 2005.

Table 5–2
ELEMENTS OF A LEAD RISK QUESTIONNNAIRE

Recommended questions

1. Does your child live in or regularly visit a house built before 1950? This could include a day care center, preschool, the home of a babysitter or relative, and so on.
2. Does your child live in or regularly visit a house built before 1978 with recent, ongoing, or planned renovation or remodeling?
3. Does your child have a sister or brother, housemate, or playmate who is being followed for lead poisoning?

Questions that may be considered by region or locality

1. Does your child live with an adult whose job (e.g., at a brass/copper foundry, firing range, automotive or boat repair shop, or furniture refinishing shop) or hobby (e. g., electronics, fishing, stained-glass making, pottery making) involves explosure to lead?
2. Does your child live near a work or industrial site (e. g., smelter, battery recycling plant) that involves the use of lead?
3. Does your child use pottery or ingest medications that are suspected of having a high lead content?
4. Does your child have exposure to burning lead-pained wood?

Reproduced, with permission, from Stead LG, Stead SM, Kaufman MS First *Aid for the Pediatrics Clerkship*. New York: McGraw-Hill, 2004:39 & 40.

through the age of 5 years. An anemic child can empirically be given a trial of an iron supplement and dietary modification. Failure to respond to iron therapy should warrant further evaluation of other causes of anemia.

Most states now mandate newborn hearing screening by auditory brainstem response or evoked otoacoustic emission. All high-risk infants, regardless of requirement, should be screened. High-risk infants include those with a family history of childhood hearing loss, craniofacial abnormalities, syndromes associated with hearing loss (such as neurofibromatosis), or infections associated with hearing loss (such as bacterial meningitis). Older infants and toddlers can be assessed for hearing problems by questioning the parents or performing office testing by snapping fingers, or by using rattles or other noisemakers. Office-based audiometry can usually be performed in children age 3 years and older. Any hearing loss should be promptly evaluated and referred for early intervention, if necessary.

Vision screening can also start in the newborn nursery. Evaluation of the neonate for red reflexes on ophthalmoscopy should be a standard part of the newborn examination. The presence of red reflexes helps to rule out the possibility of congenital cataracts and retinoblastoma. The evaluation of an older infant should include a subjective evaluation of the child's vision by the parent. Infants should be able to focus on a face by age 1 month and should move their eyes consistently and symmetrically by age 6 months. An examining light should reflect symmetrically off of both corneas; asymmetric light reflex may be a sign of strabismus. The cover–uncover test also is a screening examination for strabismus. The child focuses on an object with both eyes and the examiner covers one eye. Strabismus is suggested when the uncovered eye deviates to focus on the object. **Strabismus should be referred to a pediatric ophthalmologist as soon as it is detected,** as early intervention results in a lower incidence of amblyopia. After the age of 3 years, most children can be tested for visual acuity using a Snellen chart, modified with a "tumbling E" or pictures, instead of letters.

Other screening tests may be recommended for high-risk children. Tuberculosis (TB) screening is recommended for children who were born or live in a region of high TB prevalence or who have close contact with someone known to have TB. The Mantoux test is the screening test of choice; the multiple puncture tine test is no longer recommended. Screening for hyperlipidemia in children is controversial but may be appropriate if there is a family history of hyperlipidemia or of premature coronary artery disease.

Anticipatory Guidance

A primary feature of the well child visit should be education of the patient and family on issues that promote health and prevent illness, injury, or death. This anticipatory guidance should be focused and age appropriate. The use of preprinted handouts can reinforce issues discussed in the office, address issues that could not be discussed because of time limitations, and allow for the parent to review the information as needed at home. Subjects that should routinely be addressed include injury prevention, nutrition, development, discipline, exercise, mental health issues, and the need for ongoing care (e.g., immunization schedules, future well child visits, dental care).

Accidents and injuries are the leading cause of death in children older than age 1 year. Accidents involving motor vehicles, both traffic and pedestrian accidents, are the leading cause of these accidental deaths. All states now require the use of car safety seats for children, although the regulations vary from state to state. The general recommendation is that a child should be in the back seat of the vehicle whenever possible. If there is no back seat, the child should only ride in the front seat if there is no air bag or if the air bag can be disabled. **A child should sit in a rear-facing car seat until the child is both 1 year old and weighs at least 20 lb.** A child older than 1 year and between 20 and 40 lb should use a forward-facing car seat. When the child weighs more than 40 lb, the child may use a booster-type seat along with the lap and shoulder seatbelts. The child can stop using the booster when the child can sit with his or her back squarely against the back of the seat with the legs bent at the knees over the front of the seat. The child usually will need to be at least 4 feet tall and weigh at least 60 lb to meet these requirements.

The leading cause of death of infants younger than 1 year of age is **sudden infant death syndrome** (SIDS). The Back To Sleep campaign advises parents to place their infant on the infant's back—not abdomen or side—when the infant is put down to sleep, as this reduces the risk of dying of SIDS.

As children get older, anticipatory guidance on other safety issues become important. As children learn to crawl and walk, stairwells should be blocked to reduce the risk of injuries from falling. Cleaning supplies, medications, and other potential poisons need to be stored safely out of reach of children, preferably in locked cabinets. Similarly, firearms should be stored safely, preferably unloaded and in locked cabinets or safes. Older children should be advised regarding the importance of wearing a helmet while riding a bicycle, skateboard, scooter, or other similar vehicle. All families should be advised to have smoke detectors throughout the home, especially in rooms where people sleep, and to keep the hot water heater set at or below 120°F to reduce the risk of scald injuries.

Nutrition is another important area of anticipatory guidance. Infants younger than 1 year old should be breastfed or receive an iron-containing formula. Cereals and other baby foods can be introduced between 4 and 6 months of age. Whole cow's milk is introduced at 12 months and continued until at least the age of 2 years, before considering changing to reduced fat milk.

Immunizations

Ensuring that each child has received the child's age-appropriate immunizations is a key component of each well child visit. The child's immunization status also should be reviewed at acute care visits. Minor illnesses, even those causing low-grade fevers, are not contraindications to vaccinating children, allowing an acute care visit to be an excellent opportunity to provide this service. **True contraindications to providing a vaccination include a history of an anaphylactic reaction to a specific vaccine or vaccine component or a severe illness,** with or without a fever. Figure 5–1 shows the recommended childhood vaccination schedule. Catch-up schedules for children who are either completely unimmunized or who have missed doses of the recommended vaccines are published by the Centers for Disease Control and Prevention.

Vaccine ▼ Age ▶	Birth	1 month	2 months	4 months	6 months	12 months	15 months	18 months	24 months	4–6 years	11–12 years	13–14 years	15 years	16–18 years
Hapatitis B	Hep B	Hep B	Hep B	Hep B		Hep B					Hep B Series			
Diphtheria, Tetanus, Pertussis			DTaP	DTaP	DTaP		DTaP	DTaP		DTaP	Tdap		Tdap	
Haemophilus influenzae type b			Hib	Hib	Hib	Hib	Hib							
Inactivated Poliovirus			IPV	IPV		IPV	IPV			IPV				
Measles, Mumps, Rubella						MMR	MMR			MMR		MMR		
Varicella						Varicella	Varicella				Vericella			
Meningococcal						Vaccines within broken line are for selected populations			MPSV 4		MCV 4		MCV 4	MCV 4
Pneumococcal			PCV	PCV	PCV	PCV	PCV		PCV	PCV	PPV			
Influenza						Influenza (Yearly)	Influenza (Yearly)				Influenza (Yearly)			
Hepatitis A									Hep A Series					

Range of recommended ages   Catch-up immunization   11–12 year old assessment

This schedule indicates the recommended ages for routine administration of currently licensed childhood vaccines, as of December 1, 2005, for children through age 18 years. Any dose not administered at the recommended age should be administered at any subsequent visit when indicated and feasible. ■ Indicates age groups that warrant special effort to administer those vaccines not previously administered. Additional vaccines may be licensed and recommended during the year. Licensed combination vaccines may be used whenever any components of the combination are indicated and other components of the vaccine are not contraindicated and if approved by the Food and Drug Administration for that dose of the series. Providers should consult the respective ACIP statement for detailed recommendations. Clinically significant adverse events that follow immunization should be reported to the Vaccine Adverse Event Reporting System (VAERS). Guidance about how to obtain and complete a VAERS form is available at www.vaers.hhs.gov or by telephone, 800-822-7967.

Figure 5-1. Recommended Childhood and Adolescent Immunization Schedule. (*From the Centers for Disease Control and Prevention. Available at: www.cdc.gov/nip/recs/child-schedule-bw-print.pdf.*)

Comprehension Questions

[5.1] By what age should most children be able to sit well without support?

    A. 3 months
    B. 6 months
    C. 9 months
    D. 12 months

[5.2] A 2-year-old child weighs 34 lb. What type of car seat should the child use?

    A. A rear-facing car seat in the back seat of the vehicle.
    B. A forward-facing car seat in the back seat of the vehicle.
    C. A forward-facing car seat in the front seat of the vehicle.
    D. A booster seat in the back seat of the vehicle.

[5.3] Which of the following vaccines is routinely recommended at 4 months of age?

    A. Diphtheria, tetanus, acellular pertussis (DTaP)
    B. Oral polio vaccine (OPV)
    C. Measles, mumps, rubella (MMR)
    D. Varicella

[5.4] Which of the following is a true contraindication to vaccinating a child?

    A. Acute otitis media requiring antibiotic therapy
    B. Previous vaccination reaction that consisted of a small red knot at the vaccine site
    C. History of an allergic reaction to penicillin
    D. Previous vaccination reaction that consisted of wheezing and hypotension

Answers

[5.1] **C.** Most 6-month old children would be expected to sit without support. 6-month old children would also be expected to transfer objects from one hand to the other, roll from a prone to supine position, babble and recognize strangers.

[5.2] **B.** A child who weighs more than 20 lb and is older than 1 year of age may sit in a forward-facing car seat in the back seat of the car. A child who weighs more than 40 lb is usually big enough to use a booster seat, also in the back seat of the car.

[5.3]   **A.** DTaP is routinely recommended at ages 2, 4, 6, and 12–15 months, and at 4–6 years of age. Oral polio vaccination is no longer routinely recommended in children; the inactivated, injectable polio vaccine is recommended in its place. MMR vaccination is recommended at ages 12–15 months and 4–6 years. Varicella vaccination is recommended at age 12–15 months.

[5.4]   **D.** A previous anaphylactic reaction is a true contraindication to vaccination. A minor illness or minor vaccination reaction, such as a red knot, is not a contraindication. Penicillin is not a component of vaccines and history of allergy to this medication is not a contraindication.

CLINICAL PEARLS

❖ True contraindications to providing vaccinations are rare; acute care visits are an excellent opportunity to provide childhood vaccinations.

❖ SIDS is the leading cause of death in infants younger than age 1 year. Parents should place their children on their "Back-to-Sleep."

REFERENCES

American Academy of Pediatrics. Screening for elevated blood lead levels. Pediatrics 1998;101(6):1072.

Brayden RM. Office pediatrics. In Hay WW, Levin MJ, Sondheimer JM, et al. (eds). Current pediatric diagnosis and treatment. 15th ed, New York: McGraw-Hill, 2001:203.

Broderick P. Am Fam Physician. 1998 Sep 1;58(3):691–700, 703–4.

DeMichele AM, Ruth RA. Newborn hearing screening. Available at: www.emedicine.com/ent/topic576.htm. Last accessed December 2005.

Rakel RE. Textbook of family practice. 6th ed. Philadelphia: WB Saunders, 2002:610.

A 35-year-old female with a history of asthma presents to your office with symptoms of nasal itching, sneezing, and rhinorrhea. She states she feels this way most days but her symptoms are worse in the spring and fall. She has had difficulty sleeping because she is always congested. She states she has taken diphenhydramine (Benadryl) with no relief. She does not smoke cigarettes and does not have exposure to passive smoke but she does have 2 cats at home. On examination, she appears tired but is in no respiratory distress. Her vital signs are temperature, 98.8°F; blood pressure, 128/84 mm Hg; pulse, 88 beats/min; respiratory rate, 18 breaths/min. The mucosa of her nasal turbinates appear swollen (boggy) and have a pale, bluish-gray color. Thin and watery secretions are seen. No abnormalities are seen on ear examination. There is no cervical lymphadenopathy noted and her lungs are clear.

 What is the most likely diagnosis?

 What is your next step?

 What are important considerations and potential complications of management?

ANSWERS TO CASE 6: Allergic Disorders

Summary: A 35-year-old asthmatic female complains of chronic nasal congestion that is worse in the spring and the fall.

◆ **Most likely diagnosis:** Allergic rhinitis.

◆ **Next step in management of this patient:** Treatment with antihistamines, decongestants, or intranasal steroids. These treatments can also be used in combination with each other.

◆ **Considerations and possible complications of therapy:** Excessive use of topical decongestants can cause rebound congestion. Recognition and reduction of potential allergen exposure will yield more success in management than pharmacotherapy alone.

Analysis

Objectives

1. Understand the inflammatory nature of allergic rhinitis.
2. Recognition of physical examination findings consistent with allergic rhinitis.
3. Develop an approach to the management of allergic rhinitis, including the roles of pharmacotherapy and reduction of allergen exposure.
4. Recognition and management of asthma.
5. Identification of essential features and treatment of anaphylaxis.

Background

Rhinitis is inflammation of the nasal membranes and is characterized by any combination of the following: sneezing, nasal congestion, nasal itching, and rhinorrhea. The eyes, ears, sinuses, and throat can also be involved. Allergic rhinitis is the most common cause of rhinitis, occurring in up to 15% of the population.

Pathophysiology

Allergic rhinitis involves inflammation of the mucous membranes of the nose, eyes, eustachian tubes, middle ear, sinuses, and pharynx. Inflammation of the mucous membranes is characterized by a complex interaction of inflammatory mediators but, ultimately, is triggered by an immunoglobulin E (IgE)-mediated response to an extrinsic protein.

In susceptible individuals, exposure to certain foreign proteins leads to allergic sensitization, which is characterized by the production of specific IgE directed against these proteins. This specific IgE coats the surface of mast cells, which are present in the nasal mucosa. When the specific allergen is inhaled into the nose, it can bind to the IgE in the mast cells, leading to a delayed release of a number of mediators.

Mediators that are immediately released include histamine, tryptase, chymase, and kinase. Mast cells quickly synthesize other mediators, including leukotrienes and prostaglandin D_2. Symptoms can occur quickly after exposure. Mucous glands are stimulated, leading to increased secretions. Vasodilation occurs, causing congestion. Stimulation of sensory nerves leads to sneezing and itching. Other symptoms include the redness and tearing of eyes, postnasal drip and ear pressure.

Over the next 4–8 hours, these mediators, through a complex interplay of events, recruit neutrophils, eosinophils, lymphocytes, and macrophages to the mucosa. These inflammatory cells cause more congestion and mucus production that may persist for hours or days. Systemic effects, including fatigue, sleepiness, and malaise, can result from the inflammatory response as well.

History

Obtaining a detailed history is important in the evaluation of allergic rhinitis, as specific triggers may be identified. Evaluation should include the nature, duration, and time course of symptoms. The recent use of medications is another important consideration. Other aspects include a family history of allergic diseases, environmental exposures, and comorbid conditions.

Part of the history should include the time pattern of symptoms and whether symptoms occur at a consistent level throughout the year (**perennial rhinitis**), only occur in specific seasons (**seasonal rhinitis**), or a combination of the two. Trigger factors, such as exposure to pollens, mold spores, specific animals, or cleaning of the house, can sometimes be identified. Irritant triggers, such as smoke, pollution, and strong smells can aggravate symptoms of allergic rhinitis. Response to treatment with antihistamines supports the diagnosis of allergic rhinitis.

Symptoms

Symptoms that can be associated with allergic rhinitis include:

- Sneezing
- Itching (of nose, eyes, or ears)
- Rhinorrhea
- Postnasal drip
- Congestion
- Anosmia
- Headache
- Earache
- Tearing, red eyes
- Drowsiness

Physical Examination

Common findings on examination include "allergic shiners," which are dark circles around the eyes related to vasodilation or nasal congestion. The "nasal crease" can be seen in some cases. It is a horizontal crease across the lower half of the bridge of the nose caused by repeated upward rubbing of the tip of the nose by the palm of the hand ("allergic salute").

Examination of the nose may reveal mucosa of the nasal turbinates to be swollen (boggy) and have a pale, bluish-gray color. Assessment of the character and quantity of nasal mucus may be helpful in ascertaining a diagnosis. Thin and watery secretions are frequently associated with allergic rhinitis, whereas thick and purulent secretions are usually associated with sinusitis. The characteristic of the mucous is not always diagnostic, as thick, purulent, colored mucus can also occur with allergic rhinitis.

The nasal cavity should be inspected for growths such as polyps or tumors. Polyps are firm, gray masses that are often attached by a stalk, which may not be visible. After spraying a topical decongestant, polyps do not shrink, whereas the surrounding nasal mucosa does shrink. Examine the nasal septum to look for any deviation or septal perforation that may be present as a consequence of chronic rhinitis, granulomatous disease, cocaine abuse, prior surgery, topical decongestant abuse, or, rarely, topical steroid overuse.

Otoscopy should be performed to look for tympanic membrane retraction, air-fluid levels, or bubbles. Performing pneumatic otoscopy can be considered to look for abnormal tympanic membrane mobility. These findings can be associated with allergic rhinitis, particularly if eustachian tube dysfunction or secondary otitis media is present. Ocular examination may reveal findings of injection and swelling of the palpebral conjunctivae, with excess tear production. Dennie-Morgan lines (prominent creases below the inferior eyelid) are associated with allergic rhinitis.

"Cobblestoning" of the posterior pharynx is often observed. This is caused by the presence of streaks of lymphoid tissue on the posterior pharynx. Tonsillar hypertrophy can also be seen. The neck should be examined for the presence of lymphadenopathy. The respiratory system must be examined for findings consistent with asthma. These include wheezing, tachypnea and a prolonged expiratory phase of respiration.

Causes of Allergic Rhinitis

The causes of allergic rhinitis can differ depending on whether the symptoms are seasonal, perennial, or sporadic/episodic. Some patients are sensitive to multiple allergens and can have perennial allergic rhinitis with seasonal exacerbations. Although food allergy can cause rhinitis, particularly in children, it is rarely a cause of allergic rhinitis in the absence of gastrointestinal or skin symptoms. Seasonal allergic rhinitis is commonly caused by allergy to seasonal pollens and outdoor molds.

Pollens (Tree, Grass, and Weed)

Tree pollens, which vary by geographic location, are typically present in high counts during the spring, although some species produce their pollens in the fall. Grass pollens also vary by geographic location. Most of the common grass species are associated with allergic rhinitis. A number of these grasses are cross-reactive, meaning that they have similar antigenic structures (i.e., proteins recognized by specific IgE in allergic sensitization). Consequently, a person who is allergic to one species is also likely to be sensitive to a number of other species. The grass pollens are most prominent from the late spring through the fall, but can be present year-round in warmer climates.

Weed pollens also vary geographically. Many weeds, such as short ragweed, a common cause of allergic rhinitis in much of the United States, are most prominent in the late summer and fall. Other weed pollens are present year-round, particularly in warmer climates.

Perennial allergic rhinitis is typically caused by allergens within the home, but can also be caused by outdoor allergens that are present year-round. In warmer climates, grass pollens can be present throughout the year. In some climates, individuals may be symptomatic because of trees and grasses in the warmer months and molds and weeds in the winter.

House Dust Mites

In the United States, two major house dust mite species are associated with allergic rhinitis. These mites feed on organic material in households, particularly the skin that is shed from humans and pets. They can be found in carpets, upholstered furniture, pillows, mattresses, comforters, and stuffed toys.

Animals

Allergy to indoor pets is a common cause of perennial allergic rhinitis. Cat and dog allergies are encountered most commonly in clinical practice. However, allergies have been reported to occur with most of the furry animals and birds that are kept as indoor pets. Although cockroach allergy is most frequently considered to be a cause of asthma, particularly in the inner city, it can also cause perennial allergic rhinitis in infested households. Rodent infestation may also be associated with allergic sensitization.

Treatment

The management of allergic rhinitis consists of three major categories of treatment: allergen avoidance, pharmacologic management, and immunotherapy. All aspects of treatment are more successful when exposure to allergens is decreased. Exposure to common allergens, such as dust mites, can be enhanced by methods such as removing the carpets from homes and encasing bedding in plastic.

Pharmacotherapy can involve the use of **antihistamines, decongestants, intranasal corticosteroids, and, in severe cases, systemic corticosteroids**. **Antihistamines** competitively antagonize the receptors for histamine, which is released from mast cells. This reduces the production of symptoms mediated by the release of histamine. "First-generation" antihistamines, including diphenhydramine, chlorpheniramine, and hydroxyzine, are inexpensive and available over-the-counter. Side effects include sedation and the anticholinergic effects of dry mouth, dry eyes, blurred vision, and urinary retention. Newer, so called second-generation antihistamines, including loratadine, fexofenadine, and cetirizine, have much less penetration into the central nervous system, resulting in a lower incidence of sedation as a side effect. They also have fewer anticholinergic effects. They are, however, significantly more expensive than the older agents.

Decongestants, either given orally or intranasally, can be used to provide symptomatic relief of nasal congestion. These agents constrict blood vessels in the nasal mucosa and reduce the overall volume of the mucosa. The most commonly used agent is pseudoephedrine, an α-adrenoreceptor agonist. Oral decongestants can cause tachycardia, tremors, and insomnia. Rebound hyperemia and worsening of symptoms can occur with chronic use or upon discontinuation of nasal decongestants.

Corticosteroid nasal sprays are effective for the long-term management of allergic rhinitis. They reduce the production of inflammatory mediators and the recruitment of inflammatory cells. Systemic absorption of the steroid is relatively low, reducing the risk of complications associated with the chronic use of systemic corticosteroids. Side effects include nosebleeds, pharyngitis, and upper respiratory tract infections.

Oral corticosteroids are potent inhibitors of cell-mediated immunity. The use of systemic steroids is limited by adverse effects, including suppression of the hypothalamic–pituitary–adrenal axis and hyperglycemia. Long-term use can lead to peptic ulcer formation, increased susceptibility to infection, poor wound healing, and the reduction of bone density. Because of these significant risks, systemic steroids are used only for severe allergies and are used in the lowest effective dose for the shortest possible time.

Desensitization therapy is frequently attempted in patients who remain symptomatic despite maximal medical therapy. The first step of this treatment is to test for specific antigens to which the person is allergic. The second step is to inject the patient with highly diluted concentrations of this antigen. The concentration of the antigen(s) in the injection is gradually increased, in an effort to reduce the patient's inflammatory response to the antigen(s). Injections are typically given weekly or biweekly. This process is expensive, time-consuming, and requires numerous injections. Patients and physicians must be prepared to address severe, even anaphylactic, reactions that may occur during the process.

Anaphylaxis, Urticaria, and Angioedema

Urticaria is characterized by large, irregularly shaped, pruritic, erythematous wheals. **Angioedema** is painless, deep, subcutaneous swelling that often involves the periorbital, circumoral, and facial regions. **Anaphylaxis** is a systemic reaction with cutaneous symptoms that is associated with dyspnea, visceral edema, and hypotension. The manifestations of anaphylaxis include hypotension or shock from widespread vasodilation, respiratory distress from bronchospasm or laryngeal edema, gastrointestinal and uterine muscle contraction, and urticaria and angioedema.

At the first suspicion of anaphylaxis, aqueous epinephrine 1:1000, in a dose of 0.2–0.5 mL (0.2–0.5 mg) is injected subcutaneously or intramuscularly. Repeated injections can be given every 15–30 minutes when necessary. Rapid intravenous infusion of large volumes of fluids (saline, lactated Ringer solution, plasma or plasma expanders) is essential to replace loss of intravascular plasma into tissues. Airway obstruction may be caused by edema of the larynx or by bronchospasm. Endotracheal intubation may be required. Bronchospasm responds to subcutaneous epinephrine or terbutaline. Antihistamines may be useful as adjuvant therapy for alleviating cutaneous manifestations of urticaria or angioedema and pruritus. All patients with anaphylaxis should be monitored for a period of time; for example, 24 hours.

Asthma

Asthma is a chronic disease characterized by airway hyperresponsiveness. There are recurrent muscle spasms of the bronchi and bronchioles. Essentials of diagnosis include recurrent wheezing, shortness of breath, or cough, an increase in airway secretions, and dyspnea. A history of allergies in children is also common.

Asthma results in mild to severe obstruction to airflow in the tracheobronchial tree. Viral infections and allergens are two of the major triggers in childhood asthma. A history of wheezing, shortness of breath, dyspnea, cough, increased sputum production, and chest tightness is often found. The physical examination may reveal wheezing, increased expiratory phase, tachypnea, cyanosis, tachycardia, or use of accessory respiratory muscles.

Asthma is classified as mild intermittent, moderate intermittent, moderate persistent or severe persistent, based on the frequency of symptoms and the amount of airway obstruction (Table 6–1). **Status asthmaticus** is an obstruction that lasts for days or weeks.

Treatment involves the avoidance of triggers and the use of medications, both to reduce the frequency of exacerbation and to relieve the acute symptoms. These medications include β-adrenergic agonists, inhaled corticosteroids, leukotriene modifiers, mast cell stabilizers, and systemic corticosteroids.

The rapid acting β_2-adrenergic agonist albuterol is the mainstay treatment for acute symptomatic relief in asthma. It works to rapidly relax bronchial smooth muscle. It also reduces the release of mast cell mediators and increases mucociliary clearance. Long-acting β_2-adrenergic agonists have the same mechanism of action, but are not used for acute bronchospasm. They are effective at reducing the frequency of exacerbation in persistent asthma. The primary treatment of persistent asthma is the daily use of inhaled corticosteroids,

Table 6–1

CLASSIFICATION OF ASTHMA SEVERITY

CLASSIFICATION	DAYS WITH SYMPTOMS	NIGHTS WITH SYMPTOMS	PEF OR FEV$_1$ (PEF IS % OF PERSONAL BEST; FEV$_1$ IS % OF PREDICTED)	TREATMENT
Severe persistent	Continual	Frequent	≤60%	Preferred: high-dose inhaled steroid and long-acting β-agonist *and*, if needed, corticosteroid tablets or syrup
Moderate persistent	Daily	≥5/month	>60–<80%	Preferred: low- to medium-dose inhaled steroid and long-acting β-agonist Alternative: increase inhaled steroid within medium-dose range *or* low- to medium-dose inhaled steroid and leukotriene modifier or theophylline If needed (particularly in patients with recurring severe exacerbations): Preferred: increase inhaled steroid within medium-dose range and long-acting β-agonist Alternative: increase inhaled steroid within medium-dose range and add leukotriene modifier or theophylline

Mild persistent	3–6/week	3–4/month	≥80%	Preferred: low-dose inhaled steroid Alternative: cromolyn, nedocromil, leukotriene modifier or theophylline
Mild intermittent	≤2/week	≤2/month	≥80%	No daily medication needed Severe exacerbations may occur, separated by long periods of normal function and no symptoms, a course of systemic corticosteroids is recommended

All patients: short-acting bronchodilator as needed for symptoms. Data from National Institutes of Health. Practical guide for the diagnosis and management of asthma. Washington, DC: National Institutes of Health, National Heart, Lung and Blood Institute, 1997; and the National Asthma Education and Prevention Program (NAEPP) Expert Panel Report. Guidelines for the diagnosis and management of asthma—update on selected topics, 2002. Washington DC: National Institutes of Health, National Heart, Lung and Blood Institute, 2002.

which reduce the production of inflammatory mediators and reduce vascular permeability. They do not have an effect on smooth muscle relaxation and should not be used for an acute exacerbation. Leukotriene inhibitors, which either reduce the production of these inflammatory mediators (zileuton) or competitively antagonize their receptors (zafirlukast, montelukast), are also effective in the prevention of exacerbation in persistent asthma. Systemic corticosteroids are used in the treatment of acute exacerbation and for prophylaxis in severe persistent asthma. Table 6–1 lists the specific indications for uses of each medication.

Conjunctivitis

Conjunctivitis is an infection of the palpebral and/or bulbar conjunctiva. It is the most common eye disease seen in community medicine. Most cases are caused by bacterial or viral infection. Other causes include allergy and chemical irritants. The mode of transmission of infectious conjunctivitis is usually direct contact to the opposite eye or to other persons via fingers, towels, or handkerchiefs.

The organisms isolated most commonly in bacterial conjunctivitis are *Staphylococci, Streptococci, Haemophilus, Moraxella,* and *Pseudomonas.* There is no blurring of vision and only mild discomfort. In severe cases, examination of stained conjunctival scrapings and cultures are recommended. The disease is usually self-limited, lasting about 10–14 days if untreated. A sulfonamide instilled locally three times daily will usually clear the infection in 2–3 days.

Epidemic keratoconjunctivitis (pink eye) is highly contagious and spread by person-to-person contact or fomites. The most common cause is adenovirus. It is usually associated with pharyngitis, fever, malaise, and preauricular lymphadenopathy. Locally, the palpebral conjunctiva is red with a copious watery discharge and scanty exudates. Local sulfonamide therapy might prevent secondary bacterial infection; hot compresses reduce the discomfort of the associated lid edema; weak topical steroids may be necessary to treat the corneal infiltrates. The disease usually lasts at least 2 weeks.

Noninfectious causes of conjunctivitis include allergic and chemical irritants. Symptoms of allergic conjunctivitis include itching, tearing, redness, stringy discharge, and sometimes photophobia. Treatment can include the use of oral antihistamines or topical antihistamine or antiinflammatory eye drops.

Comprehension Questions

[6.1]   Which of the following is a chronic inflammatory disease characterized by airway hyperresponsiveness?

   A. Chronic bronchitis
   B. Emphysema
   C. Asthma
   D. Sarcoidosis

[6.2]   An 18-year-old male presents for follow-up of his asthma. He has symptoms no more than 1 day per week and 1 night per month. Which of the following is the most appropriate treatment for him?

   A. Daily inhaled corticosteroid
   B. As-needed use of a short-acting β-adrenergic agonist
   C. Daily use of a long-acting β-adrenergic agonist
   D. Daily use of leukotriene modifiers
   E. All of the above

[6.3]   Which of the following is a benefit of the second-generation antihistamines?

   A. Less expensive than the first-generation antihistamines
   B. Less sedating than the first-generation antihistamines
   C. More effective than the first-generation antihistamines
   D. They are available over-the-counter, whereas first-generation antihistamines require a prescription

Answers

[6.1]   **C.** Asthma is a chronic inflammatory disease characterized by airway hyperresponsiveness. It most commonly is triggered by allergens, infections, or irritants such as cigarette smoke.

[6.2]   **B.** This patient has mild intermittent asthma, as he has symptoms less than twice per week and less than 2 nights per month. The recommended treatment for mild intermittent asthma is the as-needed use of a short-acting inhaled β-agonist.

[6.3]   **B.** The second-generation antihistamines are less sedating and have fewer anticholinergic side effects than the first-generation antihistamines. They are, however, more expensive and no more effective at symptom relief than the first-generation antihistamines. One of the newer agents, loratadine, is available over the counter. The other second-generation antihistamines are by prescription only.

CLINICAL PEARLS

❖ The management of allergic rhinitis consists of three major categories of treatment: allergen avoidance, pharmacological management and immunotherapy.

❖ For the diagnosis of asthma look for recurrent wheezing, cough, increase in airway secretion, or dyspnea.

❖ At the first suspicion of anaphylaxis, aqueous epinephrine 1:1000 in a dose of 0.2–0.5 mL (0.2–0.5 mg) is injected subcutaneously or intramuscularly. The airway should always be assessed and patient intubated if necessary to secure breathing.

REFERENCES

Tierney LM, McPhee SJ, Papadakis MA. Current medical diagnosis and treatment. 42nd ed. New York: McGraw-Hill, 2003:195–96, 761–764.

Sheikh J. Allergic rhinitis. 2005. Available at: http://www.emedicine.com/med/topic104.htm.

Toy E, Rosenfeld G, Loose D, Briscoe D. Case files: pharmacology. New York: McGraw-Hill, 2005.

A 55-year-old male comes into your office for follow-up of a chronic cough. He also complains of shortness of breath with activity. He reports that this has been getting worse over time. As you are interviewing the patient, you note that he smells of cigarette smoke. Upon further questioning, he reports smoking 1 pack of cigarettes per day for the past 35 years and denies ever being advised to quit. On examination, he is in no respiratory distress at rest, his vital signs are normal, and he has no obvious signs of cyanosis. His pulmonary examination is notable for reduced air movement and faint expiratory wheezing on auscultation.

◆ **What would you recommend to this patient?**

◆ **What interventions are available to aid with smoking cessation?**

ANSWERS TO CASE 7: Tobacco Use

Summary: A 55-year-old male with a 35 pack/year history of smoking presents with a chronic cough and progressively worsening dyspnea.

◆ **Recommendations to this patient:** This patient should be advised to quit smoking; one strategy, using the 5 As, is discussed below.

◆ **Interventions available to help with smoking cessation:** Counseling to quit smoking along with pharmacologic assistance with bupropion and/or nicotine replacement.

Considerations

Tobacco use is the single greatest cause of preventable death. It is responsible for increased death rates from cancer, cardiac, cerebrovascular, and chronic pulmonary disease. Smoking also affects the health of those in close contact with people who smoke. Each year, 38,000 deaths from cancer and heart disease in nonsmokers are attributable to secondhand smoke. Smoking in pregnancy is associated with prematurity, intrauterine growth restriction, stillbirth, spontaneous abortion, and infant death. Smoking cessation reduces all of these risks. However, despite this evidence, it is difficult for smokers to quit. Healthcare providers are important in the effort to reduce tobacco use and its related disease burden.

Research indicates that physician intervention, even in brief encounters, increases tobacco cessation rate. Furthermore, cessation rates increase with increased physician time and frequency of encounters to address tobacco use, but the optimal duration and frequency has not been defined. **The process of discussing tobacco use and cessation involves several steps; one useful framework is the "5 As":**

Ask about tobacco use: ask the patient at each visit about current tobacco use;

Advise to quit through clear personalized messages: let the patient know of his/her specific risks of tobacco use; in the sample case, talk to the patient about how the persistent cough and dyspnea can be related to the tobacco use and how cessation might be helpful;

Assess willingness to quit: find out the patient's thoughts about quitting and if the patient is ready to proceed;

Assist to quit: including counseling and pharmacologic treatment;

Arrange follow-up and support.

Multiple factors may be part of a patient's unwillingness to quit. **A strategy to enhance motivation** includes discussing the specific *relevance* to the patient of smoking cessation, *risks* of ongoing tobacco use, *rewards* to quitting (financial, health, social), *roadblocks* to quitting (withdrawal, discouragement because of failed past attempts, enjoyment of smoking), and *repetition* (readdressing the problem at each visit and reminding patients most people attempt to quit several times before being successful).

In pregnancy, it has been found to be helpful to discuss specific risks to the mother and fetus of continued tobacco use. While cessation prior to pregnancy is ideal, cessation at any time during pregnancy is associated with health benefits for patient and fetus, so ongoing discussions are encouraged. The pregnant patient will also need ongoing support after delivery to reduce the risk of remission after delivery.

Pharmacologic Therapy

In addition to counseling and reviewing the risks and benefits of quitting, the use of pharmacologic aids can increase the likelihood of successful smoking cessation when a patient has decided to quit. The following 5 therapies are approved by the Food and Drug Administration (FDA) for smoking cessation and are considered first-line treatments for smoking cessation: bupropion sustained release, nicotine gum, nicotine patch, nicotine inhaler, and nicotine nasal spray.

Bupropion is the first nonnicotine treatment for smoking cessation approved by the FDA. It is thought to work by blocking uptake of norepinephrine and/or dopamine. It is contraindicated in patients with eating disorders, monoamine oxidase (MAO) inhibitor use in the last 2 weeks or a history of seizure disorder. The medication should be started 1–2 weeks before the quit date and the usual dose is 150 mg a day for 3 days then 150 mg twice a day. The usual course of treatment is 7–12 weeks, but it can be used for up to 6 months as maintenance therapy. This treatment can be used alone or in combination with nicotine-based treatments. In two studies comparing bupropion sustained release to placebo, the cessation rate for the bupropion group was 30%, compared to 17% in the placebo group.

Nicotine replacement therapies as a group increase smoking cessation rates over placebo. They can be used in combination therapy, which may increase cessation rates over monotherapy.

Nicotine gum is available in 2 mg and 4 mg of nicotine per piece. The patient chews a piece of the gum until the patient feels a peppery taste in the mouth, "parks" the gum in a cheek until the sensation goes away and then chews the gum again until the peppery sensation returns. The 4-mg dose is recommended for those who smoke more than 25 cigarettes per day and the 2-mg dose for those who smoke fewer than 25 cigarettes per day. Common pitfalls include not "parking" the gum (i.e., chewing constantly) and not using enough pieces per day initially. Consider advising the patient to use the gum on a scheduled basis, rather than as needed, initially, and then slowly tapering the number of pieces per day.

The nicotine cartridge inhaler is available by prescription and has also been found to be effective in increasing smoking cessation rates. Each cartridge contains 4 mg of nicotine in 80 inhalations. The recommended dose is 6–16 cartridges per day. The inhaler can be used over several months, with a gradual tapering of the dose. For both the gum and inhaler, acidic beverages can reduce absorption of the nicotine from the buccal mucosa, so the patient should avoid ingestion within 15 minutes of use of these products.

Another therapeutic option is the nicotine nasal inhaler. The inhaler provides 0.5 mg of nicotine per inhalation and can be used at a starting rate of 1–2 doses per hour, for a maximum of 40 doses per day (5 doses per hour). The inhaler can also be used over months, with gradual tapering of the dose. Nasal irritation is the most common side effect.

The nicotine patch is a passive nicotine replacement system, compared to the other methods outlined above. There are two common over-the-counter forms of the nicotine patch: Nicoderm CQ, which comes in multiple doses (21, 14, and 7 mg of nicotine per patch) and are meant to be worn for 24 hours a day, and Nicotrol, which has 15 mg of nicotine and is meant to be worn for 16 hours a day. The patch is replaced daily, and consideration should be given to starting with higher-dose patches in heavy smokers. Treatment with the patch for less than 8 weeks is as effective as longer treatment periods. The most common side effect is irritation of the skin at the site of the patch.

All of the products can be considered for use in the pregnant smoker if counseling is insufficient to promote cessation, and if, in discussion with the patient, it is determined that the risks of continued smoking outweigh the risks of the medication. The nicotine inhaler, nasal spray, and gum are pregnancy category D drugs; the patch is pregnancy category C, and bupropion is pregnancy category B.

The United States Preventive Services Task Force (USPSTF) strongly recommends screening all adults and pregnant patients for tobacco use and offering cessation intervention for those who use tobacco products (Level A recommendation). At this time there is insufficient evidence to recommend for or against screening children and adolescents for tobacco use or offering interventions to prevent tobacco use or promote cessation (Level I recommendation). However, as most smokers start in this age group, the USPSTF notes that providers may use individual discretion when discussing tobacco use in this population.

Comprehension Questions

[7.1]   A pregnant woman who smokes 1 pack of cigarettes a day asks for your advice regarding smoking cessation while she is pregnant. Which of the following statements is most appropriate?

A. She would have to quit "cold turkey," as all available pharmacologic treatments are unsafe in pregnancy.

B. It is more important for her to quit smoking after she has the baby, as the risk to her fetus is very low.

C. There is no benefit to the fetus if she quits smoking after the first trimester, as organogenesis is complete by this time.

D. Cessation at any time is beneficial both to the patient and the fetus.

[7.2] Which of the following statements regarding available treatments for smoking cessation is true?

    A. Bupropion can be used in combination with nicotine supplements.

    B. Nicotine gum is most effective if chewed continuously, to promote a constant release of the nicotine.

    C. Nicotine supplements are most effective when used as needed for withdrawal symptoms.

    D. Subcutaneous administration of nicotine supplementation is an effective regimen.

[7.3] Which of the following counseling strategies is most likely to enhance your patients' smoking cessation rates?

    A. Discuss smoking cessation techniques only with patients who ask for your advice, as others will resent your suggestions.

    B. Emphasize primarily the health risks of smoking.

    C. Note in each patient's chart that you have discussed cessation, so that you don't repeat the message to the same patient at subsequent visits.

    D. Ask about smoking cessation at each encounter.

Answers

[7.1] **D.** Cessation of smoking at any time during the pregnancy is likely to provide health benefits for the mother and the fetus. Ongoing efforts to help continue her efforts to stay off of cigarettes after the baby is born also are important. Pharmacologic aids to increase the rates of smoking cessation during pregnancy can be used, after discussion with the patient of the risks and benefits of the medications and of continued smoking.

[7.2] **A.** Bupropion can be used in combination with any of the nicotine supplementation products. The nicotine products can also be used in combination with each other. Two common pitfalls in using nicotine supplementation are using supplementation only when having withdrawal symptoms and failing to use nicotine gum correctly. The gum should be chewed briefly and then parked in the cheek. It is less effective if chewed continuously.

[7.3] **D.** Asking patients about tobacco use is a key to promoting cessation. It is important to ask each patient at each visit and to be prepared to provide advice and assistance at any time.

CLINICAL PEARLS

❖ Most smokers require multiple attempts before successfully quitting for good. Remind your patients of this if they become discouraged in their efforts.

❖ Use the 5 As—Ask, Advise, Assess, Assist, and Arrange follow-up—to help your patients quit smoking.

REFERENCES

Fiore MC, Bailey WC, Cohen SJ, et al. Treating tobacco use and dependence. Clinical practice guideline. Rockville, MD: U.S. Department of Health and Human Services, Public Health Service, June 2000.

United States Preventive Services Task Force (USPSTF). Counseling to prevent tobacco use and tobacco-caused disease. Recommendations statement. Available at: http://www.ahrq.gov/clinic/uspstf/uspstbac.htm. Last accessed November 2003.

A 16-year-old female presents to your office with the complaint of greenish vaginal discharge for the past 2 months and the recent onset of lower abdominal pain. She reports that her last period was about 2.5 months ago. She is sexually active with two partners and has never used a condom or any other contraception with either. On physical examination she is not febrile with normal blood pressure and pulse. She has greenish discharge from the cervix with friability and cervicitis. There is no cervical motion tenderness. Her urine pregnancy test is positive. A cervical sample is positive for *Chlamydia* and negative for gonorrhea. Her rapid plasma reagin (RPR) is nonreactive and an HIV test is negative. The patient is treated with appropriate antibiotics and counseled concerning safer sex practices. You also inform the patient regarding her risk for HIV conversion, even though today's test was negative. The patient asks if you are going to tell her mother that she is pregnant and has this infection. You inform the patient that because of patient confidentiality ethical considerations you will not disclose this information to her mother without her consent. She tells you that she does not want her mother to know and she does not want her boyfriends to know she is infected.

◆ **What should you do?**

◆ **What should you tell the patient?**

◆ **What are the ethical considerations?**

◆ **What are the guidelines for reporting communicable diseases?**

ANSWERS TO CASE 8: Medical Ethics

Summary: The patient is a teen who is pregnant and has a sexually transmitted infection. She engages in high-risk sexual behavior. There are several considerations involved in this case. The first issue is pregnancy. In some states, the patient would be considered emancipated. Consequently, legally she can make decisions regarding her pregnancy-related healthcare (excluding abortion) without notice to or the express consent of her parents. In addition, she has a sexually transmitted infection, which is a reportable condition; thus the physician or the physician's agent ***must*** report this to the state health department for surveillance and infection control. She is also very concerned about informing her partners about the infection. There are also issues of confidentiality.

◆   **What you should do and what you should tell the patient:** You must inform the patient that you have to contact the state health department. The department will contact her and will contact her partners without disclosing her identity. You might also advise the patient to cooperate fully with the health department to avoid phone calls or letters received at home. It is also important to stress to the patient the importance of protecting her partners as well as herself, and that by disclosing to her partners, she may avoid further exposure.

◆   **Ethical considerations include:** Teenage pregnancy, confidentiality, sexually transmitted infection reporting, and emancipation.

◆   **Guidelines for reporting communicable diseases:** The guidelines for reporting communicable disease vary slightly from state to state. However, there is usually a formal mechanism for reporting to the state department of health. The physician may do it himself/herself or may elect to use an agent, such as a nurse or other medical facility staff member. It is a federal mandate to report communicable diseases; failure to do so may result in adverse legal, civil, and even criminal actions. In the state of Texas, failure to report communicable diseases is considered a class B misdemeanor.

Definitions

Emancipation: Emancipation is a legal process in which a person who is younger than the age of 18 years petitions the court to have herself/himself declared a legal adult. Laws for emancipation vary by state. Emancipation ends the parent's legal duty to support the minor, and also ends the parents right to make decisions about the minor's residence, education, healthcare, and to control the minor's conduct. However, this does not include the ability to consume alcohol, use tobacco, or exercise voting rights.

Mature Minor Doctrine/Rule (Judicial Bypass): The mature minor exception to the need for parental consent for medical care is based on the West Virginia Supreme Court case *Belcher v. CAMC*. Statute and court decisions in many states may vary. A minor may consent to receive medical care without the consent of the parents or guardian if deemed "mature" by the judicial system.

Analysis

Objectives

1. Discuss confidentiality and its ethical and legal considerations when treating adolescent or pregnant adolescent patients.
2. Understand the legal obligations for reporting communicable diseases and informing partners.

Considerations

According to the Society for Adolescent Medicine, "the overall goal in clinical practice is to deliver appropriate high quality healthcare to adolescent patients, while encouraging communication between parents or other trusted adults without betraying the adolescent's trust in the healthcare professional." It is very important to gain the confidence of adolescent patients because if the patient does not believe that the healthcare provider will keep the patient's health information confidential, the patient is less likely to seek healthcare when needed. Confidential healthcare should be provided for all adolescent patients; however, the physician must consider some very important issues, including: Is the teen self-supporting? Is the minor mature enough to make his or her own medical care decisions? Would disclosure without consent harm the patient?

Ethics

Ethical considerations when treating adolescent patients can be complex and one should use the **moral principles of ethics,** which include **autonomy, beneficence, nonmaleficence, and justice** to guide clinical decisions to maintain confidentiality. Respect for **autonomy** should involve respect for the patient's wishes, choices, and beliefs when deciding what is best for the patient. It is important to understand the dynamics of the parent–child relationship and why the teen does not want to disclose important medical information to parents. This type of dialogue may reveal very important things about the child's current situation and help to guide your decision making. Knowing the intricacies of the family dynamic may also help the clinician and the patient develop solutions to aid in disclosure of very important health-related issues.

Nonmaleficence implies that the physician will do nothing to harm the patient, which includes emotional and psychological harm. Failure to maintain confidentiality may result in some emotional distress for the patient. Moreover, the physician should not apply the same moral standards to every patient. Some teens are more mature than others and the physician should use his or her judgment with each adolescent patient.

In addition, the treating physician should apply the principle of **beneficence,** which requires action to further a patient's welfare. In other words, do the right thing for the patient. Maintaining confidentiality may aid in full disclosure of symptoms, life situations, etc. Full disclosure of pertinent medial information can help the physician provide the most comprehensive care to the patient.

Justice implies the fair and nonbiased treatment of the patient regardless of age, sex, or ethnicity. Consequently, adolescent patients should be given the same level of care as adults, without the having fear of disclosure, when they are mentally capable of receiving care.

In most cases, every attempt should be provided to ensure confidentiality. However, **there are instances when it would be in the best interest of the patient to disclose medical information.** Examples of these situations could include patients with homicidal or suicidal ideation or serious chemical dependence, and in suspected cases of abuse. Disclosure of medical information should only be considered when the life of the adolescent must be protected. It is also important to point out that, in most cases, adolescents are not responsible for payment of medical services. The parent or the guardian usually has to assume the responsibility for payment. Thus, the maintenance of confidentiality in these cases is an issue. Because there are no clear-cut guidelines in this situation, it is important to encourage open dialogue between the patient and the patient's parent. However, in instances when this is not possible the physician must use his or her own clinical judgment while considering ethical issues and must act in the best interest of the patient.

Legal Considerations

There are laws in place to protect the confidentiality of healthcare information. In general, the law requires the consent of the parent when healthcare is provided to minors; there are, however, exceptions, such as emergencies, care for the **"mature minor,"** and when the minor is legally entitled to consent to their own medical treatment.

Laws that allow minors to consent to medical treatment vary from state to state. In some states minors are allowed to consent to medical therapy based on status, such as emancipation, marriage, pregnancy, living apart from parents, and when given the status of "mature minor." The mature minor rule was created in 1967 and is based on the West Virginia Supreme Court case *Belcher v.*

CAMC, which allowed healthcare providers to treat a youth as an adult based on an assessment and documentation of the adolescent's maturity level. According to this decision, a court must determine that a minor is deemed mature, which determination is based on various factors, including age; ability; experience; education and or training; degree of maturity and or judgment exhibited; conduct and demeanor; capacity to understand the risk and benefits of medical treatment. The process to become a mature minor is known as judicial bypass and may vary from state to state. This exception to parental consent must be received from a court.

In addition, **adolescents may consent to medical care if they are considered emancipated**. Emancipation implies that a minor must be of a certain age (which varies by state), live apart from his or her parents, and be self-sufficient. Minors are also considered emancipated if they are self-supporting, not living at home, married, pregnant or a parent, in the military, or declared emancipated by the judicial system.

In some states, **consent to healthcare may be based on the type of care the adolescent is seeking.** Examples of the types of healthcare services that may be obtained without parental consent may include maternity services; contraceptive management; treatment and diagnosis of sexually transmitted infections (including HIV) or other reportable diseases; treatment of drug or alcohol problems; and care related to sexual assault or mental health services. These provisions are very important because they allow the necessary assessment and treatment of important health-related issues. Moreover, research shows that adolescents are more likely to seek medical care if confidentiality is protected.

Reportable Diseases

Reporting sexually transmitted infections (STIs), HIV, and other reportable illnesses can be stressful for the patient. This may be particularly stressful for the adolescent. The **information may be reported by the physician or by the physician's designated appointee.** All those involved in the oversight of blood products, including clinical laboratories or blood banks, are also required to report STIs and other reportable conditions to the state's health department. It is state and federal law that these illnesses be reported in a timely fashion to the state health department.

In addition, it is **mandatory that the information be disclosed to partners.** Partner reporting is a way to control the spread of disease and to ensure prompt and proper diagnosis and treatment of all those who may be affected. Partner notification can occur in either of two ways: by patient referral or by the department of health staff. The patient can contact his/her partner(s) for referral, diagnosis, and treatment. Alternatively, the partner(s) may be notified and counseled by department of health staff, if the patient is unwilling to inform them. In the setting where a patient is unwilling to inform his/her partner(s) of a reportable illness that places the partner(s) at risk, the healthcare provider has a legal and ethical obligation to inform the partner(s) (if known by the provider) that they are at risk.

Teenage Pregnancy and Confidentiality

Issues regarding teenage pregnancy and consent to disclose information regarding pregnancy are quite controversial. Laws for reporting vary by state and the specifics may become quite daunting. For the purposes of this case, focus is limited to generalities. One must understand the laws pertaining to this issue in the state in which he or she practices. In the state of Texas, as may be the case in other states, a clinician is not required to inform the parents of issues related to the pregnancy of a minor without the child's consent, but it is not mandatory for the adolescent to give consent for a physician to disclose information related to pregnancy to parents. However, studies demonstrate that failure to maintain confidentiality in "sensitive" health-related issues may inhibit appropriate healthcare delivery to the adolescent.

In Texas, the law does not allow state funds to be used for contraception without the consent of the parent. Moreover, in most states, an adolescent younger than age 18 years cannot give consent to abortion services without the consent of one or both parents. This issue has been the subject of political debate for many years. Proponents of mandatory consent laws believe that it is in the best interest of the minor for her parent(s) or guardian to be informed of her pregnancy and decision to obtain abortion services, stating that by doing so, communication among adult and child may be improved.

Opponents of these laws, however, see them as a threat to the well being of young women by forcing them to seek abortion services from unlicensed facilities, crossing state lines to obtain abortions, and increasing medical risk. The risk to young women may be increased by enforcing mandatory wait periods, which could mean having abortions later in the pregnancy than desired.

Currently, only 6 states do not require consent from parents to obtain abortion services. In a state in which consent is required, there are some legal alternatives for young women. For example, if an adolescent is considered emancipated, then consent from parents or guardians is not required. Waivers of consent (judicial bypass) may also be obtained through the judicial system.

Conclusion

Pregnancy-related care, abortion services, and reportable illnesses are complex and a clinician should seek legal advice when appropriate. However, in general, it is preferable to protect the confidentiality of the minor unless it unreasonable or unsafe to do so. It is also important to educate teens and parents of the importance of open communication and issues related to confidentiality in medical care.

Comprehension Questions

[8.1]   A 14-year-old female is here to see you for complaints of greenish vaginal discharge. She is sexually active with one partner and does not use condoms. You do a culture and find that she has *Trichomonas vaginitis*. She asks you not to tell her mom about this diagnosis or that she is sexually active. Can you keep this information from her parents?

A. Yes, you can keep this information confidential. However, it is advisable to talk with the teen about her sexual history and discuss communication issues between her and her parents.

B. No, she is a minor; thus you must disclose this information.

C. Yes, but you can only keep this confidential for today.

[8.2]   Example(s) of reportable conditions are:

A. Tuberculosis

B. HIV/AIDS

C. Gonorrhea

D. All of the above

[8.3]   Emancipation implies that a minor is

A. Able to vote

B. Able to purchase and consume alcohol

C. Able to make their own medical decisions without parental consent

D. Legally financially independent

[8.4]   Which of the following statements regarding a minor's ability to consent for an abortion is most accurate?

A. Because of medical confidentiality, a minor is able to consent to any medical therapy she chooses without the consent of her parents or guardian.

B. Although consent requirements for abortion services vary depending on the state, most states either have some form of required consent for abortion services to minors or a mandatory wait period.

C. There are no states in which a minor can obtain an abortion without the consent of a parent or guardian.

D. A minor cannot consent to any medical therapy without her parent's approval unless she has received a court order.

Answers

[8.1]   **A.** The law does not require the disclosure of sensitive medical information to parents. However, in some states it is not forbidden to disclose that information. A clinician must use his or her best judgment when deciding whether to disclose medical information. More importantly, the physician should recognize the importance of confidentiality when treating patients and encourage open communication between adolescents and parents when it is reasonable to do so.

[8.2]   **D.** All of the listed conditions are reportable. There are numerous other reportable conditions. As the list of reportable conditions may vary from state to state, it is mandatory for each physician to check with his/her state health department for a complete listing.

[8.3]   **C.** Emancipation implies that the patient is able to make decisions regarding health-related issues but does not give the patient the right to vote, consume alcohol, or use tobacco products if the patient is not of legal age.

[8.4]   **B.** The laws regarding the consent for abortion services vary from state to state. Only 6 states currently allow a minor to have an abortion without the consent of or notification to parents.

CLINICAL PEARLS

❖   Adolescent healthcare is a complex issue. However, the clinician should attempt to administer confidential healthcare to minors seeking care for sensitive medical issues when it is safe and appropriate to do so.

❖   It is very important for clinicians to know the laws regarding consent and confidentiality when treating adolescent patients of the states in which they practice.

REFERENCES

Boonstra H, Nash E. Minors and the rights to consent to health care. The Guttmacher Report on Public Policy, Volume 3, Number 4, August 2000.0 Available at: www.guttmacher.org/pubs/tgr/03/4/gr030404.html

Center for Reproductive Rights. Mandatory parental consent and notification laws. Item F039. March 2001. Available at: www.crlpl.org.

Cundiff D. Clinical case. Available at: www.ama-assn.org/ama/pub/category/print/15548.html.

Delke I. Screening and prevention of sexually transmitted diseases including HIV infection. Available at: www.dcmsonline.org/jax-medicine/1997journals/jan97/sex-trans.htm.

Emancipated teen parents and the TANF living arrangement rules. A fact sheet. Available at: www.clasp.org/publications_teen _parents.htm.

Ford C, English A, Sigman G. Society for Adolescent Medicine position statement. Confidential health care for adolescents: position paper of the Society of Adolescent Medicine. J Adolesc Med 2004;35:160–167.

Litt I. Adolescent patient confidentiality: whom are we kidding [editorial]? J Adolesc Health 2001;29:79.

Maradiegue A. Minor's right's versus parental rights: review of legal issues in adolescent health care. J Midwifery Womens Health 2003;48(3):170–177.

A 65-year-old African-American female presented to the emergency room complaining of worsening shortness of breath and palpitations for about 1 week. She reports feeling "dizzy" on and off for the past year, which dizziness is associated with weakness that has been worsening for the past month. She has been feeling "too tired" to even walk to her backyard and water her flower bed that she used to do "all the time." She has been so dyspneic walking up the stairs at her home that she moved downstairs to the guest room about a week ago. Review of systems is significant for knee pain, for which she frequently takes aspirin or ibuprofen; otherwise the review of systems is negative. She has no significant medical history and has not been to a doctor in several years. She had a normal well woman examination and screening colonoscopy about 5 years ago. She occasionally has an alcoholic drink and denies tobacco or drug use. She is married and is a retired shopkeeper. On examination, her blood pressure is 150/85 mm Hg; her pulse is 98 beats/min; her respiratory rate is 20 breaths/min; her temperature is 98.7°F; and her oxygen saturation is 99% on room air. Significant findings on examination include conjunctival pallor, mild tenderness with deep palpation in the epigastric and left upper quadrant (LUQ) region of the abdomen with normal bowel sounds, and no organomegaly but a positive stool guaiac test. The remainder of the examination, including respiratory, cardiovascular, and nervous systems, was normal.

◆ **What is the most likely diagnosis?**

◆ **What is your next diagnostic step?**

◆ **What is the next step in therapy?**

ANSWERS TO CASE 9: Geriatric Anemia

Summary: A 65-year-old woman with worsening dyspnea on exertion, fatigue, dizziness, and palpitations. She is found to have conjunctival pallor and guaiac-positive stool.

◆ **Most likely diagnosis:** Anemia secondary to gastrointestinal bleeding; other considerations should include new-onset angina, congestive heart failure, and atrial fibrillation.

◆ **Next diagnostic step:** A complete blood count (CBC) to evaluate for the anemia. To evaluate for the other conditions on your differential diagnosis list, you should perform an electrocardiogram (EKG) and cardiac enzymes. A prothrombin time (PT) and partial thromboplastin time (PTT) to look for coagulation abnormalities would be helpful as well.

◆ **Next step in therapy:** Admission as an inpatient for further work up, including blood transfusion (if needed), completion of two more sets of cardiac enzymes, and EKGs. A gastroenterology consult for esophagogastroduodenoscopy (EGD) and colonoscopy is appropriate because of the positive guaiac findings.

Objectives

1. Know a diagnostic approach to anemia in geriatrics.
2. Be familiar with a rational work-up for anemia of different origins.

Considerations

A 65-year-old woman who has developed worsening dyspnea and palpitations over a 1-week period of time needs to be evaluated for cardiac and respiratory problems despite the gradual onset of symptoms. Specifically, in a postmenopausal woman, signs and symptoms of angina or acute myocardial infarction may not always have a typical presentation. That the patient has been feeling weak and has conjunctival pallor warrants testing for anemia. As evaluation with serial cardiac enzymes and EKGs is part of the work-up, admission into the hospital is appropriate.

Assuming that the initial work-up for cardiac and pulmonary causes is negative and that the hemoglobin and hematocrit levels are low, a thorough evaluation for the cause of the anemia is necessary. A CBC with peripheral smear, reticulocyte count, iron study, vitamin B_{12} and folic acid levels would provide clues to the type of anemia that this patient has. A gastroenterology consult for possible EGD and colonoscopy to further investigate the source of gastrointestinal bleeding should be considered. The presence of epigastric and LUQ pain, along with long-term use of nonsteroidal antiinflammatory drugs (NSAIDs), should also raise a flag for testing to rule out a bleeding ulcer.

The presence of other findings may direct your work-up toward other diagnoses. If this patient were from a developing country, the possibility of intestinal parasites would need to be considered. If the PT and PTT were abnormal, GI bleeding from a coagulopathy or liver disease would be possibilities. Weight loss, lymphadenopathy, and coagulopathy may warrant evaluation for nongastrointestinal malignancies, such as leukemias or lymphomas. In younger patients, sickle cell disease, thalassemias, glucose-6-phosphate dehydrogenase (G6PD) deficiency and other inherited causes of anemia would be on the differential diagnosis list. These are unlikely to manifest as an initial diagnosis at the age of 65 years.

APPROACH TO ANEMIA IN GERIATRIC POPULATION

Definitions

Anemia: According to the World Health Organization (WHO), a hemoglobin level <12 g/dL in women and <13 g/dL in men.
NHANES: The National Health and Nutrition Examination Surveys.

Epidemiology

The prevalence of anemia in Americans older than age 65 years is estimated at 9–45%. There is **a wide variation in the rates of anemia in different ethnic and racial groups,** with NHANES data showing the highest rates in non-Hispanic Blacks and lowest rates in non-Hispanic Whites. These differences are reportedly a result of biologic, not socioeconomic, differences. Most studies show the rate of anemia to be higher in men than women.

Clinical Presentation

Fatigue, weakness, and dyspnea are symptoms that are commonly reported by elderly persons with anemia. These vague and nonspecific symptoms are often ignored by both patients and physicians as symptoms of "old age." Anemia may result in worsening of symptoms of other underlying conditions. For example, the reduced oxygen-carrying capacity of the blood as a consequence of anemia may exacerbate dyspnea associated with congestive heart failure.

Certain signs found on examination may prompt a work-up for anemia. **Conjunctival pallor is recommended as a reliable sign of anemia in the elderly.** Other signs may suggest a specific cause of anemia. Glossitis, decreased vibratory and positional senses, ataxia, paresthesia, confusion, dementia, and pearly gray hair at an early age are signs suggestive of vitamin B_{12}-deficiency anemia. Folate deficiency can cause similar signs, except for the neurologic deficits. Profound iron deficiency may produce koilonychias.

Initial work-up of anemia should include a CBC with measurement of red blood cell (RBC) indices, a peripheral blood smear, and a reticulocyte count. Further laboratory studies would be indicated based on the results of the initial tests and the presence of symptoms or signs suggestive of other diseases.

The most common cause of anemia with a low mean corpuscular volume (MCV), microcytic anemia, is iron deficiency. Iron deficiency could be confirmed by subsequent testing that shows a low serum iron, low ferritin and high total iron-binding capacity (TIBC). Other causes of microcytic anemia include thalassemias and anemia of chronic disease. In the elderly, iron deficiency is frequently caused by chronic gastrointestinal blood loss, poor nutritional intake, or a bleeding disorder. A thorough evaluation of the gastrointestinal tract for a source of blood loss, usually requiring a gastroenterology consultation for upper and lower GI endoscopy, should be undertaken, as iron-deficiency anemia may be the initial presentation of a GI malignancy.

Anemia with an elevated MCV, macrocytic anemia, is most often a manifestation of folate or vitamin B_{12} deficiency. The presence of macrocytic anemia, with or without the symptoms previously mentioned, should lead to further testing to determine B_{12} and folate levels. An elevated methylmalonic acid (MMA) level can be used to confirm a vitamin B_{12} deficiency. Folate deficiency anemia is usually seen in alcoholics, whereas B_{12}-deficiency anemia mostly occurs in people with pernicious anemia, a history of gastrectomy, diseases associated with malabsorption (e.g., bacterial infection, Crohn disease, celiac disease), and strict vegans (rare).

In the elderly, anemia of chronic disease is the most common cause of a normocytic anemia. Anemia of chronic disease is anemia that is secondary to some other underlying condition. Along with causing a normocytic anemia, anemia of chronic disease can also present as a microcytic anemia. This type of anemia can easily be confused with iron-deficiency anemia because of its similar initial laboratory picture. **In anemia of chronic disease, the body's iron stores are normal, but the capability of using the stored iron in the reticuloendothelial system becomes decreased**. A lack of improvement in symptoms and hemoglobin level with iron supplementation are important clues indicating that the cause is chronic disease and not iron depletion, regardless of the laboratory picture. Although bone marrow iron store remains the gold standard to differentiate between iron-deficiency anemia and anemia of chronic disease, simple serum testing is still used to diagnose and differentiate these two types of anemia (Table 9–1).

Treatment

The treatment of anemia is determined based on the type and cause of the anemia. Any cause of anemia that creates a hemodynamic instability can be treated with a red blood cell transfusion. Iron-deficiency anemia is treated first by

Table 9–1

LABORATORY VALUES DIFFERENTIATING IRON-DEFICIENCY
ANEMIA FROM ANEMIA OF CHRONIC DISEASE

TEST	IRON DEFICIENCY	ANEMIA OF CHRONIC DISEASE
Serum iron	Low	Low or normal
TIBC	High	Low
Transferrin saturation	Low	Low or normal
Serum ferritin	Low	Normal or high

identification and correction of any source of blood loss. Most iron deficiency can be corrected by oral iron replacement. Various iron preparations are available; a typical treatment is ferrous sulfate 325 mg three times a day. Parenteral iron preparations are available for those with poor iron absorption and high iron replacement needs. Vitamin B_{12} deficiency traditionally has been treated by intramuscular B_{12} therapy with a regimen of 1000 µg IM daily for 7 days, then weekly for 4 weeks, then monthly for the rest of the patient's life. Newer research shows that many patients can be successfully treated with oral B_{12} therapy using 1000–2000 µg PO in a similar regimen. Folate deficiency can be treated with oral therapy of 1 mg daily until the deficiency is corrected. Anemia of chronic disease is managed primarily by treatment of the underlying condition.

Comprehension Questions

Match the following lab pictures of patients with anemia with the cases described below:

    A. Normal MMA; decreased serum folate level
    B. Elevated MMA; decreased serum B_{12} level
    C. Elevated ferritin; normal MCV; decreased serum iron level
    D. Decreased ferritin; decreased MCV; decreased serum iron level

[9.1]   A 66-year-old male with anemia and "stocking-and-glove" distribution of a burning sensation.

[9.2]   A 68-year-old male with an incidental finding of anemia while in the hospital for alcohol abuse.

[9.3]   A 65-year-old female with anemia who has chronic renal failure.

[9.4]   A 67-year-old male with dizziness and a positive stool guaiac test.

Answers

[9.1]   **B.** The presence of paresthesia suggests the finding of vitamin B_{12} deficiency and the laboratory study results of an elevated MMA and low B_{12} confirms this finding.

[9.2]   **A.** Alcohol abuse is a common cause of folate deficiency. A normal MMA level essentially rules out a concomitant vitamin B_{12} deficiency.

[9.3]   **C.** A normocytic anemia with low serum iron and high ferritin levels, along with an underlying chronic medical condition, are diagnostic of anemia of chronic disease.

[9.4]   **D.** Low serum iron, low MCV, and low ferritin levels, along with a finding of blood in the stool, are consistent with iron-deficiency anemia. A work-up for the source of the GI blood loss should ensue.

CLINICAL PEARLS

❖ Conjunctival pallor is an indication for anemia work-up in elderly patients.

❖ Clinical findings of anemia require investigation for underlying causes.

❖ GI bleeding is an important cause of iron-deficiency anemia in both female and male geriatric patients; this type of anemia mandates a GI work-up in this patient population.

❖ Investigating for vitamin B_{12} and folate deficiency is of high importance in a patient with a history of heavy EtOH (ethyl alcohol) intake and/or abuse.

REFERENCE

Smith D. Anemia in the elderly. Am Fam Physician 2000;62:1565–1572.

A 40-year-old male presents to the clinic complaining of having 10 episodes of watery, nonbloody diarrhea that started last night. He vomited twice last night but has been able to tolerate liquids today. He has had intermittent abdominal cramps as well. He reports having muscle aches, weakness, headache, and low-grade temperature. He is here with his daughter, who started with the same symptoms this morning. On questioning, he states that he has no significant medical history, no surgeries, and does not take any medications. He does not smoke cigarettes, drink alcohol, use any illicit drugs, and has never had a blood transfusion. He and his family returned to the United States yesterday, following a week-long vacation in Mexico.

On examination, he is not in acute distress. His blood pressure is 110/60 mm Hg, his pulse is 98 beats/min, his respiratory rate is 16 breaths/min, and his temperature is 99.1°F. His mucous membranes are dry. His bowel sounds are hyperactive and his abdomen is mildly tender throughout, but there is no rebound tenderness and no guarding. A rectal examination is normal and his stool is guaiac negative. The remainder of his examination is unremarkable.

◆ **What is the most likely diagnosis?**

◆ **What would you do next?**

◆ **What are potential complications?**

ANSWERS TO CASE 10: Acute Diarrhea

Summary: A 40-year-old man who recently returned from Mexico with profuse, acute, nonbloody diarrhea and dry mucous membranes on examination, which are consistent with developing dehydration. An ill family member with identical symptoms suggests an infectious cause of this acute illness.

◆ **Most likely diagnosis:** Acute gastroenteritis

◆ **Next step:** Order stool for fecal leucocytes

◆ **Potential complication:** Dehydration and electrolyte abnormalities

Analysis

Objectives

1. To clearly understand when and how to do a work-up for acute diarrhea, considering the most probable etiologies of diarrhea such us virus, *Escherichia coli, Shigella, Salmonella, Giardia,* and amebiasis.
2. To understand the role of fecal leukocytes and stool occult blood in the evaluation of acute diarrhea.
3. To understand that volume replacement and correction of electrolyte abnormalities are a key component in the treatment and prevention of diarrhea complications.

Considerations

This 40-year-old male developed severe diarrhea, nausea, and vomiting. His **most immediate problem is volume depletion,** as evidenced by his dry mucous membranes. The priority is to **replace the lost intravascular volume, usually with intravenous normal saline.** Electrolytes and renal function should be evaluated and abnormalities corrected. While correcting and/or preventing further dehydration, you need to determine the etiology of the diarrhea. Up to **90% of acute diarrhea is infectious** in etiology. He does not have any history compatible with chronic diarrhea, causes of which include Crohn disease, ulcerative colitis, gluten intolerance, irritable bowel syndrome, and parasites. He had been in Mexico recently, which predisposes him to different pathogens: *E. coli, Campylobacter, Shigella, Salmonella,* and *Giardia.* He does not have bloody stools. The **presence of blood in the stool would suggest an invasive bacterial infection,** such as hemorrhagic or enteroinvasive *E. coli* species, *Yersinia* species, *Shigella,* and *Entamoeba histolytica.*

Examination of the stool for leukocytes is a simple, inexpensive test that helps to differentiate between the types of infectious diarrhea. If leukocytes are present in the stool, the suspicion is higher for *Salmonella, Shigella, Yersinia,* enterohemorrhagic and enteroinvasive *E. coli, Clostridium difficile, Campylobacter,* and

Entamoeba histolytica. In general, ova and parasite evaluation is unhelpful, unless the history strongly points toward a parasitic source or the diarrhea is prolonged.

The majority of the diarrheas are viral, self-limited, and do not need further evaluation. In this particular patient, because of his recent travel to Mexico, traveler's diarrhea should be strongly considered and treated with the appropriate antibiotic.

APPROACH TO ACUTE DIARRHEA

Definitions

Acute diarrhea: diarrhea present for less than 2 weeks' duration
Chronic diarrhea: diarrhea present for longer than 4 weeks' duration
Diarrhea: passage of abnormally liquid or poorly formed stool in increased frequency
Subacute diarrhea: diarrhea present for 2–4 weeks' duration

CLINICAL APPROACH

Etiologies

Approximately 90% of acute diarrhea is caused by infectious etiologies, with the remainder caused by medications, ischemia, and toxins. Infectious etiologies often depend on the patient population. **Travelers to Mexico will frequently contract enterotoxigenic *E. coli*** as a causative agent. **Traveler's diarrhea** is a common entity and can be induced by a variety of bacteria, viruses, and parasites. Campers are often affected by *Giardia*.

Consumption of foods is also frequently a culprit. ***Salmonella* or *Shigella*** can be found in **undercooked chicken,** enterohemorrhagic *E. coli* from undercooked hamburger, and *Staphylococcus aureus* or *Salmonella* from **mayonnaise.** Raw seafood may harbor *Vibrio, Salmonella*, or hepatitis A. Sometimes the **timing** of the **diarrhea** following food ingestion is helpful. For example, **illness within 6 hours of eating a salad containing mayonnaise suggests *Staphylococcus aureus,* within 8–12 hours suggests *Clostridium perfringens*, and within 12–14 hours suggests *E. coli.***

Daycare settings are particularly common for *Shigella, Giardia*, and rotavirus to be transmitted. Patients in nursing homes, or who were recently in the hospital, may develop *Clostridium difficile* colitis from antibiotic use.

Clinical Presentation

Most patients with acute diarrhea have self-limited processes and do not require much workup. Exceptions to this rule include profuse diarrhea, dehydration, fever exceeding 100.4°F, bloody diarrhea, severe abdominal pain, duration of the diarrhea for more than 48 hours, and children, elderly patients, and immunocompromised patients.

Past and recent medical history should include exposures to medications and foods, travel history, and coworkers, classmates, or family members with similar symptoms. A history of a viral illness may provide a clue to the etiology. The initial evaluation should determine if the patient can tolerate oral intake. The patient who is both vomiting and having diarrhea is more prone to dehydration and more likely to need hospital admission for IV hydration.

The physical examination should focus on the vital signs, clinical impression of the volume status, and abdominal exam. Volume status is determined by observing whether the mucous membranes are moist or dry, the skin has good turgor, and the capillary refill is normal or delayed. The principal laboratory test is the stool for microscopic and microbiologic examination; usually it is sent for culture, but these results generally require several days to obtain and are not useful in the acute setting. Ova and parasite evaluation is generally unhelpful, except in selected circumstances of very high suspicion. Stool for *Clostridium difficile* toxin may yield the etiology in patients who develop symptoms after antibiotic use. Although classically associated with clindamycin, **any antibiotic can cause pseudomembranous colitis.** A complete blood count, electrolytes, and renal function tests are sometimes indicated.

Treatment

Most cases of diarrhea resolve spontaneously in a few days without treatment. Replacement of fluids and electrolytes is the first step in treating the consequences of acute diarrhea. For mildly dehydrated individuals who can tolerate oral fluids, solutions such as the World Health Organization Oral Rehydration Solution or commercially available drinks such as Pedialyte or Gatorade, often are all that is needed. Those with more serious volume deficits, elderly patients, and infants generally require hospitalization and intravenous hydration. If a parasitic infection is the cause of the diarrhea, prescription antibiotics may ease the symptoms. Antibiotics sometimes, but not always, help ease symptoms of bacterial diarrhea. However, antibiotics will not help viral diarrhea, which is the most common kind of infectious diarrhea. Over-the-counter medications may help to slow down the frequency of the stools, but they do not speed the recovery. Certain infections may be made worse by over-the-counter medications because they prevent your body from getting rid of the organism that is causing the diarrhea.

Prevention

Hand washing is a simple and effective way to prevent the spread of viral diarrhea. Adults, children, and clinic and hospital personnel should be encouraged to wash their hands. Because viral diarrhea spreads easily, children with diarrhea should not attend school or child care until their illness has resolved.

To prevent diarrhea caused by contaminated food, use dairy products that have been pasteurized. Serve food immediately or refrigerate it after it has been cooked. Do not leave food out at room temperature because it promotes the growth of bacteria.

Travelers to locations, such as developing countries, where there is poor sanitation and frequent contamination of food and water, need to be cautious to reduce their risk of developing diarrhea. They should be advised to eat hot and well-cooked foods, and to drink bottled water, soda, wine, or beer served in its original container. Beverages from boiled water, such as coffee and tea, are usually safe. Recommend the use of bottled water even for teeth brushing. Also recommend avoiding raw fruits and vegetables unless they are peeled by the consumer immediately before being eaten. Patient's should avoid tap water and ice cubes.

Traveler's Prophylaxis

The **best method for preventing traveler's diarrhea (TD) is to avoid contaminated food and water.** When antibiotics are indicated, therapy with a quinolone antibiotic should be started as soon as possible after the diarrhea begins. Most commonly, **ciprofloxacin (500 mg twice daily) is given for 1 or 2 days.** Quinolones cannot be used in children or pregnant women. Quinolones will resolve the diarrheal symptoms in the majority of patients within 1 day. **Azithromycin,** given as a single 1000-mg dose, is another effective drug for the treatment of TD. **Rifaximin** can be used in TD caused by noninvasive strains of *E. coli.* However, Rifaximin is not effective against infections associated with fever or blood in the stool.

Trimethoprim-sulfamethoxazole and ampicillin were popular drugs used in the past to treat TD, but increased resistance limits their use at this time. Bismuth subsalicylate is not recommended because, to be effective, it needs to be taken in large amounts that can cause salicylate toxicity.

Comprehension Questions

Match the following etiologies to the clinical situations described below:

    A. Rotavirus
    B. *Giardia*
    C. *E. coli*
    D. *Staphylococcus aureus*
    E. *Cryptosporidium*
    F. *Vibrio*

[10.1] Several friends develop vomiting and diarrhea 6 hours after eating food at a private party.

[10.2] A 40-year-old man travels to Mexico and develops diarrhea 1 day after coming back.

[10.3] A young woman eats raw seafood and 2 days later develops fever, abdominal cramping, and watery diarrhea.

[10.4] During the winter, a young daycare worker develops watery diarrhea.

[10.5] An HIV-positive patient develops diarrhea.

Answers

[10.1] **D.** *Staphylococcus aureus* toxin usually causes vomiting and diarrhea within a few hours of food ingestion.

[10.2] **C.** *E. coli* is the most common etiology for traveler's diarrhea.

[10.3] **F.** *Vibrio* is a common cause of diarrhea among people who eat raw sea food.

[10.4] **A.** Rotavirus is a common etiology for watery diarrhea, especially in the winter.

[10.5] **E.** Suspect *Cryptosporidium* in an immunocompromised host.

CLINICAL PEARLS

❖ Most acute diarrheas are self-limited.
❖ Be cautious when assessing diarrhea in a child, elderly patient, or immunosuppressed host.
❖ Dehydration, bloody diarrhea, high fever, and diarrhea that do not respond to therapy after 48 hours are warning signs of possible complicated diarrhea.
❖ In general, acute, uncomplicated diarrhea can be treated with oral electrolyte and fluid replacement.

REFERENCES

Centers for Disease Control and Prevention. Travelers' health. 2005. Available at: http://www.cdc.gov/travel/diarrhea.htm.

Toy E, Simon B, Liu TH, Trujillo J, Takenaka K. Case files: emergency medicine. New York: McGraw-Hill, 2005.

A 50-year old Caucasian female, new to your practice, presents for an "annual physical examination." She reports that she is generally very healthy, feels well and has no specific complaints. She has a history of having had a "partial hysterectomy," by which she means that her uterus and cervix were removed but her ovaries were left in place. The surgery was performed because of fibroids. She has had a pap smear every year since the age of 18, all of which have been normal. She has had annual mammograms since the age of 40, all of which have been normal. She has no other significant medical or surgical history. She takes a multivitamin pill daily but no other medications. Her family history is significant for breast cancer that was diagnosed in her maternal grandmother at the age of 72. The patient is married, monogamous, does not smoke cigarettes or drink alcohol. She tries to avoid dairy products because of "lactose intolerance." She walks 3 miles 4-times a week for exercise. Her physical examination is normal.

◆ **For this patient, how often should a Pap smear be performed for cervical cancer screening?**

◆ **What could you recommend to reduce her risk of developing osteoporosis?**

◆ **What is the recommended interval for screening mammography?**

ANSWERS TO CASE 11: Health Maintenance in Adult Female

Summary: A 50-year old woman with a history of having had a hysterectomy for a benign indication comes to your office for a routine health maintenance visit.

◆ **Interval for cervical cancer screening in this patient:** Based upon her history of having a hysterectomy for benign disease and her overall low risk status, cervical cancer screening can be discontinued in this patient

◆ **Interventions to reduce her risk of developing osteoporosis:** Supplementation with at least 1200 mg calcium and 400-800 IU vitamin D daily; regular weight-bearing exercise

◆ **Recommended interval for screening mammography in 50-year old woman:** Annual

Analysis

Objectives

1. Discuss age appropriate preventive health measures for adult women.
2. Review evidence in support of specific health maintenance measures.

Considerations

When evaluating patients for preventive health measures, there should not be a "one size fits all" approach to care. Some interventions are appropriate across age groups; some are age or risk factor specific and should be tailored accordingly. Interventions to consider include screening for cardiovascular disease, breast cancer, cervical cancer, osteoporosis and domestic violence. Other health maintenance measures, such as screening for colon cancer (Chapter 1), routine adult immunizations (Chapter 1) and tobacco use (Chapter 7) are discussed elsewhere. The interventions discussed in this chapter are primarily based upon recommendations of the United States Preventive Services Task Force (USPSTF); recommendations of other expert panels or advocacy organizations are included where appropriate.

Cardiovascular Disease in Women

Cardiovascular diseases are the number one killer of women in the United States. Many of the cardiovascular disease risk factors in women are the same as those in men: hypertension, high LDL-cholesterol, tobacco use, Diabetes Mellitus, family history of cardiovascular disease. As such, the **USPSTF screening recommendations for cardiovascular disease for women are similar to those for men.** All women aged 18 and older should be screened for hypertension by the measurement of blood pressure (Level A recommendation). Further, all women aged 45 and older should be screened for lipid disorders (Level A recommendation). Abnormally elevated blood pressure or serum lipids should be managed appropriately.

An area of cardiovascular disease risk unique to women is in post-menopausal hormone replacement. Many women have taken hormone replacement therapy for relief of vasomotor symptoms ("hot flashes") and reduction of risk of developing osteoporosis. Recent studies, most notably the Women's Health Initiative, have shown **increased rates of adverse cardiovascular outcomes in women taking either estrogen alone or combined estrogen and progesterone.** These risks include an increased risk of coronary heart disease, stroke and venous thromboembolic disease. For this reason, the use of hormone replacement therapy for the prevention of chronic conditions is not advised (Level D recommendation) and **any use of hormone replacnt should be of the lowest effective dose for the shortest effective time period.**

Screening for Breast Cancer

Breast cancer is second to lung cancer in number of cancer related deaths in women. There are approximately 190,000 new cases and over 40,000 deaths per year from breast cancer in the United States. The incidence increases with age; other risk factors include having the first child after the age of 30, a family history of breast cancer (particularly if in the mother or sister), personal history of breast cancer or atypical hyperplasia found on a previous breast biopsy, or a known carrier of the BRCA-1 or BRCA-2 gene.

The process of screening for breast cancer generally includes consideration of three modalities: the breast self exam (BSE), the clinical breast exam (CBE) performed by a health care professional and mammography. Other modalities, including ultrasonography and magnetic resonance imaging, are available but currently are not widely recommended for screening purposes. Upon review of the available studies, the USPSTF has determined that, at this time, there is insufficient evidence to recommend either the CBE or SBE (Level I recommendation). Both SBE and CBE may be associated with increased risks of false positive results and subsequent need for biopsies while evidence is lacking that they reduce breast cancer mortality. Studies regarding both are ongoing.

Mammography screening every 12-33 months has been shown to reduce mortality from breast cancer. The **benefits of routine mammographic screening increase with age,** as the incidence of breast cancer is higher in older women. There is not an age cut off to stop screening, but a discussion about continuing screening can be considered in the older woman with significant co-morbid conditions that may limit her life expectancy. Part of the discussion regarding mammography also includes the risk of false positive or false negative (less common) results and need for additional interventions, such as breast biopsy. **Most abnormalities found on mammography are not breast cancer** but require further evaluation to make that determination. The USPSTF advises screening with mammography, beginning at the age of 40 for the general population, with a recommended interval of every 1-2 years (Level B recommendation). Recommendations are also available from other organizations, including the American Cancer Society, American Academy of Family Physicians and American College of Obstetrics and Gynecology, that advocate annual mammography after the age of 50. Their recommendations for women age 40-49 vary, but generally advise screening every 1-2 years.

Screening for Cervical Cancer

Cervical cancer is the tenth leading cause of cancer death in women in the United States, with 4100 deaths in 2002. **The incidence of cervical cancer has fallen dramatically since the introduction of the Pap smear as part of routine screening.** Risk factors for cervical cancer include early onset of sexual intercourse, multiple sexual partners, human papilloma virus (HPV) infection with high risk subtype of HPV (HPV viral types 16, 18, 45, 56) and tobacco use.

The optimal age to begin screening is unclear, but the USPSTF recommends starting at age 21 or within three years of the onset of sexual activity, whichever comes first (Level A recommendation). While there is limited utility in screening for cervical cancer in a person who has never been sexually active, many organizations will advocate an age based approach because of high rates of sexual activity by a certain ages and because health care providers may not always get accurate sexual histories.

Most cases of cervical cancer occur in women who either have not been screened in over 5 years or did not have follow up after an abnormal pap smear. The optimal screening interval between pap smears is not known. Based upon the available studies, the USPSTF has not found evidence that annual screening is better at reducing morbidity and mortality from cervical cancer than screening ever 3 years. The American Cancer Society recommends annual pap smears until age 30 and then spacing out the interval to every two to three years; other groups suggest spacing out the interval after three consecutive normal pap smears.

The purpose of a pap smear is to detect precancerous cervical changes or possible cases of cervical cancer early, in order to improve the odds of survival. Keeping this in mind, the USPSTF recommends against pap smears for women who have had a hysterectomy (including removal of the cervix) for benign indications (Level D recommendation). It is prudent to ask a woman who has had a hysterectomy why the surgery was performed and to confirm (either by reviewing the operative report or on exam) the absence of the cervix. A woman who had a hysterectomy for cancerous indications falls out of the general screening parameters discussed here.

The optimal age to stop screening is subject to debate. The USPSTF discusses discontinuing cervical cancer screening after the age of 65 both if no new risk factors have been identified (i.e., new partner) and there has been adequate recent screening. The incidence of cervical cancer falls with age; the false positive rate increases, thus potentially subjecting women to additional unnecessary procedures. The American Cancer Society recommends that screening may be stopped at the age of 70 if a woman has had three consecutive normal pap smears and no abnormal pap smears in the last 10 years.

Screening for Osteoporosis

Osteoporosis is a condition of decreased bone mineral density associated with an increased risk of fracture. **Half of all postmenopausal women will have an osteoporosis related fracture in their lifetime.** These include hip fractures, which are associated with higher risks of loss of independence, institutionalization and death. The risk of osteoporosis is increased with advancing age, tobacco use, low body weight, Caucasian or Asian ancestry, family history of osteoporosis, low calcium intake and sedentary lifestyle.

Osteoporosis may also occur in men, although with a lower incidence than it does in women. Along with the risk factors noted above, the prolonged use of corticosteroids, presence of diseases that alter hormone levels (such as chronic kidney or lung disease) and undiagnosed low testosterone levels increase the risk of osteoporosis in men.

Screening for osteoporosis is done by measurement of bone density. Measurement of the hip bone density by Dual energy X-ray Absorptiometry (DXA) is the best predictor of hip fracture. Measurement of bone density is compared to the bone density of young adults and the result is reported as standard deviation from the mean bone density of the young adult (T-score). Osteoporosis is present if the patient's T-score is at or below -2.5 (i.e., measurement of the patient's bone density is more than 2.5 standard deviations below the young adult mean); osteopenia is present if the T-score is between -1.0 and -2.5. Other modalities, such as measurement of wrist or heel density, single energy x-ray aborptiometry and ultrasound are being evaluated and may have some short term predictive value. The USPSTF recommends screening for osteoporosis via DXA in women after the age of 65 and considering screening in women over age 60 with higher risk of osteoporosis related fractures (Level B recommendation).

Calcium and vitamin D intake have a role in the prevention and treatment of osteoporosis. The National Osteoporosis Foundation (NOF) recommends at least **1200 mg of calcium and 400-800 IU of vitamin D per day for all women over the age of 50.** If dietary intake is not sufficient, supplements may be used. Weight-bearing and muscle strengthening exercise is also recommended both for its direct effects on increasing bone density and for its benefits in strength, agility and balance, which may reduce the risk of falls.

When osteoporosis is diagnosed, patients should be treated with calcium, vitamin D, exercise and strategies should be implemented to reduce the risk of falls. These strategies include evaluation and treatment, if needed, of vision and hearing deficits, management of medical disorders that can promote falls (movement disorders, neurological disorders, etc) and periodic evaluation of medications taken that may affect balance or movement. Hip protectors may be beneficial in those at high risk for falls.

Medications used for the prevention and treatment of osteoporosis are included in Table 11.1.

Table 11–1

MEDICATIONS FOR THE PREVENTION AND TREATMENT OF OSTEOPOROSIS

CLASS/ MEDICATION	BRAND NAME	OSTEOPOROSIS-RELATED INDICATIONS	DOSAGE	SIDE EFFECTS
Bisphosphonates				Esophagitis, gastritis, swallowing difficulty; all bisphosphonates should be taken on an empty stomach with a full glass of water and the patient should stay upright for at least 30 minutes after taking the pill
Alendronate	Fosamax	Prevention and treatment	Prev: 5 mg daily or 35 mg weekly Tx: 10 mg daily or 70 mg weekly	
Risedronate	Actonel	Prevention and treatment	Prev:	
Ibandronate	Boniva	Prevention and treatment	Prev and Tx: 150 mg monthly	
Calcitonin	Miacalcin (inj or nasal spray)	Treatment	IM/SC: 100 units daily Nasal: 1 spray (200 units) daily	Inj: flushing, injection site reaction NS: nosebleeds, nasal irritation

Estrogen	Numerous	Prevention	Varies	Potential increased risk of DVT, MI, stroke, PE
Parathyroid Hormone Teriparatide	Forteo	Treatment	20 μ SC daily	Leg cramps, dizziness, transient hypercalcemia
Selective Estrogen Receptor Modulator Raloxifene	Evista	Prevention and treatment	60 mg daily	Hot flashes, weight gain, DVT/PE

Abbreviations: DVT, deep venous thrombosis; Inj, injection; MI, myocardial infarction; NS, nasal spray; PE, pulmanary embolism; Prev, prevention; Tx, treatment.

Screening for Domestic Violence

Estimates indicate that between 1 and 4 million women are sexually, physically, or emotionally abused by an intimate partner each year. Women are also much more likely to be abused by an intimate partner than men. Multiple factors are associated with intimate partner violence and include young age, low income status, pregnancy, mental illness, alcohol or substance use by victims or partner, separated or divorced status, and a history of childhood sexual/physical abuse. Multiple rating scales are available to assess for presence of domestic violence which are of variable quality. The USPSTF found insufficient evidence to recommend for or against routine screening for intimate partner abuse, or that screening affects outcomes (Level I recommendation). Other groups, including the American Academy of Family Physicians and American Medical Association, recommend awareness and advocate asking about domestic violence. Documentation and treatment of injuries, counseling and information regarding protective services are part of the evaluation when domestic violence is suspected. Reporting of domestic violence is mandatory in several states; be aware of the requirements of your state.

Comprehension Questions

[11.1] Which of the following screening tests would be recommended in a 50-year-old woman with hypertension and who had a total abdominal hysterectomy at the age of 35 for endometriosis?

    A. Exercise stress test
    B. Pap smear
    C. DXA scan
    D. Stool occult blood

[11.2] Which of the following situations is associated with an increased risk of intimate partner violence?

    A. Pregnancy
    B. Older age
    C. Higher income
    D. Married status

[11.3] Which of the following statements regarding osteoporosis is true?

    A. Fewer than 25% of women will have an osteoporosis related fracture in their lifetime.
    B. Long-term therapy with a combination of estrogen and progesterone is recommended for the treatment of postmenopausal osteoporosis.
    C. Asian and African-American women have an increased risk of osteoporosis.
    D. 1200 mg of calcium and 400-800 IU vitamin D, through diet or supplement, is recommended for all women over the age of 50.

Answers

[11.1] **D.** Screening for colon cancer is recommended for all adults over the age of 50. Acceptable regiments include stool occult blood testing, flexible sigmoidoscopy, colonoscopy or barium enema. Heart disease screening by stress testing and cervical cancer screening by Pap smear in a patient with a history of hysterectomy for benign disease are not routinely indicated, but may be appropriate if other high risk status is known. DXA screening may be considered routinely starting at the age of 60 in a woman with higher risk; it is routinely advised at the age of 65 or above.

[11.2] **A.** Intimate partner violence can occur in any relationship, but the risk is increased in certain situations, which include young age, low income status, pregnancy, mental illness, alcohol or substance use by victims or partner, separated or divorced status, and a history of childhood sexual/physical abuse.

[11.3] **D.** Women over the age of 50 should be advised to have a daily intake of 1200 mg or more of calcium and 400-800 IU of Vitamin D and to participate in regular weight-bearing and muscle-building exercise. Approximately half of all women will have an osteoporosis related fracture. Hormone replacement therapy should be of the lowest effective dose for the shortest effective time, due to the increased risk of adverse cardiovascular and thromboembolic complications. Asian and Caucasian women are at higer risk of osteoporosis than African-American women.

CLINICAL PEARLS

❖ Most abnormalities found on mammography are not breast cancer.
❖ The number one killer of women in America is cardiovascular disease. Risk factors for cardiovascular diseases in women need to be managed as aggressively as they are in men.

REFERENCES

Ullom-Minnich P. Prevention of osteoporosis and fractures. Am Fam Physician 1999;60:194–202.

United States Preventive Services Task Force (USPSTF). Screening for breast cancer. Available at http://www.ahrq.gov/clinic/uspstf/uspsbrca.htm. February 2002.

United States Preventive Services Task Force (USPSTF). Screening for cervical cancer. Available at http://www.ahrq.gov/clinic/uspstf/uspscerv.htm. January 2003.

United States Preventive Services Task Force (USPSTF). Osteoporosis - screening. Available at http://www.ahrq.gov/clinic/uspstf/uspsoste.htm. September 2002.

United States Preventive Services Task Force (USPSTF). Screening for family and intimate partner violence. Available at http://www.ahrq.gov/clinic/uspstf/uspsfamv.htm. March 2004.

National Osteoporosis Foundation. Physicians guide to prevention and treatment of osteoporosis. Washington, D.C.: National Osteoporosis Foundation, 2003.

A 25-year-old male presents to your office on a Monday morning with ankle pain. He was playing in his usual Saturday afternoon basketball game when he injured his right ankle. He says that he jumped for a rebound and landed on another player's foot. His right ankle "rolled over," he fell to the floor, and his ankle immediately started to hurt. He did not hear or feel a pop. He was able to stand and walk with a limp, but was unable to continue playing. His ankle swelled over the next day in spite of rest, icing, and elevation. He suffered no other injury from the fall. On examination, he is a healthy-appearing man with normal vital signs. The lateral aspect of the right ankle is swollen. The right ankle has normal dorsiflexion and plantar flexion and there is no focal tenderness to palpation of the fibula, malleoli, or foot. No ligamentous laxity is noted on testing. He can bear weight with minimal pain. There is normal sensation and capillary refill in the foot. The remainder of his examination is normal.

◆ **What is the most likely diagnosis of this injury?**

◆ **What further diagnostic testing is needed at this time?**

◆ **What is the most appropriate therapy?**

ANSWERS TO CASE 12: Musculoskeletal Injuries

Summary: A 25-year-old male presents with an inversion injury of his right ankle that occurred during a basketball game. His ankle is swollen, but he is able to bear weight, and has no focal tenderness and no ligament laxity.

◆ **Most likely diagnosis:** Sprain of the right ankle.

◆ **Further diagnostic testing needed:** None at this time.

◆ **Most appropriate initial therapy:** "PRICE" therapy: **P**rotection, **R**est, **I**ce, **C**ompression, and **E**levation; a nonsteroidal antiinflammatory drug (NSAID) or acetaminophen as needed for pain and early mobilization.

Analysis

Objectives

1. Learn an approach to the diagnosis of musculoskeletal injuries.
2. Know when to order imaging tests and which test to order to evaluate musculoskeletal complaints.
3. Be able to manage common joint sprains and strains.

Considerations

Ankle sprains are the most common acute, sports-related injury, and are a common reason for visits to primary care physicians, urgent care centers, and emergency rooms. As in this case, **most ankle sprains are the result of inversion of an ankle that is plantar flexed**—landing on another player's foot in basketball, stepping in a hole or on uneven ground when running, missing a curb while walking. The lateral ankle is injured much more commonly than the medial ankle, as the bony anatomy of the tibiotalar joint and the very strong deltoid ligament complex protect the medial ankle from injury. The lateral ligaments—anterior talofibular ligament (ATFL), calcaneofibular ligament (CFL), and posterior talofibular ligament (PTFL)—are relatively weaker and more commonly injured. The **ATFL is the most commonly injured ligament,** followed by the CFL.

Ankle sprains are graded as grade 1, 2, or 3 injuries. A grade 1 sprain is stretching of the ATFL, which causes pain and swelling, but no mechanical instability and little to no functional loss. The patient can usually bear weight with, at most, mild pain. The history and examination of the patient in the case presented is consistent with a grade 1 ankle sprain. A grade 2 sprain represents a partial tear of the ATFL and stretching of the CFL. This injury causes more severe pain, swelling, and bruising. There is mild to moderate joint instability, significant pain with weight bearing, and loss of range of motion. A grade

3 sprain is a complete tear of the ATFL and CFL with partial tearing of the PTFL. This injury causes significant joint instability, loss of function, and inability to bear weight.

The Ottawa Ankle Rules are a decision model designed to aid a physician in determining which patients with ankle injuries need an x-ray. These decision rules have been validated for nonpregnant adults who have a normal mental status, no other significant concurrent injury, and who are evaluated within 10 days of the injury. When properly applied, the **Ottawa Ankle Rules have a sensitivity approaching 100% in ruling out significant malleolar and midfoot fractures.** These rules show that x-rays of the ankle should be performed if there is bony tenderness of the posterior edge or tip of the distal 6 cm of either the medial or lateral malleolus, or if the patient is unable to bear weight immediately or when examined. Foot x-rays should be performed if there is bony tenderness over the navicular bone (medial midfoot), the base of the fifth metatarsal (lateral midfoot) or if the patient is unable to bear weight. The patient presented, who has no bony tenderness, no limitation in weight bearing, and no contraindication to the application of the decision rules, does not need imaging of his ankle or foot.

The management of ankle sprains should follow the pneumonic "PRICE"— Protection, Rest, Ice, Compression, and Elevation. Protection by appropriate splinting or casting can help to prevent further injury. Relative rest from activity also helps to promote ligament healing, although weight bearing can be allowed as tolerated and early, functional rehabilitation exercises are crucial. Ice applied as soon as possible after the injury helps to minimize swelling and relieve pain. Compression and elevation also promote reduction of swelling. In most cases, NSAIDs or acetaminophen are adequate for pain relief.

Definitions

Sprain: A stretching or tearing injury of a ligament.
Strain: A stretching or tearing injury of a muscle or tendon.

APPROACH TO SPRAINS AND STRAINS

History

As in all areas of medicine, the history of the presenting illness will guide the diagnostic work-up. In the history of a patient with musculoskeletal complaints, important information to gather includes whether the primary symptom is pain, limited movement, weakness, instability, or a combination of symptoms. The onset of the symptoms—whether acute, chronic, or an acute worsening of a chronic problem—can be significant. The location, severity, and pattern of radiation of pain should be delineated. Associated symptoms, such as numbness, should be identified. Efforts should be made to identify as specifically as possible the mechanism of any injury that led to the complaint. Interventions that have already been made, such as ice or heat, medications, splinting, and whether or not the interventions helped, should be noted.

Joint Examination

Examination of the musculoskeletal system should include documentation of inspection, palpation, range of motion, strength, neurovascular status, and, where appropriate, testing specific for the involved joint. Inspection should note the presence of swelling, bruising, deformity, and the use of any supports or assistive devices (e.g., splints, crutches, bandages) that the patient is already using. **Examination of the unaffected limb can provide a good comparison and allow for subtle changes to be more easily identified.** Documentation should also be made of the patient's general functioning and mobility—does the patient walk with a limp, can the patient easily rise from a chair, is there difficulty getting on the examining table, is the patient's arm moving freely or held tightly to the patient's chest, and so on.

Palpation of the affected and surrounding areas can help to localize and confirm the presence of a specific injury. A focal area of bony tenderness may lead to the consideration of a fracture, whereas a tender, tight muscle may be more suggestive of a strain. The presence of joint effusions or soft-tissue swelling should be documented and may lead to consideration of specific injuries. Notation should be made of sensation, peripheral pulses, and capillary refill in the involved extremity. Absent pulses and delayed capillary refill, especially if the extremity is cool or cold, should prompt emergent evaluation and management of vascular insufficiency.

Range of motion should be tested both passively and actively. Active range of motion tests the patient's ability to move a joint. It tests the structural integrity of the joint, muscles, tendons, and neurologic impulses to the area and can be limited by problems with any of them or by the presence of pain. Passive range of motion tests the movement that an examiner can elicit in a relaxed patient. The presence of a dislocated joint or significant joint effusion may lead to limitations in both passive and active range of motion, where a torn tendon or muscle injury may have limited active, but preserved passive, range of motion.

Each joint or body area has specific examination maneuvers that can help to identify injury to specific structures. Table 12–1 lists some common maneuvers that are used to examine the shoulder, knee, and ankle.

Imaging

Following the history and examination, the physician must decide when it is necessary to perform x-rays or other imaging tests. Validated decision rules are available to aid in some of these decisions. The Ottawa Ankle Rules for the determination of when an x-ray is necessary in an ankle injury were discussed

Table 12–1

SPECIFIC TESTS FOR SHOULDER, KNEE, AND ANKLE
EXAMINATIONS

TEST	STRUCTURE TESTED	RESULT IDENTIFIED (COMPARE TO UNAFFECTED SIDE)
Shoulder/Rotator Cuff		
Empty Can Test—with arm abducted, elbow extended, and thumb pointing down, patient elevates arm against resistance	Supraspinatus	Rotator cuff injury or tear
External Rotation—with elbows at sides and flexed at 90 degrees, patient externally rotates against resistance	Infraspinatus Teres minor	Rotator cuff injury or tear
Lift-off Test—patient places dorsum of hand on lumbar back and attempts to lift hand off of back	Subscapularis	Rotator cuff injury or tear
Ankle		
Anterior Drawer—examiner pulls forward on patient's heel while stabilizing lower leg with other hand	Anterior talofibular ligament	Excessive translation of joint suggests ATFL tear
Inversion Stress Test—examiner inverts ankle with one hand while stabilizing lower leg with other hand	Calcaneofibular ligament	Excessive translation or palpable "clunk" of talus on tibia suggests ligament tear
Squeeze Test—examiner compresses tibia/fibula at midcalf	Syndesmosis	Pain at anterior ankle joint (below where examiner is squeezing) suggests syndesmotic injury
Knee		
Lachman Test—knee in 20-degree flexion, examiner pulls forward on upper tibia while stabilizing upper leg	Anterior cruciate ligament	Excessive translation with no solid end point suggests tear

(Continued)

Table 12–1

SPECIFIC TESTS FOR SHOULDER, KNEE, AND ANKLE
EXAMINATIONS (*CONTINUED*)

TEST	STRUCTURE TESTED	RESULT IDENTIFIED (COMPARE TO UNAFFECTED SIDE)
Anterior Drawer—knee in 90-degree flexion, examiner pulls forward on upper tibia while stabilizing upper leg	Anterior cruciate ligament	Excessive translation with no solid end point suggests tear
Valgus Stress—in full extension and at 30-degree flexion, medial-directed force on knee, lateral-directed force on ankle	Medial collateral ligament	Excessive translation suggests tear
Varus Stress—in full extension and at 30-degree flexion, lateral-directed force on knee and medial-directed force on ankle	Lateral collateral ligament	Excessive translation suggests tear

earlier in this case. Similarly, the Ottawa Knee Rules can aid in the determination of when to perform an x-ray in a knee injury. The Ottawa Knee Rules recommend performing a knee x-ray on patients with a knee injury who have any one of the following five criteria:

1. Age 55 years or older
2. Isolated patella tenderness
3. Tenderness of the head of the fibula
4. Inability to flex the knee to 90 degrees
5. Inability to bear weight for 4 steps immediately and in the examination room (regardless of limping)

These rules were validated for, and should only be applied to, adults older than age 18 years, although further study suggests that they may be valid in younger ages.

When a decision is made to perform an imaging test, whether to acutely rule out a fracture or to evaluate an injury that is failing to improve, the **initial imaging study of choice is the plain x-ray.** At minimum, an x-ray series should include at least two views at 90-degree angles to each other. In patients with normal x-rays and continued symptoms, or with suspected ligament or tendon injuries of the shoulder, ankle, knee, or hip, magnetic resonance imaging (MRI) has largely supplanted other modalities as the imaging method of choice. MRI is highly sensitive and specific for articular or soft-tissue abnormalities, including ligament, tendon, and cartilage tears.

Management Principles

The initial management of most acute sprains and sprains is "PRICE"— Protection from further injury, relative Rest, Ice to reduce swelling and pain, Compression, and Elevation to reduce edema. In most cases, NSAIDs or acetaminophen are adequate for pain control, with narcotics used only when necessary.

Numerous studies show that early mobilization of injured ligaments actually promotes healing and recovery. Range-of-motion exercises should be started as early as possible in patients with sprains and strains. For lower-extremity injuries, protected weight bearing with orthotics is allowable, with advancement to unsupported weight bearing as tolerated. Crutches may be necessary initially because of painful weight bearing.

The **most common cause of persistently stiff, painful, or unstable joints following sprains are inadequate rehabilitation.** All patients with sprain or strain injuries should be educated on the importance of rehabilitative exercises. When possible, handouts with a specific exercise program should be given to the patient when the patient is evaluated. If the patient is unsuccessful in accomplishing this themself, referral for a formal physical therapy program can be beneficial.

Comprehension Questions

[12.1]   In which of the following settings is it appropriate to apply the Ottawa Ankle Rules to determine whether to have x-rays taken?

A. A 6-year-old boy injures his ankle riding a scooter.
B. A 33-year-old woman injures both ankles and knees in a motor vehicle accident.
C. A 43-year-old man injured his ankle yesterday while playing volleyball.
D. A 22-year-old woman injures her ankle after falling while drunk.

[12.2]   A 32-year-old male comes for evaluation of right shoulder pain that he's had for the past 3 weeks. He thinks that he injured it playing softball but does not remember a specific injury. There is no bruising or swelling. He gets pain in the joint on external rotation and abduction, but has preserved range of motion. Which of the following is the initial imaging test of choice?

A. X-ray
B. MRI
C. CT scan
D. Arthrogram

[12.3] A 45-year-old woman comes in for follow-up of an ankle sprain that occurred while she was jogging. X-rays done at your initial visit were negative for fracture. She has been unable to run because of persistent stiffness. Examination reveals no joint instability or focal tenderness. Your most appropriate management at this time is:

A. MRI of the ankle to evaluate for ligament tear
B. Referral to orthopedic surgeon
C. Repeat the plain x-rays
D. Increase her dose of ibuprofen
E. Refer her for physical therapy

Answers

[12.1] **C.** The Ottawa Ankle Rules apply in adult patients who have a normal mental status, who don't have other painful injuries, and who are seen within 10 days of their injury. The only setting in which all of these criteria apply is C.

[12.2] **A.** Plain film x-rays are the diagnostic imaging test of choice for the initial evaluation of the painful joint. In patients who have normal x-rays and who have a suspected soft-tissue (ligament, tendon, cartilage) injury, MRI scanning is usually the next most appropriate imaging study to perform.

[12.3] **E.** The most common cause of a stiff or painful joint following a sprain is inadequate rehabilitation. When a patient is unable to adequately self-rehabilitate an injury, a physical therapy referral can be beneficial. If the patient continues to have symptoms after that, consideration of advanced imaging or orthopedic referral is appropriate.

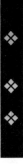

CLINICAL PEARLS

❖ If you suspect that a patient's limited active range of motion is primarily a result of pain, you can numb the joint by injecting lidocaine into it and then reexamine the joint.

❖ Use the uninjured, contralateral extremity as a comparison for your examination of an injured extremity.

❖ An adequate x-ray series must include at least two views at 90 degrees to each other.

REFERENCES

Hockenberry RT, Sammarco GJ. Evaluation and treatment of ankle sprains. Phys Sports Med 2001;29(2). Available online at: www.physsportsmed.com/issues/2001/02_01/feb01.htm

Trojian TH, McKeag DB. Ankle sprains: expedient diagnosis and management. Phys Sports Med 1998;26(10). Available online at: www.physsportsmed.com/issues/1998/10Oct/oct98.htm

Wolfe MW, Uhl TL, McCluskey LC. Management of ankle sprains. Am Fam Physician 2001;63:93–104.

Woodward TW, Best TM. The painful shoulder: part I. Clinical evaluation. Am Fam Physician 2000;61:3079–3088.

A 45-year-old White female presents to your office concerned about a "mole" on her face. She says that it has been present for year but her husband has been urging her to have it checked. She denies any pain, itching, or bleeding from the site. She has no significant past medical history, takes no medications, and has no allergies. She has no history of skin cancer in her family. She is an accountant by occupation.

On examination, the patient is normotensive, afebrile, and appears slightly younger than her stated age. A skin examination reveals a nontender, symmetric, 4-mm papule that is uniformly reddish-brown in color. The lesion is well circumscribed, and the surrounding skin is normal in appearance. There are no other lesions in the area.

◆ **What is the most likely diagnosis?**

◆ **What features are reassuring of a benign condition?**

◆ **What is your next step?**

ANSWERS TO CASE 13: Skin Lesions

Summary: A 45-year-old healthy woman with no significant past medical history presents for evaluation of a skin lesion. She does not have a family history of skin cancer. The lesion is symmetric, with well-defined borders, relatively small (<6 mm), and uniform coloration. She is not able to assess whether the lesion has changed recently (i.e., become larger), and does not give a history of itching or bleeding at the site of the lesion.

◆ **Most likely diagnosis:** benign nevus

◆ **Reassuring features:** size <6 mm, symmetric, uniform color, well-defined borders

◆ **Next step in treatment:** Reassurance and surveillance

Analysis

Objectives

1. Describe an approach to the evaluation of skin lesions.
2. Be able to describe the features of a skin lesion in dermatologic terms.
3. Know which features of a lesion are typically benign and which are concerning for malignancy or potential malignancy.

Considerations

This case represents a typical scenario seen in primary care medicine: "I have this mole. Is it cancer?" Although simplified, this is what the patient is most concerned about and wants to know. The **role of the physician is to determine the likelihood of malignancy or premalignancy and to define a course of action that is appropriate.** In this particular case, there are several features that reassure a benign condition that can be monitored without the need for a biopsy. There was neither a family medical history of skin cancer nor history of skin cancer in the patient. She has an occupation that does not expose her to harmful chemicals or the sun on a regular basis. On examination, the lesion has typically benign features (size <6 mm, symmetric, uniform color, well-defined borders). In this case, it would be appropriate to make a note (or possibly even a photograph) in the patient's chart describing the characteristic features of the lesion and monitor for changes in the lesion at periodic health evaluations. The patient should also be educated in self-examination of the skin, with an emphasis on what to look for and when to come to the physician's office for an evaluation of a new or changing skin lesion. Finally, it should be understood that many otherwise benign-appearing moles might have an atypical characteristic that warrants further investigation. The **criteria that are used to predict the likelihood of a benign versus malignant lesion are only guidelines;** to be sure, not all malignant skin lesions present in the same manner and a malignant melanoma is not always visibly pigmented. The bottom line is that the physician should use all of the tools at his disposal: the history of present illness (HPI), medical history of the patient, the family medical history (FMH), social and occupational history, and a pertinent review of systems so as to arrive at a conclusion that is consistent with the physical exam.

Definitions

Abscess: A closed pocket containing pus.

Bulla: A blister greater than 0.5 cm in diameter (plural: bullae).

Cyst: A closed, saclike, membranous capsule containing a liquid or semisolid material.

Macule: A discoloration on the skin that is neither raised nor depressed.

Nodule: A small mass of rounded or irregular shape that is greater than 1.0 cm in diameter.

Papule: A small, circumscribed *elevated* lesion of the skin that is less than 0.5 cm in diameter.

Plaque: A plateaulike, raised, solid area on the skin that covers a large surface area in relation to its height above the skin.

Ulcer: A lesion through the skin or mucous membrane resulting from loss of tissue.

Vesicle: A small blister less than 0.5 cm in diameter.

APPROACH TO SKIN LESIONS

Incidence and Risk Factors

There has been an increase in the morbidity and mortality of skin cancer in the past few decades in the United States. In 2005, an estimated 21 persons per day died from malignant melanoma and nearly 60,000 new cases were diagnosed. This figure does not include the 2005 cases of basal cell carcinoma or squamous cell carcinoma, which raise the total to more than 1 million new cases.

The **single most important risk factor for the development of skin cancer is exposure to ultraviolet radiation.** Other risk factors include a prior history of skin cancer, a family history of skin cancer, fair skin, red or blonde hair, a propensity to burn easily, chronic exposure to toxic compounds such as creosote, arsenic, or radium, and a suppressed immune system.

Four Basic Types of Melanoma

Superficial Spreading Melanoma

This is the **most common type of melanoma** in both sexes. As its name implies, this lesion spreads superficially along the top layers of skin before penetrating into the deep layers. The superficial, or radial, growth phase is slower than the vertical phase, which is when the lesion grows into the dermis

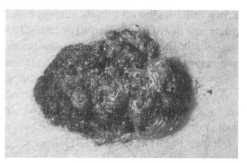

Figure 13–1. Nodular melanoma. (*Reproduced with permission from Kaspar DL, Braunwald E, Fauci A, et al., Harrison's principles of internal medicine. 16th ed. New York: McGraw-Hill, 2005:499.*)

and can invade other tissues or metastasize. Men are more commonly affected on the upper torso, whereas women are affected mostly on the legs.

Lentigo Maligna

Similar to the superficial spreading type, this lesion is **most often found in the elderly,** usually on chronic sun-damaged skin such as the face, ears, arms, and upper trunk. Although it is the **least common of the four types of melanoma,** this is the most common form of melanoma found in Hawaii.

Acral Lentiginous Melanoma

Similar to the other two superficial melanomas in that it begins in situ, this lesion is different in many ways. This is the **most common melanoma found in African-Americans and Asians.** This melanoma is usually found under the nails, on the soles of the feet, and on the palms of the hands.

Nodular Melanoma

This melanoma, unlike the other three, is usually invasive at the time of diagnosis. This is the **most aggressive type of melanoma (Fig. 13–1).**

Physical Examination

In 1985, it was noted by clinicians studying melanoma that there were several characteristic features of skin lesions that correlated with melanoma. Specifically, color variegation, border irregularity, asymmetry, and size greater than 6 mm in diameter were consistently observed with melanoma. This led to the **ABCD acronym** which has been used extensively to determine the likelihood of a cancerous skin lesion (Table 13–1).

One other criterion that is often used is the change in the size or appearance of the skin lesion. This is sometimes cited as E in the above ABCD criteria, and referred to as Evolving. Benign lesions may present at birth, or any time thereafter, and several benign lesions may also present near the same point in

Table 13–1
CLASSIC ABCD CRITERIA OF SUSPICIOUS SKIN LESIONS

ACRONYM	CHARACTERISTIC	LIKELY BENIGN	LIKELY MALIGNANT
A	Asymmetry	Symmetric (right half looks like left half)	Asymmetric
B	Borders	Well defined	Ragged or blurred
C	Color	Uniform color	Variegated
D	Diameter	Less than 6 mm	Greater than 6 mm

time. However, a benign lesion, once present, will usually remain stable in size and appearance, whereas a malignancy will present as increasing in size or changing in appearance. Thus, it is useful to ask whether a "mole" has recently changed in appearance or has grown in size.

Treatment

Benign nevi need only be monitored visually. The patient can accomplish this after education on what to look for and when to come back for reevaluation. In general, any preexisting nevus that has changed or any new pigmented lesion that exhibits any of the ABCDE signs should be excised completely with a 2–3-mm margin around the lesion. Larger lesions that may be cosmetically difficult to completely excise may be biopsied in several areas. If the pathology indicates a malignancy, the lesion should then be completely excised with 5-mm margins by a physician trained in plastic surgical technique. Complete excision of malignant melanomas requires at least a 5-mm margin. Once a patient has been identified as having a malignant skin lesion, the patient should be observed on an annual basis for any new or changing skin lesions.

Prognosis

The single most important piece of information for prognosis in melanoma is the thickness of the tumor, known as the Breslow measurement. **Melanomas <1-mm thick have a low rate of metastasis** and a high cure rate with excision. Thicker melanomas have higher rates of metastases and poorer outcomes.

Prevention

Prevention is aimed at reducing exposure to ultraviolet radiation. When possible, avoid the sun between 10 A.M. and 4 P.M.; wear sun-protective clothing when exposed to sunlight; wear a sunscreen with a sun protection factor (SPF) of at least 15; and avoid artificial sources of ultraviolet (UV) radiation.

Nonmelanoma Skin Cancers

Both basal cell and squamous cell carcinomas arise from the epidermal layer of the skin. The primary risk for these types of skin cancers is exposure to ultraviolet radiation, especially sun exposure but also tanning bed use. A history of actinic keratoses and human papillomavirus infection of the skin also raises the risk of squamous cell carcinomas.

Basal cell carcinomas are the most common of all cancers. They typically appear as pearly papules, often with a central ulceration or with multiple telangiectasias. Patients typically present with a growing lesion and sometimes complain that it bleeds or itches. Basal cell carcinomas rarely metastasize but can grow large and can be locally destructive. The primary treatment is excision.

Squamous cell carcinomas have a higher rate of metastasis than basal cell carcinomas, but the risk is still low. These lesions are often irregularly shaped plaques or nodules with raised borders. They are frequently scaly, ulcerated, and bleed easily. Complete excision is the treatment of choice.

Comprehension Questions

Match the following characteristics to the correct type of skin lesion as described below (answers may be used once, more than once, or not at all):

    A. Benign nevus
    B. Superficial spreading melanoma
    C. Lentigo maligna
    D. Nodular melanoma
    E. Acral lentiginous melanoma

[13.1] Most common type of melanoma in both males and females; it has two growth phases.

[13.2] Skin lesion that is usually invasive at the time of diagnosis.

[13.3] Most common type of melanoma found in African-Americans and Asians.

[13.4] Skin lesion that may appear at any age, and remains stable in size and appearance.

Answers

[13.1] **B.** Superficial spreading melanomas are the most commonly occurring melanomas.

[13.2] **D.** Nodular melanomas are the most aggressive melanomas and are usually invasive at the time of diagnosis.

[13.3] **E.** Acral lentiginous melanomas are found on the palms of hands, soles of feet, and under finger- and toenails.

[13.4] **A.** Benign nevi (moles) may appear at any age. A hallmark of their diagnosis is their stability over the course of time.

CLINICAL PEARLS

❖ The preventable risk factor common to all skin cancers is sun exposure. Recommend to your at-risk patients limiting exposure to sunlight in the middle of the day, wearing appropriate protective clothing, and using sun screen.

❖ Contrary to popular belief, the use of tanning beds is also a risk factor for skin cancer.

❖ There is no such thing as a "healthy tan."

REFERENCES

Abbasi NR, Shaw HM, Rigel DS, et al. Early diagnosis of cutaneous melanoma: revisiting the ABCD criteria. JAMA 2004;292:2771–2776.

Fitzpatrick TB, Johnson RA, Wolf K, et al. in Cooke D, Englis M, Morriss J, ed. Color atlas and synopsis of clinical dermatology. 4th ed. New York: McGraw-Hill, 2001.

Goldstein BG, Goldstein AO. Diagnosis and management of malignant melanoma. Am Fam Physician 2001;63:1359–1368, 1374.

Pierson JC. Pigmented skin lesions (nevi and melanoma). Best Practice of medicine. November 2001. Available at: http://merck.micromedex.com/index.asp?page= bpm_brief&article_id=BPM01DE07.

Rose LC. Recognizing neoplastic skin lesions: a photo guide. Am Fam Physician 1998;4:58.

Saraiya M, Glanz,K, Briss P, et al. Preventing skin cancer: findings of the task force on community preventative services on reducing exposure to ultraviolet light. MMWR _ October 17, 2003:52(RR15);1–12_.

Stulberg DL, Crandell B, Fawcett RS. Diagnosis and treatment of basal cell and squamous cell carcinomas. Am Fam Physician 2004;70:1481–1488.

A 40-year-old male with no past medical history presents to the clinic to establish care. He reports that he had a prior urinalysis that revealed blood as an incidental finding. The urinalysis was done as a standard screening test by his former employer. He denies ever seeing any blood in his urine and denies any voiding difficulties, dysuria, sexual dysfunction, or any history or risk factors for sexually transmitted diseases. His review of systems is otherwise negative. He has smoked a half-pack of cigarettes per day for the past 10 years and exercises by jogging 15 minutes and light weight training daily. On examination, his vital signs are normal and the entire physical examination is unremarkable. A complete blood count (CBC) and a chemistry panel (electrolytes, blood urea nitrogen, and creatinine) are normal. The results of a urinalysis done in your office are: specific gravity, 1.015; pH 5.5; leukocyte esterase, negative; nitrites, negative; white blood cell count (WBC), 0; red blood cell count (RBC), 4–5 per high-power field (HPF).

◆ **What is your diagnosis?**

◆ **How would you approach this patient?**

◆ **What is the work-up and plan for this patient?**

◆ **What are the concerns and how would you counsel the patient?**

ANSWERS TO CASE 14: Hematuria

Summary: A 40-year-old male smoker is found incidentally to have red blood cells in his urine sample on a urinalysis.

◆ **Current diagnosis:** Asymptomatic microscopic hematuria

◆ **Initial approach to this patient:** Repeat the urinalysis, assess for risk factors, image the upper and lower urinary tract.

◆ **Work-up and plan:** Rule out infection by performing a urine culture; evaluate for malignancy by imaging of the upper urinary tract, cystoscopy, and voided cytology.

◆ **Concerns and counseling for the patient:** The primary concern is to rule out malignancy, including renal cell carcinoma and transitional cell carcinoma. Counsel the patient on the importance of an appropriate work-up, but reassure the patient about the low prevalence of the condition.

Analysis

Objectives

1. Learn about the significance of microscopic hematuria.
2. Learn an evidence-based approach to work-up asymptomatic microscopic hematuria.
3. Be familiar with recommendations for follow-up on patients with hematuria after a negative work-up.

Definitions

Gross hematuria: The presence of enough blood in a urine sample to be visible to the naked eye.
Lower urinary tract: The urinary bladder and urethra.
Microscopic hematuria: The presence of 3 or more red blood cells per HPF on 2 or more properly collected urinalyses.
Upper urinary tract: The kidneys and ureters.

Considerations

This patient has asymptomatic microscopic hematuria, as opposed to gross hematuria. Although he is asymptomatic, this patient deserves a thorough work-up in order to determine an etiology, if possible, and to rule out malignancy.

The patient's history should be reviewed with specific questions to determine any risks for sexually transmitted diseases (STDs), occupational exposures to

chemicals, strenuous exercise, drugs, medications, and herbal/nutritional supplements. The work-up should begin with a repeat urinalysis. If the condition
persists, the patient should have imaging studies of both the upper and lower
urinary tract. The **upper tract can be imaged by either an intravenous pyel-
ogram (IVP) or computed tomography (CT) scan**. The **lower tract is most
commonly evaluated by cystoscopy,** an endoscopic procedure. Urine should
also be sent for cytology and culture. Urologic consultation should be requested
if the work-up reveals an abnormality that cannot be treated in a primary care
office or if the condition persists. Inform the patient that a complete work-up
is necessary to evaluate for the presence of conditions such as infections or
tumors, but he should be reassured that the **incidence of cancer presenting as
asymptomatic microscopic hematuria is low.**

APPROACH TO HEMATURIA

Hematuria is divided into glomerular, renal (nonglomerular), and urologic etiologies. Glomerular hematuria typically is associated with significant proteinuria, erythrocyte casts, and dysmorphic RBCs. Renal (nonglomerular) hematuria
is secondary to tubulointerstitial, renovascular, and metabolic disorders. Like
glomerular hematuria, it often is associated with significant proteinuria; however,
there are no associated dysmorphic RBCs or erythrocyte casts. Urologic causes
of hematuria include tumors, calculi, infections, trauma and benign prostatic
hyperplasia (BPH). Urologic hematuria is distinguished from other etiologies by
the absence of proteinuria, dysmorphic RBCs, and erythrocyte casts.

Hematuria in adults should first be defined as gross hematuria or microscopic hematuria. Gross hematuria denotes that the patient is able to visualize
blood in his voided specimen. Patients most often describe their urine as having
a reddish or brownish color. They commonly are concerned about malignancy or
kidney stones. In contrast, microscopic hematuria is usually asymptomatic and
often discovered incidentally. Although a thorough work-up of microscopic
hematuria is advocated, many **authorities do not recommend routine screening for hematuria.**

Microscopic hematuria is defined as 3 or more red blood cells per high-
power field on microscopic evaluation of urinary sediment from two of three
properly collected urinalysis specimens. The initial determination of microscopic hematuria should be based on microscopic examination of urinary sediment from a freshly voided, early morning, clean-catch, midstream urine
specimen. Urine must be refrigerated if it cannot be examined promptly, as
delays of more than 2 hours between collection and examination often cause
unreliable results.

Hematuria can be measured quantitatively by any of the following methods:
(a) determination of the number of red blood cells per milliliter of urine excreted
(chamber count); (b) direct examination of the centrifuged urinary sediment (sediment count); or (c) indirect examination of the urine by dipstick (the simplest

way to detect microscopic hematuria). Given the limited specificity of the dip-stick method (65–99% for 2–5 red blood cells per high-power microscopic field), however, the initial **finding of hematuria by the dipstick method should be confirmed by microscopic evaluation of urinary sediment.**

Despite the recommendation that two positive urinalyses are needed prior to work-up, it is important to consider the individual patient's risk factors. If a patient has significant risk factors, even one properly collected urine specimen with 1–2 RBCs is sufficient to warrant a work-up. Risk factors include smok-ing, occupational exposure to chemicals or dyes (benzenes or aromatic amines), history of gross hematuria, older than age 40 years, history of urologic disorder or disease, history of irritative voiding symptoms, history of urinary tract infec-tion, analgesic abuse, or history of pelvic irradiation.

The prevalence of asymptomatic hematuria is roughly 0.20% in the adult population in the United States. There are myriad possible causes; risk factors should guide the specific work-up for the individual patient. Although some elements of the work-up are standard for everyone, other more detailed and expensive tests can be deferred for those at low risk. The presence of signifi-cant proteinuria, red cell casts, or renal insufficiency, or a predominance of dys-morphic red blood cells in the urine should prompt an evaluation for renal parenchymal disease or referral to a nephrologist. In general, glomerular bleed-ing is associated with more than 80% dysmorphic red blood cells, whereas lower urinary tract bleeding is associated with more than 80% normal red blood cells.

Evaluation of the **urinary sediment** can allow for the diagnosis of patients with renal parenchymal disease. This analysis **will often also allow for dis-tinction between glomerular disease and interstitial nephritis.** The pres-ence of red cell casts and dysmorphic red blood cells is suggestive of renal glomerular disease. Interstitial nephritis, often caused by analgesics or other drugs, is suggested by the presence of eosinophils in the urine.

A complete evaluation for microscopic hematuria starts with a detailed his-tory and physical examination, appropriate laboratory testing (including uri-nary cytology), and imaging of the upper and lower urinary tract. In all patients, the urinalysis should be repeated. If the repeat urinalysis is negative and the patient remains asymptomatic, no further work-up is required for low-risk patients. However, if the hematuria persists, a full work-up is warranted regardless of a benign history or physical exam. The repeat urinalysis should be done after avoidance of any potential confounders such as menses, med-ications, exercise, drugs, and nutritional/herbal products. Exercise-induced hematuria usually resolves spontaneously in 72 hours in the absence of other coexisting conditions. In addition, careful attention should be taken in women to ensure the blood is not from the vaginal or rectal areas. In men, one should also exclude local trauma to the foreskin. If in doubt, a catheterized specimen should be obtained, taking care not to induce trauma during the procedure.

The laboratory studies should start with urinalysis with microscopy and evaluation of centrifuged urinary sediment. The urine should be examined for number of RBCs per high power field, dysmorphic RBCs, and presence of casts and eosinophils. Urinary tract infection (UTI) should be ruled out by urine culture. If an infection is present, it should be appropriately treated and the urinalysis repeated in 6 weeks. If the **hematuria resolves with treatment of the UTI, no further work-up is needed.**

A serum creatinine should also be obtained to assess renal function, with comparison to old records if available. If the laboratory evaluation reveals elevated creatinine or red cell casts, work-up should focus on renal parenchymal disease and possible etiologies such as hypertension, diabetes, or autoimmune diseases. Renal biopsy may be appropriate for certain individuals. Patients with risk factors should also undergo cytologic evaluation of the urine to assess for transitional cell carcinoma. Although voided urine cytology may not pick up low-grade carcinoma, it is fairly reliable for high-grade lesions, especially if repeated.

Numerous options exist for imaging of the upper urinary tract. An IVP is x-ray imaging of the upper urinary tract after the administration of an intravenous contrast dye. It is a widely available and relatively low-cost procedure, but it can miss small renal masses and may not distinguish solid from cystic lesions. Ultrasonography is also widely available and does not require the use of contrast dye but also may miss small lesions. CT scanning has a high sensitivity and specificity for detecting masses, renal stones, renal or perirenal infections, and obstruction. The CT scan should be initially performed as a noncontrast study to detect calculi, and then a contrast study should be obtained. Both CT scanning and IVP may lead to nephropathy caused by IV contrast dye. Premedication with N-acetylcysteine may be used reduce the risk contrast nephropathy. In patients with renal insufficiency or who are at high risk of contrast nephropathy, a retrograde pyelography combined with a renal ultrasound may be an option. Retrograde pyelography is an invasive procedure in which a catheter is placed in the bladder and dye injected up the ureters to the kidneys. There is little risk of contrast nephropathy because no contrast dye is given IV.

The lower urinary tract should be examined for transitional cell carcinoma by cystoscopy performed by a urologist. In the absence of risk factors in selected patients with a negative history, examination, laboratory work-up, and upper tract imaging, cystoscopy may be deferred or individualized at the discretion of the treating physician.

In patients with a thorough but negative work-up, the American Urological Association recommends follow-up blood pressure measurements, urinalyses, and voided urine cytologic studies at 6, 12, 24, and 36 months. The reason for the regular follow-up is to assess for the possibility of an underlying lesion, despite a low likelihood of there being one. If the work-up remains negative for 36 months and the patient continues to be asymptomatic, no further follow-up is recommended. However, if the patient develops gross hematuria, voiding difficulties, pain, or any abnormal cytology, immediate urologic reevaluation and urologic consultation is warranted. Patients who develop hypertension, proteinuria, glomerular casts, or abnormal renal function should be referred to a nephrologist for consultation.

Comprehension Questions

[14.1] A 24-year-old male bodybuilder with no significant medical history presents with gross hematuria. He was told by his trainer that exercise can induce hematuria and that this is nothing to worry about. He comes to you for a second opinion. You advise the patient:

A. The trainer is correct, no further work-up is needed.
B. To check a urinalysis and, if it is normal, no other work-up is needed.
C. That if it resolves after 72 hours of not exercising, no work-up is needed.
D. That gross hematuria should always be worked up.

[14.2] A 78-year-old male with multiple medical problems presents with dysuria and is found to have microscopic hematuria. His examination is only positive for a very tender and boggy prostate. You next step is:

A. Stat urology referral.
B. Treat the prostatitis with 1 month of antibiotics and reevaluate the patient with a follow up urinalysis and culture posttreatment.
C. Obtain an IVP followed by cystoscopy.
D. Obtain a CT of the abdomen and pelvis, followed by cystoscopy.

[14.3] A 45-year-old female with a history of cancer, currently receiving radiation therapy, presents as a new patient. On a routine urinalysis, you discover 2 RBCs per HPF, 15–20 WBCs per HPF, nitrites, and leukocyte esterase. What is the next logical approach?

A. Repeat a clean-catch midstream specimen, send for culture, and treat the UTI. Repeat urinalysis after the UTI treatment.
B. Treat the UTI and also refer the patient for an IVP and cystoscopy.
C. Check urine for cytology.
D. Inform the patient that the urinalysis results are a result of the radiation treatment and no further work-up is needed.

Answers

[14.1] **D.** Gross hematuria always deserves a full work-up. Although exercise-induced hematuria resolves in 72 hours, gross hematuria, especially in a person with risk factors, must have a thorough evaluation.

[14.2] **B.** A tender/boggy prostate alludes to the diagnosis of prostatitis. Reevaluation should be done after adequate treatment of the prostatitis. If the hematuria persists following treatment, further work-up is necessary.

[14.3] **A.** True microscopic hematuria is the presence of 3 or more RBCs per HPF in a midstream clean-catch specimen after exclusion of a UTI. If there is evidence of a UTI, it should be cultured, treated, and urinalysis repeated after treatment.

CLINICAL PEARLS

❖ Hematuria in adults always should be evaluated. If no source is found, patients should be followed for at least 3 years if no further hematuria is found.

❖ Patients should be thoroughly instructed in the proper technique for a "clean-catch" urine sample. This will reduce the number of false-positive findings.

REFERENCES

Cohen RA, Brown RS. Microscopic hematuria. N Engl J Med 2003;348:2330–2338.

Simerville JA, Maxted WC, Pahira JJ. Urinalysis: a comprehensive review. Am Fam Physician. 2005;71(6):1153–1162.

Grossfeld GD, Wolf JS Jr, Litwan MS, et al. Asymptomatic microscopic hematuria in adults: summary of the AUA best practice policy recommendations. Am Fam Physician. 2001;63(6):1145–1154.

Grossfeld GD, Litwin MS, Wolf JS, et al. Evaluation of asymptomatic microscopic hematuria in adults: the American Urological Association best practice policy— part I: definition, detection, prevalence, and etiology. Urology 2001;57(4):599–603.

Grossfeld GD, Litwin MS, Wolf JS Jr, et al. Evaluation of asymptomatic microscopic hematuria in adults: the American Urological Association best practice policy— part II: patient evaluation, cytology, voided markers, imaging, cystoscopy, nephrology evaluation, and follow-up. Urology 2001;57(4):604–610.

Thaller TR, Wang LP. Evaluation of microscopic hematuria in adults. Am Fam Physician 1999;60(4):1143–1152, 1154.

A 27-year-old woman presents to your office complaining of progressing nervousness, fatigue, palpitations, and the recent development of a resting hand tremor. She also states that she is having difficulty concentrating at work and has been more irritable with her coworkers. The patient also notes that she has developed a persistent rash over her shins that has not improved with the use of topical steroid creams. All of her symptoms have come on gradually over the past few months and continue to get worse. Review of systems also reveals an unintentional weight loss of about 10 pounds, insomnia, and amenorrhea for the past 2 months (the patient's menstrual cycles are usually quite regular). The patient's past medical history is unremarkable and she takes no oral medications. She is currently not sexually active and does not drink alcohol, smoke, or use any illicit drugs. On examination, she is afebrile. Her pulse varies from 70–110 beats per minute. She appears restless and anxious. Her skin is warm and moist. Her eyes show evidence of exophthalmos and lid retraction bilaterally, although funduscopic examination is normal. Neck examination reveals symmetric thyroid enlargement, without any discrete palpable masses. Cardiac examination reveals an irregular rhythm. Her lungs are clear to auscultation. Extremity examination reveals an erythematous, thickened rash on both shins. Neurologic examination is normal except for a fine resting tremor in her hands when she attempts to hold out her outstretched arms. Initial lab tests include a negative pregnancy test and an undetectable level of thyroid-stimulating hormone (TSH).

◆ **What is the most likely diagnosis?**

◆ **What imaging study is most appropriate at this time?**

◆ **What is the definitive nonsurgical treatment of this condition?**

ANSWERS TO CASE 15: Thyroid Disorders

Summary: A 27-year-old female with progressively worsening anxiety, palpitations, tremor, menstrual irregularities, and weight loss. Her TSH level is suppressed, confirming the presence of hyperthyroidism.

◆ **Most likely diagnosis:** Hyperthyroidism secondary to Graves disease

◆ **Most appropriate imaging study:** Nuclear medicine thyroid scan with uptake

◆ **Definitive nonsurgical treatment:** Thyroid ablation with radioactive iodine

Analysis

Objectives

1. Know the most common conditions that cause hyper- and hypothyroidism.
2. Be able to interpret the common tests used to evaluate thyroid function.
3. Learn the modalities of treatment for disorders of the thyroid.

Considerations

This patient has symptoms and signs consistent with hyperthyroidism, including warm, moist skin caused by excessive sweating and cutaneous vasodilation; a resting tremor; an enlarged thyroid gland; weight loss; and tachycardia. Her irregular heart beat may be a manifestation of atrial fibrillation, which occurs in approximately 10% of hyperthyroid patients. Eye abnormalities are common in hyperthyroid states. Retraction of the upper lid, resulting in the "thyroid stare" is common. Graves disease has a unique ophthalmopathy that may cause a prominent exophthalmos **(Fig. 15–1). The most common cause of noniatrogenic hyperthyroidism is Graves disease,** an autoimmune thyroid disorder. Autoantibodies to the TSH receptors on the thyroid gland result in hyperfunctioning of the gland, with the result that the thyroid gland functions outside the usual control of the hypothalamic–pituitary axis. Graves disease commonly occurs in reproductive-age females and is much more common in women than men. The treatment of Graves disease includes antithyroid drugs (such as propylthiouracil and methimazole) and/or β-blockers to block some of the peripheral effects of the excessive thyroxine. However, these are only temporary measures used to give patients symptomatic relief. The definitive treatment is radioactive iodine, which destroys the thyroid gland. **At least 40% of patients who receive radioactive iodine eventually become hypothyroid** and will need thyroid hormone replacement. Radioactive iodine therapy is contraindicated in pregnant women, as the isotope can cross the placenta and cause

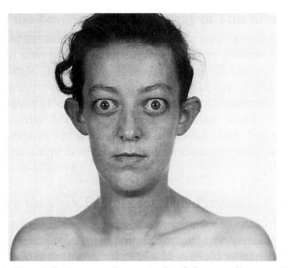

Figure 15–1. Exophthalmos and proptosis of Graves disease. (*Reproduced with permission from Kasper, et al. Harrison's principles of internal medicine. 16th ed. New York: McGraw-Hill, 2005:2114.*)

fetal thyroid ablation. Surgical removal of the thyroid gland is another option for the treatment of Graves disease, but it is often reserved for pregnant patients.

Hyperthyroidism

Signs and Symptoms

Hyperthyroidism usually presents with progressing nervousness, palpitations, weight loss, fine resting tremor, dyspnea on exertion, and difficulty with concentration. Physical findings include a rapid pulse rate and elevated blood pressure, with the systolic pressure increased to a greater extent than the diastolic pressure, creating a widened pulse–pressure hypertension. Examination findings can include atrial fibrillation and a fine resting tremor.

Thyroid storm is an acute hypermetabolic state associated with the sudden release of large amounts of thyroid hormone into circulation. It occurs most often in patients with Graves disease, but can also occur in acute thyroiditis conditions. Symptoms include fever, confusion, restlessness, and psychoticlike behavior. Examination may demonstrate tachycardia, elevated blood pressure, fever, and dysrhythmias. Patients can also have other signs of high-output heart failure, such as dyspnea on exertion and peripheral vasoconstriction, and may exhibit signs of cerebral or cardiac ischemia. **Thyroid storm is a medical emergency** that requires prompt attention and reversal of the metabolic demands of the acute hyperthyroidism.

Pathogenesis

Graves disease is the most common cause of hyperthyroidism and is more commonly found in women. It is an autoimmune disorder caused by immunoglobulin (Ig) G antibodies that bind to TSH receptors, initiating the production and release of thyroid hormone. In addition to the usual findings, approximately **50% of patients with Graves disease also have exophthalmos.** The second most common cause of hyperthyroidism is an autonomous thyroid nodule that secretes thyroxine. These nodules do not rely on TSH stimulation and continue to excrete large amounts of thyroxine despite low, or nonexistent, circulating TSH levels. Hyperthyroidism can also be caused by the acute release of thyroid hormone in the early stages of thyroiditis. In such cases, symptoms are generally transient and resolve within weeks of onset. Iatrogenic hyperthyroidism can occur secondary to the overuse of thyroxine supplementation.

Laboratory and Imaging Evaluation

Hyperthyroidism can be diagnosed by an elevated free thyroxine level, usually with a corresponding low TSH level. Once it has been identified, further testing for autoimmune antibodies and radionucleotide scanning of the thyroid can help to determine whether the problem is Graves disease, an autonomous nodule, or thyroiditis. Radionucleotide imaging provides a direct scan of the gland and an indication of its functioning. Imaging is performed using either an isotope of technetium-99m (^{99m}Tc) or iodine-123 (^{123}I). After the administration of one of these agents, imaging the thyroid allows visualization of active and inactive areas, as well as an indication as to the level of activity in a particular area. In patients with Graves disease, there will be diffuse hyperactivity with large amounts of uptake. In contrast, thyroiditis demonstrates patchy uptake with overall reduced activity, reflecting the release of existing hormone rather than the overproduction of new thyroxine. The detection of serum thyroid-receptor antibodies is a specific diagnostic test for Graves disease.

Treatment

Radioactive iodine is the treatment of choice for Graves disease in adult patients who are not pregnant. It should not be used in children or breast-feeding mothers. Antithyroid drugs are also well tolerated and successful at blocking the production and release of thyroid hormone in patients with Graves disease. Some examples of these drugs include propylthiouracil (PTU), methimazole, and carbimazole. These drugs work by inhibiting the organification of iodine, although PTU also prevents the peripheral conversion of thyroxine (T_4) to triiodothyronine (T_3), its more active form. The most serious potential side effect of these drugs is agranulocytosis, which occurs in 3 per 10,000 treated patients per year. All of these drugs are relatively safe during pregnancy, although PTU is the preferred agent. **Antithyroid drugs are especially useful in treating adolescents, in whom Graves disease may go into spontaneous remission after 6–18 months of therapy.** Surgery is reserved for patients in whom medications and radioactive iodine ablation are unacceptable treatment modalities, or in whom a large goiter is present that is either compressing nearby structures or is disfiguring. For patients presenting with thyroid storm, aggressive initial therapy is essential to prevent complications. Treatment should include the administration of high doses of PTU and β-blockers (to control tachycardia and other peripheral symptoms of thyrotoxicosis). Hydrocortisone is given to prevent possible adrenal crisis.

Hypothyroidism

Signs and Symptoms

Patients with hypothyroidism can present with a wide range of symptoms, including lethargy, weight gain, hair loss, dry skin, slowed mentation or forgetfulness, constipation, intolerance to cold, and a depressed affect. **In older patients, hypothyroidism can be confused with Alzheimer disease** and other conditions that cause dementia. In women, it is often confused with depression. Physical findings that can present in hypothyroid patients include low blood pressure, bradycardia, nonpitting edema, hair thinning or loss, dry skin, and a diminished relaxation phase of reflexes.

Pathogenesis

Several different conditions can cause hypothyroidism. The **most common noniatrogenic condition causing hypothyroidism in the United States is Hashimoto thyroiditis,** an autoimmune thyroiditis. Iatrogenic causes include post-Graves disease thyroid ablation and surgical removal of the thyroid gland. Another cause is secondary hypothyroidism related to hypothalamic or pituitary dysfunction. These conditions are primarily found in patients who have received intracranial irradiation or surgical removal of a pituitary adenoma.

Laboratory and Imaging Evaluation

In primary hypothyroidism, the TSH level is elevated, indicating insufficient thyroid hormone production to meet metabolic demands. Free thyroid levels are low. In contrast, patients with secondary hypothyroidism have low or undetectable TSH levels. **Once the diagnosis of primary hypothyroidism is made, further imaging or serologic testing is unnecessary if the thyroid gland is normal on physical examination.** In cases of secondary hypothyroidism, however, further testing is needed to determine whether the cause is a hypothalamic or pituitary problem. This can be done by using a thyroid-releasing hormone (TRH) test. Endogenous TRH is released by the hypothalamus and stimulates the pituitary to release TSH. When TRH is injected intravenously, a normally functioning pituitary will result in an increase of TSH that can be measured in about 30 minutes. No increase in TSH after injection of TRH suggests a malfunctioning pituitary gland. In cases where pituitary dysfunction is suspected, imaging of the pituitary gland to detect microadenomas and testing of other hormones that are dependent on pituitary stimulation are indicated.

Treatment

Most healthy adults with hypothyroidism require about 1.7 μg/kg of thyroid hormone replacement daily, with requirements falling to about 1 μg/kg for the elderly. This usually amounts to between 0.10 and 0.15 mg/d of levothyroxine. Children with hypothyroidism may require higher doses for full replacement. In young patients without cardiovascular risk factors, replacement can start close to the estimated daily requirement. Older patients or those with risks for cardiovascular compromise that could occur with a rapid increase in resting heart rate and blood pressure should be started on lower doses and gradually increased over time. Doses can be increased in increments of 0.025–0.050 mg every 4–6 weeks until TSH levels return to normal. Thyroxine is usually dosed once daily, although some evidence suggests that weekly dosing may also be effective. In patients with an intact hypothalamic–pituitary axis, the adequacy of thyroid replacement can be followed with serial TSH measurements. Evaluation of TSH levels should be performed no earlier than 4 weeks after an adjustment in medication has been made. Full effects of thyroid replacement on TSH level may not be present until after 8 weeks of treatment. With increased age, thyroid binding decreases as a consequence of a drop in serum albumin level and medication dosage may need to be reduced by up to 20%. Annual monitoring of the TSH level in the elderly is necessary to avoid overreplacement.

Nodular Thyroid Disease

Thyroid nodules, both solitary and multiple, are common and are often found incidentally on physical examination, ultrasonography, or computed tomography. They are more prevalent in women and increase in frequency with age. Although their pathogenesis is not clear, nodules are known to be associated with iodine deficiency, higher gravidity, and the ingestion of goitrogens. **Further work-up of identified nodules is indicated, as the incidence of malignancy in solitary nodules is estimated at 5–6%.** The incidence of malignancy is higher in children, adults younger than 30 or older than 60 years, and patients with a history of head or neck irradiation. Other historical risk factors include a family history of thyroid cancer, the presence of cervical lymphadenopathy, and the recent development of hoarseness of the voice, progressive dysphagia, or shortness of breath.

Initial assessment should include evaluation of thyroid function. **Functional adenomas that present with hyperthyroidism are rarely malignant.** These represent less than 10% of all nodules. These patients are best evaluated with a radioactive iodine uptake study to confirm functionality of the nodule. Hyperfunctioning nodules are treated with surgery or radioactive ablation therapy, depending on the level of hyperthyroidism.

Nonfunctioning nodules measuring greater than 1 cm by examination or ultrasonography require biopsy. This can be done by fine-needle aspiration (FNA), which is a highly sensitive test. Ultrasound findings suggestive of malignancy include irregular margins, intranodular vascular spots, and microcalcifications. Results of the FNA determine further management and treatment. Cytologic evaluation of FNA specimens are reported as being nondiagnostic, benign, indeterminate, or malignant. **Follicular cell malignancy cannot be distinguished cytologically from its benign equivalent,** and thus is often read as indeterminate. These patients should be referred to surgery to obtain a definitive evaluation. Papillary, medullary, and anaplastic thyroid carcinomas can be diagnosed accurately by FNA. Patients with thyroid malignancy are treated by thyroidectomy followed by radioactive ablation. These patients will require long-term follow-up by an endocrinologist.

Thyroid nodules discovered during pregnancy are handled similarly, except that radioisotope scanning is contraindicated. Fine-needle aspiration is safe during pregnancy, and thyroidectomy can be performed relatively safely during the second trimester. However, because thyroid cancer is relatively indolent, it may be wise to defer definitive diagnosis and treatment until the postpartum period in patients with indeterminate lesions on FNA.

Comprehension Questions

[15.1] Hyperthyroidism is generally characterized by:

    A. Normal TSH and elevated T_4/T_3 levels
    B. Low T_4/T_3 and elevated TSH levels
    C. Normal T_4/T_3 and elevated TSH levels
    D. Low TSH and elevated T_4/T_3 levels

[15.2] Primary hypothyroidism is generally treated using:

    A. Glucocorticoids
    B. Radioactive iodine treatment
    C. Levothyroxine (T_4)
    D. TSH injections

[15.3] During the first trimester of pregnancy, thyroid cancer usually should be:

    A. Confirmed using radioisotope scanning
    B. Treated with immediate thyroidectomy
    C. Followed until after delivery of child
    D. Treated with radioactive iodine ablation

[15.4] When the diagnosis of primary hypothyroidism is made in a patient with a normal examination, which of the following tests should be performed?

    A. Thyroid ultrasound
    B. Fine-needle aspiration
    C. Nuclear medicine thyroid scan
    D. No further testing is required

Answers

[15.1] **D.** Most cases of hyperthyroidism will result in a suppressed level of TSH and elevated T_4/T_3 levels. An exception to this would be a secondary hyperthyroid state, such as with a pituitary tumor that secretes TSH, resulting in both a high TSH level and high serum hormone levels (caused by overstimulation of the thyroid gland).

[15.2] **C.** Most cases of hypothyroidism are treated with thyroxine given orally. T_4 given in pill form will convert to the more metabolically active T_3.

[15.3] **C.** Thyroid cancer detected during pregnancy can usually be observed until after the pregnancy is complete. If needed, thyroid surgery can be performed safely in the second and third trimesters. The use of radioactive iodine is contraindicated in pregnancy.

[15.4] **D.** No further testing is need in the setting of primary hypothyroidism with a normal examination. Treatment can be instituted with thyroxine supplementation.

CLINICAL PEARLS

❖ The most common forms of both hyper- and hypothyroidism are autoimmune: Graves disease causing hyperthyroidism and Hashimoto thyroiditis causing hypothyroidism.

❖ Hyperfunctioning ("hot") thyroid nodules are rarely malignant. Hypofunctioning ("cold") nodules >1 cm in diameter should be biopsied.

❖ Thyroid disease is more common in women than men.

REFERENCES

Davis A, Shahla N. A practical guide to thyroid disease in women. Female patient (Primary care ed). 2005;30(9):38–47.

Rakel RE. Essentials of family practice. Philadelphia: WB Saunders, 1993.

Singer PA, Cooper DS, Levy EG, et al: Treatment guidelines for patients with hyperthyroidism and hypothyroidism. JAMA 1995;273:808.

South-Paul JE, Matheny SC, Lewis EL (eds.). Current diagnosis and treatment in family medicine. New York: McGraw-Hill, 2004.

A 25-year-old gravida$_2$, para$_1$ woman at 39 weeks estimated gestational age presents to the labor and delivery triage unit stating that her "bag of water has broken." She reports having had a large gush of clear fluid followed by a constant leakage of fluid from her vagina. She subsequently started having uterine contractions approximately every 4 minutes. She has had an uncomplicated prenatal course with good prenatal care since 8 weeks' gestation. Her prenatal records are available for review in the triage unit. Her first pregnancy resulted in the full-term delivery of a 7 lb 8 oz, healthy boy.

In the triage unit, she is placed on an external fetal monitor. Her blood pressure is 110/70 mm Hg, her pulse is 90 beats/min, and her temperature is 98.7°F. Her general examination is normal. Her abdomen is gravid, with a fundal height of 38 cm. The fetus has a cephalic presentation by Leopold maneuvers and an estimated fetal weight of 8 lb.

◆ **What signs and tests could confirm the presence of rupture of membranes?**

◆ **On the fetal monitoring strip shown (Fig. 16–1), what is the approximate baseline fetal heart rate? How often is she having uterine contractions?**

◆ **Her prenatal records reveal that she had a positive group B streptococcus (GBS) vaginal culture at 36 weeks' gestation. What therapy should be instituted at this time?**

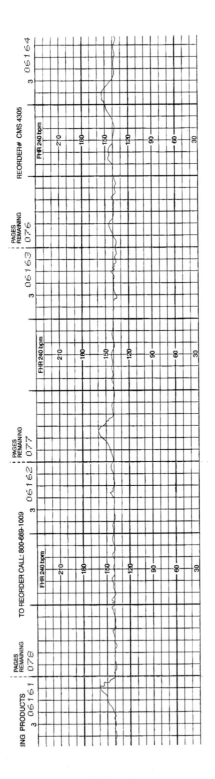
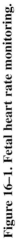

Figure 16–1. Fetal heart rate monitoring.

ANSWERS TO CASE 16: Labor and Delivery

Summary: A 25-year-old pregnant woman at term presents with the spontaneous rupture of membranes and subsequent uterine contractions, signaling the onset of labor.

 Signs that could confirm the rupture of membranes: visualization of amniotic fluid leaking from the cervix; the presence of pooling of amniotic fluid in the posterior vaginal fornix; demonstration of a pH above 6.5 in fluid collected from the vagina using Nitrazine paper; or visualization of "ferning" on a sample of fluid on an air-dried microscope slide

Baseline fetal heart rate: 140 beats/min; **Contraction interval:** approximately every 3 minutes

Recommended antibiotic prophylaxis for GBS colonization during labor: penicillin 5 million units IV loading dose followed by 2.5 million units IV every 4 hours; alternative treatments include IV ampicillin, cephalothin, erythromycin, clindamycin, and vancomycin.

Analysis

Objectives

1. Know the definition of labor, including the three stages of labor, and know the normal progression of labor in nulliparous and multiparous women.
2. Understand the types of fetal monitoring that are routinely performed during labor and how monitoring correlates with the physiologic processes occurring during labor.
3. Be familiar with the abnormal progression of labor and some of the interventions that can be made to address these problems.

Considerations

This woman arrives at the labor and delivery triage unit in need of evaluation for the possibility that she is in labor and that she has ruptured her membranes (broken her bag of water). The accurate and appropriate diagnosis of labor is extremely important in obstetrical care. Incorrectly diagnosing a woman as being in labor may result in unnecessary interventions, whereas not diagnosing labor may result in complications or delivery occurring without access to appropriate personnel and facilities. Furthermore, the diagnosis of rupture of membranes is critical for several reasons. First, especially at term, the spontaneous rupture of membranes may signify the impending onset of labor. Second, if the presenting part is not well applied in the pelvis, prolapse of the umbilical

cord with resultant compression of the cord and disruption of the oxygen supply to the fetus may occur. Finally, the prolonged rupture of membranes, especially after 24 hours or longer, may predispose to the development of infection.

The physician also must promptly make assessments of both maternal and
fetal well-being. A careful history and physical examination should be performed. When available, prenatal records should be reviewed to evaluate for
any problems during this, or previous, pregnancies and to confirm the gestational age of the pregnancy. In this case, the presence of GBS colonization
requires the institution of appropriate antibiotic prophylaxis to reduce the risk
of fetal infection with GBS, a common cause of neonatal morbidity and mortality. In GBS-colonized women, the recommended antibiotic prophylaxis is IV
penicillin. When this is not available, ampicillin is often substituted. In penicillin-
allergic women, cephalothin, erythromycin, clindamycin, or vancomycin can be
used. Fetal well-being is monitored most commonly using external, electronic
fetal-monitoring equipment, although other options are available. With this
equipment, the baseline fetal heart rate, heart rate variability, accelerations and
decelerations, along with the presence and frequency of uterine contractions,
may be evaluated. Determination of the presentation of the fetus (cephalic,
breech, or shoulder [i.e., transverse lie]) is also critical, as this may play a significant role in the determination of route of delivery (vaginal or cesarean).

APPROACH TO LABOR AND DELIVERY

Definitions

Fetal lie: The relationship of the long axis of the fetus to the long axis of
the mother; either longitudinal or transverse.

Fetal presentation: The part of the fetus that is either foremost in the birth
canal or in closest proximity to the birth canal.

Labor: Regular uterine contractions that lead to the effacement and dilation of the cervix.

Premature rupture of membranes: Rupture of the fetal membranes prior
to the onset of labor.

Clinical Approach

Labor usually begins spontaneously and occurs normally within 2 weeks of
the estimated date of confinement (280 days after the first day of the last menstrual period). The onset of labor more than 4 weeks before the estimated date
of confinement (EDC) is considered preterm labor. If labor has not started
spontaneously by 2 weeks after the EDC, the pregnancy is considered post-
term. Labor is typically divided into 3 stages. The **first stage of labor is from
the onset of labor until the cervix is completely dilated.** This stage can further be divided into a latent phase and an active phase. During the latent phase

of labor, the contractions become stronger, longer lasting, and more coordinated. The active phase of labor, which usually starts at 3–4 cm of cervical dilation, is when the rate of cervical dilation is at its maximum. Contractions are usually strong and regular. In active labor in a woman without an epidural, the minimum expected rates of cervical dilation are 1.2 cm per hour for a nulliparous woman and 1.5 cm per hour for a parous woman. The **second stage of labor is from complete cervical dilation (10 cm) until the delivery of the fetus.** The combination of the force of the uterine contractions and the pushing efforts of the mother results in the delivery of the baby. A normal second stage lasts less than 2 hours in a nulliparous patient and less than 1 hour in a parous patient. The presence of epidural anesthesia can prolong these times by up to 1 hour. The **third stage of labor begins after the delivery of the baby and ends with the delivery of the placenta and membranes.** The third stage is typically short and is considered prolonged if it lasts longer than 30 minutes.

The progress of labor usually depends upon the **"3 Ps."** The **Power** is the strength of the uterine contractions during the active phase of labor and of the maternal pushing efforts during the second stage of labor. The power of the contractions can be assessed subjectively by an examiner palpating the uterus during a contraction or objectively by placing an intrauterine pressure catheter, which directly measures pressure within the uterine cavity. The **Passenger** is the fetus. Its size, lie presentation, and position within the birth canal all play a role in the progression of labor and rate of fetal descent. Finally, the shape and size of the **Pelvis** can result in delay or failure of descent of the fetus because of the relative disproportion between the fetal and pelvic sizes.

The diagnosis of active labor is an indication for admission to the birthing unit for labor management and monitoring. The presence of ruptured membranes is also an indication for admission. The rupture of membranes can be confirmed by a careful vaginal examination performed with a sterile speculum and gloves. The visualization of fluid leaking from the cervical os, either spontaneously or with the patient performing a Valsalva maneuver, and the presence of amniotic fluid pooling in the posterior vaginal fornix are confirmatory. The detection of fluid in the vagina with a pH >6.5 is consistent with amniotic fluid, as normal vaginal secretions typically have a pH <5.5. Using a sterile applicator to sample vaginal fluid and applying it to Nitrazine paper can make this determination. The presence of semen, blood, or bacterial vaginosis can cause elevated pH in vaginal secretions and a false-positive Nitrazine test. The visualization of ferning of vaginal fluid under microscopic magnification of an air-dried sample also suggests the presence of amniotic fluid.

When the pregnant patient is admitted to the labor and delivery unit, **fetal well-being is assessed by either continuous or intermittent fetal heart rate monitoring.** Continuous external fetal heart rate monitoring is the more commonly used procedure in the United States. A Doppler ultrasound device is used to continuously trace the fetal heart rate. Continuous monitoring can also be accomplished using an internal device, by attaching an electrode to the fetal scalp that directly measures and amplifies fetal cardiac electrical activity. This procedure requires that the membranes are ruptured. With either of these two techniques, a continuous graphic recording of the fetal heart rate is recorded. Alternatively, intermittent auscultation using a stethoscope or handheld Doppler can be performed. The American College of Obstetricians and Gynecologists (ACOG) recommends that, in intermittent auscultation of low-risk pregnancies, the fetal heart should be monitored after a contraction at least every 30 minutes during the first stage of labor and every 15 minutes in the second stage. In at-risk pregnancies, the monitoring frequency is increased to at least every 15 minutes during the first stage and to every 5 minutes in the second stage.

Important considerations in interpreting fetal heart rate data are the **baseline heart rate, variability,** and **periodic heart rate changes.** The baseline heart rate is the approximate average heart rate during a 10-minute tracing. A baseline heart rate of 110–160 beats/min is considered normal, less than 110 beats/min is considered to be bradycardia, and greater than 160 beats/min is considered to be tachycardia. Fetal bradycardia may occur with maternal hypothermia, certain medications given to the mother, or congenital heart block, or may be a sign of significant fetal distress. Bradycardia may also be a normal variant. The most common cause of fetal tachycardia is maternal fever. Other common causes include medications and fetal arrhythmias.

Variability is regulated by the balance of sympathetic and parasympathetic control of the sinoatrial node. **Short-term (or beat-to-beat) variability** is the change in fetal heart rate from one beat to the next and can only be accurately determined when an internal scalp electrode is placed. Normal short-term variability is 6–25 beats/min. **Long-term variability** is the waviness of the baseline heart rate over 1 minute, with normal oscillations occurring at a rate of 3 to 5 cycles per minute. As variability is largely a manifestation of the autonomic nervous system, anything that affects nervous system functioning can affect it. Common causes of decreased variability are fetal sleep cycles, CNS depressant drugs (such as narcotic analgesics) given to the mother, congenital neurologic abnormalities, and prematurity. Fetal acidemia secondary to hypoxemia can impair CNS function and reduce variability. The presence of normal variability makes fetal acidemia unlikely.

Periodic heart rate changes are the **accelerations** and **decelerations** from the baseline heart rate that occur, often related to uterine contractions. An acceleration is an increase in the fetal heart rate of ≥15 beats/min for ≥15 seconds and is a reassuring finding. The presence of accelerations, whether occurring spontaneously or in response to contractions, fetal movement or stimulation of the fetus (either scalp stimulation during a cervical examination or vibroacoustic stimulation using an artificial larynx) virtually ensures that the fetal arterial pH is greater than 7.2. Decelerations are generally defined as **early, late,** or **variable** based on the timing of the deceleration in relation to a contraction. An **early deceleration** coincides with a contraction in onset of the fetal heart rate decline and return to the baseline. Early decelerations are thought to be a result of increased vagal tone caused by compression of the fetal head and are not associated with fetal hypoxia or acidemia. A **late deceleration** is a gradual reduction in the fetal heart rate that starts at or after the peak of a contraction and has a gradual return to the baseline. Late decelerations are a manifestation of uteroplacental insufficiency and can be caused by numerous circumstances. Common among these are maternal hypotension, as is often seen with epidural anesthesia and uterine hyperstimulation caused by oxytocin administration. Conditions that impair placental circulation, including maternal hypertension, diabetes, prolonged pregnancy, and placental abruption, often contribute to late decelerations. A **variable deceleration** is an abrupt decrease in fetal heart rate, usually followed by an abrupt return to baseline, that occurs variably in its timing, relative to a contraction. Variable decelerations are the most common types of decelerations seen during fetal heart monitoring and are considered to be due to umbilical cord compression during contractions. Variable decelerations, particularly when there is also the presence of normal variability and accelerations, are usually not associated with fetal hypoxemia.

Current fetal monitoring equipment also allows for contraction monitoring along with the fetal heart rate assessment. An external tocodynamometer is most commonly used. It allows for evaluation of the presence and timing of contractions but does not measure the strength of the contractions. To assess the strength of contractions, an internal intrauterine pressure catheter (IUPC) can be placed. Like the fetal scalp electrode, this requires the presence of ruptured membranes. An IUPC can be useful when the first stage of labor is not progressing at an expected rate, as the frequency and power of contractions can be directly measured. Contractions that are inadequate in frequency or power may be augmented with an oxytocic agent. Intravenous oxytocin is the drug of choice, as it is effective, inexpensive, and most practitioners are familiar with its usage. Oxytocin has a short half-life, which allows it to be given by continuous infusion and allows for the rapid cessation of its activity when it is discontinued. Labor augmentation with oxytocin can cause uterine hyperstimulation, defined as the presence of 6 or more contractions in a 10-minute period that causes nonreassuring fetal heart rate abnormalities (such as late decelerations). This would be managed by reduction in dose or discontinuation of the oxytocin, repositioning of the patient, and providing oxygen via face mask to the mother.

During labor, the fetal head descends through the birth canal and undergoes four **cardinal movements.** During initial descent, the head undergoes **flexion,** bringing the fetal chin to the chest. As descent progresses **internal rotation** occurs, causing the fetal occiput to move anteriorly towards the maternal symphysis pubis. As the head approaches the vulva it undergoes **extension,** to allow the head to pass below the symphysis pubis and through the upward-directed vaginal outlet. Further extension leads to the delivery of the head, which then restitutes via **external rotation** to face either to the maternal right or left side. This corresponds with rotation of the fetal body, aligning one shoulder anteriorly below the symphysis pubis and the other posterior towards the sacrum. Maternal pushing, along with gentle downward traction on the fetal head, will deliver the anterior shoulder, and upward traction similarly delivers the posterior shoulder. Delivery of the remainder of the body will quickly follow. Occasionally, the anterior shoulder will not readily pass below the pubic symphysis. This is called a **shoulder dystocia** and is an obstetrical emergency, requiring a coordinated effort by the entire medical team to reduce the dystocia. Maneuvers, including hyperflexion of the hips (McRoberts maneuver), suprapubic pressure, cutting an episiotomy, or rotation of the fetal body in the vaginal canal, are attempted and are usually successful.

Of deliveries in the United States, 20% or more are accomplished via cesarean delivery. The most common indications are a history of prior cesarean delivery, arrest of labor or descent, fetal distress necessitating immediate delivery, and breech presentation. Operative vaginal delivery can be performed using either forceps or vacuum assistance. These can only be used when the cervix is completely dilated, membranes are ruptured, the presenting part is the vertex of the scalp, and there is no disproportion between the size of the fetal head and maternal pelvis. If any of these conditions are not met and delivery must be accomplished urgently, a cesarean delivery is indicated.

Comprehension Questions

[16.1] A 21-year-old gravida$_1$ woman is admitted to the labor unit with spontaneous rupture of membranes. On initial examination, her cervix is 5 cm dilated. Four hours later, her cervix remains unchanged. Which of the following is the most likely diagnosis?

A. Prolonged latent phase
B. Arrest of active phase
C. Arrest of descent
D. Prolonged third stage of labor

[16.2] Which of the following are thought to be a result of compression of the fetal head?

A. Early decelerations
B. Variable decelerations
C. Late decelerations
D. Sinusoidal heart rate pattern

[16.3] A pregnant woman with an estimated gestational age of 34 weeks presents to the labor triage unit with a clear vaginal discharge. On sterile speculum examination you see a pool of watery fluid in the vagina. Microscopic examination reveals "ferning." Which of the following is the most likely diagnosis?

A. Urinary incontinency
B. Rupture of membranes
C. Bacterial vaginosis
D. *Candida* vaginitis

Answers

[16.1] **B.** The cervical dilation beyond 4 cm means active phase. No cervical change for 2 hours is defined as arrest of active phase.

[16.2] **A.** Early decelerations are thought to be caused by fetal head compression. Variable decelerations are caused by cord compression and late decelerations by uteroplacental insufficiency.

[16.3] **B.** A pool of clear fluid with ferning noted on an air-dried microscopic slide is diagnostic of rupture of fetal membranes. In this case, as she is 34 weeks' gestation, it represents preterm rupture of membranes.

CLINICAL PEARLS

❖ The presence of accelerations on a fetal heart tracing is very reassuring and consistent with a fetal pH of ≥7.2.

❖ The use of universal, prenatal screening for group B streptococcus and provision of intrapartum antibiotics to women who are colonized can reduce the risk of GBS disease in infants by approximately 50%.

❖ Fetal heart rate tracings must be interpreted within the overall clinical situation. Reduction in variability shortly after giving a narcotic pain medication may represent fetal sleep cycle; reduction in variability along with repetitive late decelerations may be an ominous sign of fetal distress.

REFERENCES

Cunningham FG, Gant NF, Leveno KJ, Gilstrap LC, Hauth JC, Wenstrom KD. Williams obstetrics. 21st ed. New York: McGraw-Hill, 2001.

Garite TJ. Intrapartum fetal evaluation. In: Gabbe SG, Niebyl JR, Simpson JL (eds). Obstetrics: normal and problem pregnancies. 4th ed. New York: Churchill Livingstone, 2002, pp. 395–427.

Rouse DJ, St. John E. Normal labor, delivery, newborn care, and puerperium. In: Scott JR, Gibbs RS, Karlan BY, Haney AF (eds). Danforth's obstetrics and gynecology. Philadelphia: Lippincott, Williams & Wilkins, 2003, pp. 36–57.

A 58-year-old female presents to your office for follow-up of an emergency department visit. She was seen 1 week earlier in the emergency department for abdominal pain and was diagnosed with nephrolithiasis. Ultimately, she was sent home with pain medications and given instructions to strain her urine for stones and to follow up with her primary care physician. Today, she is asymptomatic. She takes no medications on a regular basis. Her family history is significant only for a father with high blood pressure. She had several routine labs drawn in the emergency department, copies of which she brings with her. Upon your review of the labs, you note the following (normal values are in parenthesis): sodium 142 mEq/L (135–145); potassium 4.0 mEq/L (3.5–5.0); chloride 104 mg/dL (95–105); bicarbonate 28 mEq/L (20–29); blood urea nitrogen (BUN) 20 mg/dL (7–20); creatinine 0.9 mg/dL (0.8–1.4); **calcium 12.5 mg/dL (8.5–10.2);** albumin 4.2 g/dL (3.4–5.4). The complete blood count (CBC) was within normal limits.

The renal calculus was detected by helical CT scanning without contrast and was midureter on the right.

Your patient has brought with her the stone that she has strained from the urine. Upon questioning, you learn that she has had multiple episodes of "kidney stones" in the past 2 years. You send the stone to the lab for analysis and order a repeat serum calcium level. The results show that the stone is made of calcium oxalate the serum calcium is still elevated at 11.9 mg/dL.

◆ **What is your diagnosis?**

◆ **What is the most likely cause?**

◆ **What is the next step?**

ANSWERS TO CASE 17: Calcium Disorders

Summary: This is a 58-year-old female with a history of recurrent nephrolithiasis, presenting for follow-up and found to have calcium oxalate stones. She had an initial serum calcium level that was elevated, as was the repeat serum calcium 1 week later. At the time of her follow up, she was completely asymptomatic. She takes no medications, and has a family history only significant for hypertension.

◆ **Diagnosis:** Hypercalcemia and recurrent nephrolithiasis

◆ **Most likely cause:** Hyperparathyroidism

◆ **Next step:** Further laboratory work-up, including serum parathyroid hormone (PTH)

Analysis

Objectives

1. Be familiar with the differential diagnosis of hypercalcemia, especially the most common etiologies.
2. Understand the work-up of hypercalcemia.
3. Learn the basics of calcium regulation.
4. Learn about management options of hyperparathyroidism.

Considerations

This patient illustrates one common presentation of hypercalcemia. Many times, patients with hypercalcemia are asymptomatic and an elevated calcium level is found unexpectedly on routine labs. The diagnostic work-up begins with a careful review of the patient's history, as clues to its etiology may often be elicited here. The diagnostic work-up is designed to distinguish parathyroid dysfunction from other etiologies so that optimal treatment and management can be pursued.

Discussion

Pathophysiology of Calcium Homeostasis

Before discussing the differential diagnosis of hypercalcemia, it is essential to review the basic mechanism by which normal calcium levels are maintained in the body. **Most of the calcium in the body is found in the skeleton** (approximately 98%). The remaining calcium is found in circulation. Of this remaining 2%, about half is bound to albumin and other proteins, and half is "free," or ionized. It is the ionized calcium that has physiologic effects. Because the serum calcium is partially bound to albumin, abnormally low serum albumin levels will affect the measurement of calcium, thus causing a misinterpretation of an abnormal calcium level. With patients found to have a concomitant hypoalbuminemia, the ionized calcium can be measured directly. However, there is a useful formula that can correct for this error. A "corrected" serum calcium is provided by the formula:

"corrected" serum calcium = [(normal albumin) − (patient's albumin level)]
× [0.8 × (serum calcium)]

PTH, calcitonin, and 1,25-dihydroxyvitamin D_3 (calcitriol) are responsible for regulating calcium levels and maintaining calcium homeostasis. **An increase of calcium resorption from bone, an increase in exogenous calcium from the gastrointestinal tract, or decreased renal excretion will cause hypercalcemia.** When calcium levels increase, calcitonin, produced by the thyroid parafollicular cells, attempts to lower calcium levels through renal excretion of calcium and by opposing osteoclast activation. When calcium is excreted through this pathway, phosphate is also excreted. Conversely, low levels of circulating calcium normally result in PTH secretion. This promotes osteoclast activation, which mobilizes calcium from bone and effects calcium resorption at the kidneys, thereby retaining circulating calcium. PTH also increases calcitriol levels, which act at the gastrointestinal tract to promote both calcium and phosphate absorption.

Etiology of Hypercalcemia

Any process that increases gastrointestinal calcium absorption, decreases renal excretion, or activates osteoclastic activity will raise serum calcium levels. If this occurs beyond the normal bounds of maintaining calcium homeostasis, hypercalcemia will occur. **The most common cause of hypercalcemia in the ambulatory patient is hyperparathyroidism.** Cancer ranks as the second leading cause, and is a common etiology among hospitalized patients with hypercalcemia. Given the many etiologies that exist, it is useful to categorize them (Table 17–1).

Clinical Manifestations of Hypercalcemia

Mild hypercalcemia frequently is asymptomatic. As calcium levels increase, physical manifestations may become apparent. The classic mnemonic, "stones, bones, psychic groans, and abdominal moans" is useful to categorize the constellation of physical symptoms associated with hypercalcemia (Table 17–2). Other clinical manifestations include the cardiac sequelae of shortening QT interval and arrhythmias.

APPROACH TO HYPERCALCEMIA

The diagnostic approach to hypercalcemia begins with a careful history, including the manifestations of elevated calcium levels. When the aforementioned etiologies are taken into consideration, it becomes clear that the history should include family history of calcium disorders, such as renal stones or malignancy. The patient's risk factors for malignancy, such as smoking, should be investigated. A careful review of medications should also take place, to include not only prescription medications but also over-the-counter supplements. At this

Table 17–1
COMMON CAUSES OF HYPERCALCEMIA

Increased Bone Resorption	*Specific Example*	*Pathophysiology*
Primary hyperparathyroidism	Sporadic or familial; Multiple endocrine neoplasia (types I and II)	
Malignancy	Solid tumors of lung; squamous carcinoma of head and neck; renal carcinoma	Tumor secretion of PTH-rP
	Breast cancer; multiple myeloma; prostate cancer	Direct osteolysis
Hypervitaminosis A (vitamin A intoxication)	Includes both vitamin A and its analogs (used to treat acne)	Increased bone resorption
Immobilization	Less common than above causes	Increased risk when underlying disorder of high bone turnover (e.g., Paget disease)
Increased Calcium Absorption		
Hypervitaminosis D (vitamin D intoxication)		Increased calcitriol level leads to increased GI absorption of calcium and phosphate
Granulomatous disease	Tuberculosis; sarcoidosis; Hodgkin disease	Increase extrarenal conversion of 25-hydroxyvitamin D_3 to calcitriol
Milk alkali syndrome		Excessive intake of calcium-containing antacids
Miscellaneous		
Medications	Thiazide diuretics Lithium	Reduced urinary excretion of calcium Increased PTH secretion
Rhabdomyolysis		Calcium released from injured muscle
Adrenal insufficiency		Increased bone resorption and increased protein binding of calcium
Thyrotoxicosis (usually mild hypercalcemia)		Increased bone resorption

Table 17–2
PHYSICAL MANIFESTATIONS OF HYPERCALCEMIA

SYMPTOM/SIGNS	
Stones	Renal calculi
Bones	Bone pain, including arthritis and osteoporosis
Psychic groans	Poor concentration, weakness, fatigue, stupor, coma
Abdominal moans	Abdominal pain, constipation, nausea, vomiting, pancreatitis

point, if the hypercalcemia is mild and the patient asymptomatic, it is acceptable to stop the suspect medication and repeat the serum calcium level.

The next step, if a causative medication is not found, is to measure a serum intact PTH level. This level will either be suppressed, normal, or elevated. As with many endocrine disorders, **it is useful not to think of normal or abnormal values; rather, one should understand what is appropriate for a given situation.** For example, in normal subjects, an increased calcium load will normally depress the PTH hormone level, thus a low PTH level in this situation is *normal,* or appropriately suppressed. If a patient has an elevated calcium level and the PTH is "normal," it is said to be inappropriately normal, because in the face of hypercalcemia it should be low, or suppressed.

If our patient with hypercalcemia has a normal or elevated PTH level, then the normal feedback loop is not responding. In this situation, the pituitary is producing PTH without check, which, in turn, is elevating the calcium level. This is hyperparathyroidism. Primary hyperparathyroidism occurs when the parathyroid gland overproduces PTH and does not respond to the negative feedback of elevated calcium levels. **The vast majority of primary hyperparathyroidism is caused by an adenoma (benign tumor) of one of the four parathyroid glands.**

Secondary hyperparathyroidism occurs as the parathyroid glands overproduce PTH to respond to low serum calcium levels. This may occur as a response to low dietary calcium intake or a deficiency of vitamin D. Tertiary hyperparathyroidism occurs in patients who have renal failure. Patients in renal failure usually present with *hypo*calcemia, hyperphosphatemia, and low vitamin D levels. If this is untreated, it leads to hyperplasia of the parathyroid glands, an increased PTH secretion, and subsequent hypercalcemia.

There is a condition that can produce inappropriately high PTH levels unrelated to the parathyroid production. This is familial hypocalciuric hypercalcemia (FHH), a genetic disorder related to a defect in a gene that codes for a calcium-sensing receptor. Consequently, simply measuring PTH alone may confound this diagnosis, which may be mistaken for primary hyperparathyroidism.

To distinguish these entities, a 24-hour urinary calcium level is obtained. In hyperparathyroidism, the kidneys spill calcium into the urine at a normal or elevated level. With FHH the urinary calcium level is low.

A PTH level that is low with an elevated serum calcium suggests that the parathyroid gland is responding appropriately to the high calcium environment. The etiology in this scenario must be some process that causes calcium to be released from bone or calcium to be absorbed from the gut despite the suppressed PTH. This is seen when tumors produce a hormone that mimics the active site of the PTH molecule, but that have no counter regulatory mechanism for suppression when calcium levels rise. This molecule is called parathyroid hormone-related peptide (PTH-rP). PTH-rP is produced by lung cancers, squamous cell cancers of the head and neck, and renal cell cancer. PTH-rP effects osteoclastic bone resorption, increases calcitriol, and promotes calcium resorption from the kidneys, resulting in increased levels of serum calcium. The continued production of PTH-rP effectively takes the parathyroid gland out of the loop in calcium homeostasis. Because cancer is a common etiology for hypercalcemia, the **search for malignancy is paramount at this step in diagnosis, before other, less common, disorders are considered.**

If a malignancy is not found, other etiologies must be considered. These fall into the category of endocrine disorders other than parathyroid and include hyperthyroidism, adrenal insufficiency, and acromegaly. The work-up thus includes thyroid-stimulating hormone (TSH), a cortisol level, and a pituitary imaging study, respectively.

Treatment of Hypercalcemia

The **treatment of hypercalcemia is directed at the underlying disorder.** Patients with mild hypercalcemia may be treated with preventative measures aimed at avoiding aggravating factors. These measures include adequate hydration (dehydration aggravates nephrolithiasis), avoiding thiazide diuretics or other offending medications, encouraging physical activity, and avoiding prolonged inactivity. Other interventions for mild hypercalcemia are disease specific.

For the treatment of primary hyperparathyroidism, surgical parathyroidectomy is the definitive treatment. Surgery is appropriate for patients with symptomatic hyperparathyroidism. Surgery may be an option for selected asymptomatic patients, including those who have developed osteoporosis or renal insufficiency, who have markedly elevated calcium levels, or who are younger than age 50 years.

Comprehension Questions

[17.1] A 60-year-old male comes into your office with the complaint of fatigue and constipation. He has had no dietary changes recently. A history reveals that he has hypertension, treated with medications, and an inguinal hernia that was repaired 10 years earlier without complications. The examination was nonspecific. You decide to obtain an electrolyte panel and find that the calcium level is elevated at 11.5 mg/dL (normal 8.5–10.2). Other labs were normal. What is the next step?

A. Consult vascular surgery for placement of a dialysis catheter and schedule for dialysis.
B. Advise the patient to drink plenty of fluids and repeat the labs in 1 month.
C. Explore the patient's hypertension, including what medications he takes.
D. Obtain a chest x-ray, looking for possible malignancy

[17.2] A 48-year-old male presents for follow-up of an elevated calcium level of 12.3 mg/dL found on routine screening labs at his last well-male visit. He takes no medications other than an occasional antihistamine for allergies. He recently started smoking a half-pack of cigarettes per day. He was prompted to attend to his well-male visit by his wife who claims that he has become forgetful, has a decreased appetite, and has had a 10-pound weight loss over the past 2 months. As part of his follow-up labs, you obtain a serum PTH, which comes back within the normal range. What is the next step in diagnosis?

A. Chest x-ray
B. Repeat calcium after hydration
C. Measurement of PTH-rP levels
D. Measurement of urinary calcium excretion

[17.3] You obtain follow-up labs for a hypercalcemic patient and find that the PTH level is suppressed. There are no suspect medications. You suspect lung cancer based on a 30 pack-year smoking history, but the chest x-ray is normal. What do you do next?

A. Continue a malignancy work-up.
B. Check TSH, as a thyroid disorder may be the cause.
C. Refer the patient to an endocrinologist, as hypercalciuric hypercalcemia is an exceedingly rare genetic cause of an elevated calcium that requires specialist care.
D. Measure urinary calcium excretion.

Answers

[17.1] **C.** When presented with a patient who has elevated calcium levels, the first step is to determine if there are any causative medications. Hydrochlorothiazide is a commonly used antihypertensive medication that may contribute to elevated calcium levels (thiazide diuretic).

[17.2] **D.** This patient has symptomatic hypercalcemia. He has an inappropriately normal PTH level, which should be suppressed with this degree of hypercalcemia. The next step is to measure a 24-hour urinary calcium excretion to determine if this condition represents primary hyperparathyroidism (most common) or familial hypocalciuric hypercalcemia (rare).

[17.3] **A.** In a hypercalcemic patient, a suppressed PTH first should be considered a sign of malignancy until proven otherwise. A chest x-ray is insufficient to rule out malignancy, as there are other malignancies that can cause hypercalcemia, mediated either by way of PTH-rP or through direct osteoclastic bone resorption. Multiple myeloma, granulomatous disease such as tuberculosis, sarcoidosis, and Hodgkin lymphoma, breast cancer, and squamous cell cancers of the head and neck can cause an elevated calcium with an appropriately suppressed PTH.

CLINICAL PEARLS

❖ Be sure to question any patient with hypercalcemia regarding all medications—both prescription and over-the counter—as both megadose vitamins (A and D) and excessive use of calcium carbonate antacids may play a role.

❖ Most cases of primary hyperparathyroidism occur in postmenopausal women, who are often already at increased risk of osteoporosis. Be sure to check their bone density with a dual-energy x-ray absorptiometry (DEXA) scan.

❖ Hypercalcemia with a suppressed PTH should be considered malignancy until you can prove otherwise.

REFERENCES

Agus Z. Diagnostic approach to hypercalcemia. 2005. Available at:www.Uptodate.com.

Agus Z. Etiology of hypercalcemia. 2003. Available at: www.Uptodate.com.

Agus Z, Fuleihan G. Management of asymptomatic primary hyperparathyroidism. 2005. Available at: www.Uptodate.com.

Al Zarani A, Levine MA. Primary hyperparathyroidism. Lancet 1997;349: 1233–1238.

Carroll M, Schade D. A practical approach to hypercalcemia. Am Fam Physician 2003;67:1959–1966.

Taniegra ET. Hyperparathyroidism. Am Fam Physician 2004;69:333–340.

A 75-year-old white male presents for a health maintenance check-up. The patient has stable hypertension but has not seen a physician in more than 2 years. He denies any particular problems. He lives alone. He takes an aspirin a day and is compliant with his blood pressure medication (hydrochlorothiazide). His son fears that his father is either experiencing a stroke or getting Alzheimer disease because his father is having trouble with speech discrimination and understanding what family members are saying during social events. The son reported no noticeable weakness or gait impairment. On physical examination, the patient's blood pressure was 130/80 mm Hg. Examination of the ears showed no cerumen impaction and normal tympanic membranes. His general examination is normal. Laboratory studies, including thyroid-stimulating hormone (TSH), are normal.

◆ **What is the most likely diagnosis?**

◆ **What is the next step?**

ANSWERS TO CASE 18: Geriatric Health Maintenance

Summary: A 75-year-old man who presents with loss of speech discrimination and complains of difficulty understanding speech and conversation in noisy areas most likely has presbycusis. Presbycusis is age-related sensorineural hearing loss typically associated with both selective high-frequency loss and difficulty with speech discrimination. Physical examination of the ears in patients with presbycusis is normal.

◆ **Most likely diagnosis:** Presbycusis.

◆ **Next step:** Presbycusis is a diagnosis of exclusion. Hearing aids are underused in presbycusis but are potentially beneficial for most types of hearing loss, including sensorineural hearing loss. Consequently, referral to an audiologist for testing and consideration of amplification with a hearing aid may be an important next step.

Analysis

Objectives

1. To be familiar with geriatric health maintenance.
2. To describe the importance of geriatric screening.

APPROACH TO HEALTH MAINTENANCE IN THE ELDERLY

By the year 2030 the number of people ages 65 years and older is expected to double from what it was in 1999, increasing from 34 million to 69 million. Geriatric health maintenance provides screening and therapy with the goal of enhancing function and preserving health in the elderly. Screening is not indicated unless early therapy for the screened condition is more effective than late therapy or no therapy. **Preventive services for the elderly include as goals the optimization of quality of life, satisfaction with life, and maintenance of independence and productivity.** Most recommendations for patients older than age 65 years overlap recommendations for the general adult population. Certain categories are unique to older patients, including sensory perception and accident. The primary care physician can perform effective health screening using simple and relatively easily administered assessment tools **(Fig. 18–1).**

Functional Assessment

Functional assessment gauges a patient's ability to manage tasks of self-care, household management, and mobility. Impairment in activities of daily living results in an increased risk of falls, hip fracture, depression, and institutionalization.

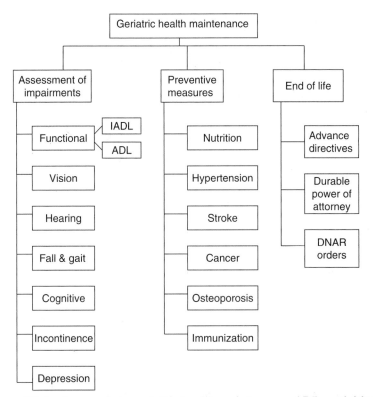

Figure 18–1. Approach to geriatric health maintenance. ADL, activities of daily living; DNAR, do not attempt resuscitation; IADL, instrumental activities of daily living.

An estimated **25% of patients older than age 65 years have impairments in their instrumental activities of daily living (IADL) or activities of daily living (ADL) (Table 18–1)** Persons who are unable to perform IADL independently are far more likely to have dementia than their independent counterparts.

Vision Screening

Visual impairment is an independent risk factor for falls, which has a significant impact on quality of life. Direct visual testing with a Snellen chart or Jaeger card is the most sensitive and specific approach to visual screening. Referring all older people for a complete eye examination has the advantages of improving the quality of the examination and allowing for cataract and glaucoma screening. The majority of conditions leading to vision loss in the elderly are presbyopia, macular degeneration, glaucoma, cataract, and diabetic retinopathy.

Table 18–1
INSTRUMENTAL ACTIVITIES OF DAILY LIVING (IADL)
AND ACTIVITIES OF DAILY LIVING (ADL)

IADL	ADL
Transportation	Bathing
Shopping	Dressing
Cooking	Eating
Using the telephone	Transferring from bed to chair
Managing money	Continence
Taking medications	Toileting
Housecleaning	
Laundry	

The incidence of presbyopia increases with age. Patients have difficulty focusing on near objects while their distant vision remains intact. **Age-related macular degeneration (AMD) is the leading cause of severe vision loss in the elders.** AMD is characterized by atrophy of cells in the central macular region of the retinal pigment epithelium, resulting in the loss of central vision. Glaucoma is characterized by a group of optic neuropathies that can occur in all ages. Although glaucoma is most often associated with elevated intraocular pressure, it is the optic neuropathy that defines the disease. Cataract is any opacification of the lens. Age-related, or senile, cataracts account for 90% of all cataracts. **Cataract disease is the most common cause of blindness worldwide.** Diabetic retinopathy is the leading cause of blindness in working-age adults in the United States. It is important to consider diabetic retinopathy in geriatric vision screening.

Hearing Screening

More than one-third of persons older than age 65 and half of those older than age 85 years have some hearing loss. This deficit is correlated with social isolation and depression. The whispered voice test has sensitivities and specificities ranging from 70% to 100%. The initial office screening for general hearing loss can be reliably performed with questionnaire such as the HHIE-S (Hearing Handicap Inventory for the Elderly). Limited office-based pure-tone audiometry is more accurate in identifying patients who would benefit from a more formal audiometry.

The majority of patients with hearing impairment will present with complaints unrelated to their sensory deficit. In a quiet examination room with face-to-face conversation, patients can overcome significant hearing loss and avoid detection from a physician. Family members are often more concerned about the hearing loss than the patient. **Common causes of geriatric hearing impairments are presbycusis, noise-induced hearing loss, cerumen impaction, otosclerosis, and central auditory processing disorder.** Presbycusis is age-related sensorineural hearing loss usually associated with both selective high-frequency loss and difficulty with speech discrimination. Presbycusis is the most common form of hearing loss in the elderly. Because it often goes unrecognized, exact prevalence data are lacking. Presbycusis is a diagnosis of exclusion. Complete deafness is not an expected end result of presbycusis. Noise-induced hearing loss is essentially a wear-and-tear phenomenon that can occur with either industrial or recreational noise exposure. Patients will typically present with tinnitus, difficulty with speech discrimination, and problems hearing background noise. Cerumen impaction in the external auditory canal is a common, frequently overlooked problem in the elderly, that may produce a transient, mild conductive hearing loss. It is estimated that 25–35% of institutionalized or hospitalized elderly are affected by impacted cerumen. Otosclerosis is an autosomal dominant disorder of the bones in the inner ear. It results in progressive conductive hearing loss with onset most commonly in the late 20s to the early 40s. Speech discrimination is typically preserved. Geriatric patients with hearing loss may have otosclerosis complicating their presentation. Central auditory processing disorder (CAPD) is the general term for conditions involving hearing impairment that results from CNS dysfunction. The patient with CAPD will have difficulty understanding spoken language, but may be able to hear sounds well.

Fall Assessment

Falls are the leading cause of nonfatal injuries in the elderly. The associated complications are the leading cause of death from injury in those older than age 65 years. Hip fractures are common precursors to functional impairment and nursing home placement. Approximately **30% of the noninstitutionalized elderly fall each year.** The annual incidence of falls approaches 50% in patients older than 80 years of age. Factors contributing to falls include age-related postural changes, alterations in visual ability, certain medications, and diseases affecting muscle strength and coordination. Every older person should be asked about falls, as many will not volunteer such information. Gait impairments commonly coexist with falls.

Cognitive Screening

The prevalence of dementia doubles every 5 years after age 60, so that by age 85 approximately 30–50% of individuals have some degree of impairment. Patients with mild or early dementia frequently remain undiagnosed because their social graces are retained. **The combination of the "clock draw" and the "three-item recall" is a rapid and fairly reliable office-based screening for dementia**. When patients fail either of these screening tests, further testing with the Folstein Mini-Mental State questionnaire should be performed.

Incontinence Screening

Incontinence in the elderly is common. Incontinence is estimated to affect 11–34% of elderly men and 17–55% of elderly women. Continence problems are frequently treatable, have major social and emotional consequences, but are often not raised by patients as a concern.

Depression Screening

Depressive symptoms are more common in the elderly despite major depressive disorder being slightly lower in prevalence when compared with younger populations. **Unlike dementia, depression is usually treatable.** Depression significantly increases morbidity and mortality, and is often overlooked by physicians. A simple two-question screen (*Have you felt down/depressed/hopeless in the last 2 weeks?* and *Have you felt little interest or pleasure in doing things?*) shows high sensitivity. Positive responses can be followed up with a Geriatric Depression Scale, a 30-question instrument that is sensitive, specific, and reliable for the diagnosis of depression in the elderly.

Nutrition Screening

Approximately 15% of older outpatients and half of the hospitalized elderly are malnourished. **A combination of serial weight measurements obtained in the office and inquiry about changing appetite are likely the most useful methods of assessing nutritional status in the elderly.** Adequate calcium intake for women is advised. Supplementation with a multivitamin formulated at about 100% daily value can decrease the prevalence of suboptimal vitamin status in older adults and improve their micronutrient status to levels associated with reduced risk for several chronic diseases. Malnutrition is common in nursing homes, and protein undernutrition has a prevalence of 17–56% in this setting. Protein undernutrition is associated with an increased risk of infections, anemia, orthostatic hypotension, and decubitus ulcers.

Hypertension Screening

Treatment of hypertension is of substantial benefit in the elderly. Heart disease and cerebrovascular disease are leading causes of death in the elderly. Treatment of hypertension has contributed to a reduction in mortality from both stroke and coronary artery disease. Lifestyle modifications are recommended for all hypertensive patients. Thiazides are the drugs of choice unless a comorbid condition makes another choice preferable.

Stroke Prevention

The incidence of stroke in older adults roughly doubles with each 10 years of age. The greatest risk factor is hypertension followed by atrial fibrillation.

Anticoagulation with warfarin reduces the risk of strokes in people with atrial fibrillation, but many elderly patients are not anticoagulated because of the fear of injuries from falls. In most instances, the benefits of anticoagulation are likely to outweigh the increased risk of fall-related bleeding, unless the patient has multiple falls, high-risk falls, or a very low risk of stroke.

Cancer Screening

Screening elderly men for prostate cancer is not routinely recommended, as it has not been definitively shown to prolong life and because of the risk of incontinence or erectile dysfunction caused by the treatments. An older woman should undergo annual mammography until her life expectancy falls below 5–10 years. Screening for colon cancer (either with colonoscopy every 10 years or with annual fecal occult testing plus flexible sigmoidoscopy every 5 years) can be stopped when a patient's life expectancy is less than 5–10 years.

Osteoporosis Screening

The prevalence of low bone mineral density in the elderly is high, with osteopenia found in 37% of postmenopausal women. Primary prevention of osteoporosis begins with identification of risk factors (older age, female gender, White or Asian race, low calcium intake, smoking, excessive alcohol use, and chronic glucocorticoid use). Calcium carbonate (500 mg three times daily) and vitamin D (400–800 IU/d) reduce the risk of osteoporotic fractures in both men and women. Bone mineral density testing using dual-energy x-ray absorptiometry (DEXA) of patients with multiple risk factors may uncover asymptomatic osteoporosis.

Immunizations

Individuals older than age 65 years should receive annual influenza vaccination. Similarly, persons older than age 65 should receive at least one pneumococcal immunization. A single booster dose of tetanus and diphtheria vaccine should be given at age 65 or older.

End of Life Issue

Advance Directives

Well-informed, competent adults have a right to refuse medical intervention, even if refusal is likely to result in death. To further patient autonomy, physicians are obligated to inform patients about the risks, benefits, alternatives, and expected outcomes of end-of-life medical interventions such as cardiopulmonary resuscitation, intubation and mechanical ventilation, vasopressor medication, hospitalization and ICU care, and artificial nutrition and hydration. **Advance directives are oral or written statements made by patients when they are competent that are intended to guide care should they become incompetent.** Advance directives allow patients to project their autonomy. Although oral statements about these matters are ethically binding, they are not legally binding in all states. Written advance directives are essential so as to give effect to the patient's wishes in these matters.

Durable Power of Attorney for Health Care (DPOA-HC)

A Durable Power of Attorney allows the patient to designate a surrogate decision maker. The responsibility of the surrogate is to provide "substituted judgment" to decide as the patient would, not as the surrogate wants. In the absence of a designated surrogate, physicians turn to family members or next of kin, under the assumption that they know the patient's wishes.

Do Not Attempt Resuscitation (DNAR) Orders

Physicians should encourage patients to express their preferences for the use of cardiopulmonary resuscitation (CPR). Despite the favorable portrayal of CPR in the media, **only approximately 15% of all patients who undergo CPR in the hospital survive to hospital discharge.** DNAR ("do not attempt resuscitation") is the preferred term over DNR ("do not resuscitate) to emphasize the low likelihood of successful resuscitation. In addition to mortality statistics, patients deciding about CPR preferences should also be informed about the possible consequences of surviving a CPR attempt. CPR may result in fractured ribs, lacerated internal organs, and neurologic disability. There is also a high likelihood of requiring other aggressive interventions if CPR is successful. For some patients at the end of life, decisions about CPR may not be about whether they will live but about how they will die.

Comprehension Questions

[18.1] Which of the following statements is most accurate?

A. The American Urological Association (AUA) and United States Preventive Services Task Force (USPSTF) recommend annual prostate cancer screening with digital rectal examination (DRE) and prostate-specific antigen (PSA).

B. All men older than age 50 years should have a PSA drawn each year, regardless of other health conditions.

C. Compared to DRE alone, the combination of DRE and PSA increases the sensitivity and specificity of prostate cancer screening.

D. Transrectal ultrasound offers the greatest sensitivity and specificity for detecting prostate cancer.

E. For healthy men older than age 70 years, the AUA discourages any prostate cancer screening.

[18.2] Regarding presbycusis, which of the following is true?

A. Sensorineural presbycusis does not respond to hearing aid use.
B. Presbycusis usually results in major depression.
C. Presbycusis usually results in loss of speech discrimination.
D. Presbycusis usually results in unilateral hearing loss.
E. Presbycusis usually results in low-frequency hearing loss.

[18.3] Which of the following statements is accurate?

A. Glaucoma is the leading cause of severe vision loss in older Americans.
B. Vitamin A deficiency is the most common cause of blindness worldwide.
C. Ninety percent of cataracts are age-related, or senile, cataracts.
D. Diabetic retinopathy is the leading cause of blindness worldwide.

Answers

[18.1] **C.** The combination of DRE and PSA is known to increase the sensitivity and specificity of prostate cancer detection. However, the benefit of routine use of rectal examination to detect prostate cancer is questionable.

[18.2] **C.** Up to one-third of persons older than age 65 years suffer from hearing loss. Presbycusis typically presents with symmetric high-frequency hearing loss. There is loss of speech discrimination, so that patients complain of difficulty understanding rapid speech, foreign accents, and conversation in noisy areas.

[18.3] **C.** The vast majority of cataracts are age related, although there are other causes. Cataracts are the leading cause of blindness worldwide. Diabetic retinopathy is the leading cause of blindness in working-age adults in the United States. Age-related macular degeneration is the most common cause of severe vision loss in the elderly.

CLINICAL PEARLS

❖ Protein undernutrition is associated with an increased risk of infections, anemia, orthostatic hypotension, and decubitus ulcers.

❖ Smoking is associated with osteoporosis.

❖ If "osteoporotic" fractures, such as vertebral compression fractures, occur in conjunction with osteopenia on x-ray, the diagnosis of osteoporosis is almost certain.

❖ Hearing loss, and sensory impairments in general, can be confused with cognitive impairment or an affective disorder.

❖ Presbyopia, macular degeneration, glaucoma, cataracts, and diabetic retinopathy account for the majority of conditions leading to vision loss in the elderly.

REFERENCES

Golding J. Geriatric health maintenance. April 2005. Available at: UpToDate website.
Johnston CB, Lyons WL. Geriatric medicine. In: Tierney LM, McPhee SJ, Papadakis MA (eds). Current medical diagnosis and treatment. New York: McGraw-Hill, 2003, pp. 41–44.
Rabow MW, Pantilat SZ. Care at the end of life. In: Tierney LM, McPhee SJ, Papadakis MA (eds). Current medical diagnosis and treatment. New York: McGraw-Hill, 2003, pp. 60–74.
Rosenfeld KE, Wenger NS, Kagawa-Singer M et al. End-of-Life decision making: a qualitative study of elderly individuals. J Gen Intern Med 2000;15:620.
State-specific advance directives forms. Available at: www.partnershipforcaring.org.
The American Geriatric Society. Available at: www.americangeriatrics.org.
Tulsky JA, Fischer, GS, Rose, MR et al. Opening the black box: how do physicians communicate about advance directives? Ann Intern Med 1998;129:441.
Williams PM, Williams A. Hearing and vision impairment in the elderly. In: South-Paul JE, Matheny SC, Lewis EL (eds). Current diagnosis and treatment. Family medicine. New York, NY: McGraw-Hill, 2004:573.

A 45-year-old male presents to the clinic with a cough productive of purulent sputum of 3 weeks' duration. He says that he had just gotten over a cold a few weeks prior to this episode. He occasionally has fevers and he coughs so much that he has chest pain. He reports having a mild sore throat and nasal congestion. He has no history of asthma or of any chronic lung diseases. He denies nausea, vomiting, diarrhea, and any recent travel. He denies any smoking history. On examination, his temperature is 98.6°F, his pulse is 96 beats/min, his blood pressure is 124/82 mm Hg, his respiratory rate is 18 breaths/min, and his oxygen saturation is 99% on room air. Head, ears, eyes, nose, and throat (HEENT) examination reveals no erythema of the posterior oropharynx, tonsillar exudates, uvular deviations, or significant tonsillar swelling. Neck examination is negative. The chest examination yields occasional wheezes.

◆ **What is the most likely diagnosis?**

◆ **What is your next step?**

◆ **What are some common noninfectious causes of cough?**

ANSWERS TO CASE 19: Acute Bronchitis

Summary: A 45-year-old male, who has no history of lung disease and does not smoke, with 3 weeks of productive cough following an upper respiratory infection.

◆ **Likely diagnosis:** Acute bronchitis

◆ **Next step:** Bronchodilators, analgesics, antitussives; antibiotics have not been consistently shown to be beneficial. The illness is usually self-limited.

◆ **Common noninfectious causes of cough:** Asthma, chronic obstructive pulmonary disease (COPD), malignancy, postnasal drip, gastroesophageal reflux disease (GERD), medication side effect (e.g., angiotensin-converting enzyme inhibitors), congestive heart failure

Analysis

Objectives

1.   Develop a differential diagnosis of cough persisting for 3 weeks or more.
2.   Understand that most upper respiratory infections are self-limited illnesses.
3.   Develop an approach for rational prescription of antibiotics for respiratory infections.

Considerations

Acute bronchitis refers to inflammation of the tracheobronchial tree. The inflammatory response to the trigger, whether infectious, allergic, or irritant, leads to increased mucous production and airway hyperresponsiveness. As bronchitis most commonly occurs in the setting of an upper respiratory illness, it is seen more frequently in the winter. Influenza, parainfluenza, adenovirus, rhinovirus, other viruses, *Mycoplasma pneumoniae,* and *Chlamydia pneumoniae* have been implicated as causes.

As the primary symptoms are nonspecific, other etiologies can be mistakenly diagnosed as acute bronchitis. In one study, one third of patients who had been determined to have recurrent bouts of acute bronchitis were eventually identified as having asthma. Occupational history may be important in determining whether irritants play a role.

There are no specific diagnostic criteria for acute bronchitis, although cough productive of purulent sputum is the most common presentation. Other symptoms are often present, including fever, malaise, rhinorrhea or nasal congestion, sore throat, wheezing, dyspnea, chest pain, myalgias, or arthralgias. The sputum produced can be of variable color and consistency; **the color of sputum is not diagnostic of the presence of a bacterial infection.**

The physical examination in bronchitis is typically nonspecific and, frequently, is normal. The presence of fever, tachypnea, tachycardia, and hypo- or hypertension should be noted. In persons with underlying pulmonary or cardiac conditions, or in persons with more severe symptoms, an oxygen saturation by pulse oximetry may be warranted. Examination of the lungs may reveal rales, rhonchi, or wheezes, but in most cases is unremarkable.

Occasionally, findings on examination may suggest a particular etiology or an alternate diagnosis. Prolonged fever and signs of consolidation on pulmonary examination may suggest a diagnosis of pneumonia. When pneumonia is suspected, a chest radiograph should be obtained to confirm the diagnosis. Conjunctivitis and adenopathy suggest adenoviral infection, although these findings are not specific.

Bronchitis is nearly always self-limited in an otherwise healthy individual. Although most acute bronchitis lasts for less than 2 weeks, in some cases the cough can last for 2 months or more. Severe cases occasionally produce deterioration in patients with significant comorbid conditions.

APPROACH TO UPPER RESPIRATORY INFECTIONS

Treatment

The use of antibiotics has not been shown consistently to alter the natural history of acute bronchitis, except in the uncommon case of infection with *Bordetella pertussis*. Patients with abnormal vital signs (pulse ≥100 beats/min, respiration ≥24 breaths/min, temperature ≥100.4°F) and examination findings consistent with pulmonary consolidation should be evaluated further for the diagnosis of pneumonia and treated appropriately, if confirmed. Pneumonia may present atypically in the elderly and in persons with chronic lung disease. Physicians must have a higher index of suspicion in these populations.

As some of the symptoms of bronchitis are caused by airway hyperreactivity, bronchodilator therapy has been shown in some studies to offer benefit in reducing symptoms. Antitussives, such as dextromethorphan and codeine, may have modest benefits in reducing the cough associated with this illness.

Other Infections of the Upper Respiratory Tract

Rhinosinusitis

Rhinosinusitis is the inflammation/infection of the nasal mucosa and of one or more paranasal sinuses. Sinusitis occurs with obstruction of the normal drainage mechanism. It is traditionally subdivided into acute (symptoms lasting <4 weeks), subacute (symptoms lasting 4–12 weeks), chronic (symptoms lasting >12 weeks), and acute exacerbation of chronic sinusitis.

The signs and symptoms of rhinosinusitis are nonspecific and similar to other general upper respiratory tract infection symptoms. As most viral upper respiratory tract infections improve in 7–10 days, expert opinion suggests considering a diagnosis of bacterial rhinosinusitis after 7 days of symptoms in adults and 10 days in children. The diagnosis is suggested by the presence of purulent nasal discharge, maxillary tooth or facial pain, unilateral maxillary sinus tenderness, and worsening of symptoms after initial improvement.

Streptococcus pneumoniae and *Haemophilus influenzae* are the organisms most commonly responsible for acute bacterial sinusitis in adults; *S. pneumoniae, H. influenzae,* and Moraxella catarrhalis are most common in children. In chronic sinusitis, the infecting organisms are variable, with a higher incidence of anaerobic organisms seen (e.g., *Bacteroides, Peptostreptococcus,* and *Fusobacterium species*).

Treatment of acute sinusitis should be directed at the likely causative agents. Amoxicillin and trimethoprim-sulfamethoxazole are widely used first-line agents, typically for 10–14-day regimens. Second-line antibiotics, for those who fail to improve on the initial regimen or who have recurrent or severe disease, include amoxicillin-clavulanic acid, second- or third-generation cephalosporins (cefuroxime, cefaclor, cefprozil, others), fluoroquinolones, or second-generation macrolides (azithromycin, clarithromycin). Adjunctive therapy with oral or topical decongestants may provide symptomatic relief. Topical decongestants should not be used for more than 3 days, to avoid the risk of rebound vasodilation with resultant worsening of symptoms. Nonsteroidal antiinflammatory drugs (NSAIDs) and acetaminophen may provide symptomatic relief of pain and fever.

Pharyngitis

Pharyngitis is an inflammation or irritation of the pharynx and/or tonsils. In adults, the **vast majority of pharyngitis is viral.** It can also be bacterial or allergic in origin; trauma, toxins, and malignancy are rare causes. As most cases of pharyngitis in adults are benign and self-limited, a focus of the examination of a patient with symptoms of pharyngitis should be to rule out more serious conditions, such as epiglottitis or peritonsillar abscess, and to diagnose group A β-hemolytic *Streptococcus* (GAS) infection.

Pharyngitis occurs with much greater frequency in the pediatric population, with a peak incidence between 4 and 7 years of age. *Mycoplasma pneumoniae, Chlamydia pneumoniae,* and *Arcanobacterium haemolyticus* are common causes of pharyngitis in teens and young adults. GAS causes 15% of all adult pharyngitis and approximately 30% of pediatric cases.

The cause of pharyngitis cannot always be distinguished based on history or examination. Sore throat associated with cough and rhinorrhea is more likely to be viral in origin. The presence of tonsillar exudates does not distinguish bacterial from viral causes, as GAS, Epstein-Barr virus (infectious mononucleosis), mycoplasma, chlamydia, and adenoviruses, among others, can all cause exudates. **Findings frequently associated with GAS infections include an abrupt onset of sore throat and fever, tonsillar and/or palatal petechiae, tender cervical adenopathy and absence of cough.** GAS can also cause an erythematous, sandpaperlike (scarlatiniform) rash.

Infectious mononucleosis, caused by infection with Epstein-Barr virus, is extremely difficult to distinguish clinically from GAS infection. Exudative pharyngitis is prominent. Features suggestive of mononucleosis include retrocervical or generalized adenopathy and hepatosplenomegaly. Atypical lymphocytes can be seen on peripheral blood smear. The associated splenomegaly can be significant, as it predisposes to splenic rupture in response to trauma (even minor trauma). A patient with splenomegaly from mononucleosis should be restricted from activities, such as sports participation, in which abdominal trauma may occur.

On examination, the **patency of the airway must be addressed first.** The presence of stridor, drooling, and a toxic appearance suggest epiglottitis. Patients with epiglottitis are sometimes seen leaning forward on their outstretched arms, the so-called tripod position. Patients with suspected epiglottitis need to be managed in a setting where the airway can be emergently secured, via intubation or cricothyroidotomy. Epiglottitis is a rare infection and is becoming even rarer, with near universal immunization for *H. influenzae, type B.*

Swelling of the peritonsillar region, with the associated tonsil pushed toward the midline and with contralateral deviation of the uvula, is consistent with a peritonsillar abscess. This can be seen either as the initial complaint of sore throat, frequently with associated trismus (pain with chewing), or as a complication of streptococcal pharyngitis. Suspicion of peritonsillar abscess should prompt immediate referral for surgical drainage of the abscess.

The diagnosis of GAS infection can be made by rapid antigen testing or throat culture. **Rapid antigen tests** can be conducted in a few minutes in the office or emergency department setting. They are **highly specific but have a lower sensitivity than throat culture.** A positive rapid antigen test would prompt antibiotic treatment; a negative test should be followed by a throat culture. **Throat cultures are considered the gold standard** for diagnosis of GAS infections. Cultures can take 24–48 hours; this is acceptable in most instances, as the risk of complication from GAS infections is low if treatment is instituted within 10 days of onset of symptoms.

Complications from untreated GAS infections are rare, but include rheumatic fever, glomerulonephritis, toxic shock syndrome, peritonsillar abscess, meningitis, and bacteremia. Rheumatic fever, which may complicate up to 1 in 400 untreated cases of GAS pharyngitis, can cause permanent cardiac and neurologic sequelae. Glomerulonephritis results from antigen/antibody complex deposition in the glomeruli. **Poststreptococcal glomerulonephritis may occur whether or not the patient receives appropriate antibiotic treatment.**

Penicillin is the antibiotic of choice for GAS pharyngitis. Oral therapy requires a 10-day course of penicillin V. Intramuscular therapy of penicillin G benzathine for adults and children weighing more than 27 kg is 1.2 million units. Children who weigh less than 27 kg can receive 600,000 units of penicillin IM. In penicillin-allergic patients, treatment options include cephalosporins and macrolides.

Infections of the Ear

Otitis externa (OE) is an infection of the external auditory canal. Patients with OE complain of ear pain and, sometimes, itching. The pain from OE can be severe. Examination shows an inflamed, swollen, external ear canal, often with exudates and discharge. Movement of the external ear is usually quite painful. The tympanic membrane may be uninvolved. The most common pathogens include staphylococci, streptococci, and other skin flora. Some cases have been associated with the use of swimming pools or hot tubs. This infection (swimmer's ear) is usually caused by *Pseudomonas aeruginosa*. Irrigation and administration of topical antibiotics, frequently combined with steroid, is usually successful. **Patients with diabetes mellitus are at risk for an invasive external otitis** (malignant OE) caused by *P. aeruginosa*. Treatment for this condition involves surgical debridement of necrotic tissue and 4–6 weeks of IV antibiotics, if cranial bones are involved.

Otitis media (OM) is an infection of the middle ear seen primarily among preschool children, but occasionally in adults as well. Infection of the middle ear space, caused by upper respiratory tract pathogens, is promoted by obstruction to drainage through edematous, congested eustachian tubes. Viral infection with serous otitis may predispose to acute bacterial otitis media. Fever, ear pain, diminished hearing, vertigo, and tinnitus are common presenting symptoms. On examination, the tympanic membrane may appear red, but the presence of decreased mobility of or fluid behind the tympanic membrane are necessary for the diagnosis. *S. pneumoniae, H. influenzae,* and *M. catarrhalis* are the most common bacterial pathogens. **Most cases of acute OM will resolve spontaneously.** Indications for treatment with antibiotics include prolonged, recurrent or severe symptoms. Numerous antibiotics can be used for treatment. Amoxicillin remains the recommended initial therapy. Alternative treatments include amoxicillin-clavulanic acid, trimethoprim-sulfamethoxazole, or second- and third-generation cephalosporins. Complications are uncommon, but include mastoiditis, bacterial meningitis, brain abscess, and subdural empyema.

Comprehension Questions

[19.1] A 25-year-old healthy female presents with a cough productive of yellowish sputum for the past week. She has also had a runny nose and sore throat. Her 2-year-old son has been sick with a similar illness. In your office she is afebrile, has a normal ear, nose, and throat (ENT) examination and clear lungs. Which of the following statements is most accurate about this patient?

   A. She most likely has a viral infection.
   B. Because she has a cough productive of yellow sputum, she most likely has a bacterial infection.
   C. This is probably the initial presentation of asthma.
   D. This is probably related to a seasonal allergy.

[19.2] A 40-year-old male presents with severe unilateral ear pain for the past
3 days. He swims laps daily at the YMCA for exercise. Which of the
following are you most likely to find on examination?

A. A bulging tympanic membrane
B. A high fever
C. An inflamed external ear canal
D. Tenderness over the mastoid process

[19.3] An 18-year-old female comes to the office with a sore throat, fever, and
fatigue. On examination, she has an exudative pharyngitis, bilateral
cervical lymphadenopathy, and an enlarged spleen. Which of the following statements is most likely to be true?

A. She will require treatment with IM penicillin.
B. She may return to playing for the school basketball team when her
fever has resolved.
C. She is at risk for developing acute rheumatic fever.
D. A complete blood count (CBC) is likely to show atypical lympho-
cytes.

Answers

[19.1] **A.** This patient has an upper respiratory infection that is most likely
viral. The color of her sputum does not necessarily indicate the presence
of a bacterial infection. The absence of signs of consolidation on her
pulmonary examination makes pneumonia unlikely. That her child has
a similar illness also makes a contagious, viral infection more likely.

[19.2] **C.** This patient has symptoms suggestive of "swimmer's ear," otitis
externa, probably caused by *P. aeruginosa*. The most common examination finding consistent with this is an inflamed external auditory
canal. Other findings might be pain with movement of the external ear
and exudates in the auditory canal.

[19.3] **D.** Her symptoms and examination findings are consistent with infectious
mononucleosis caused by Epstein-Barr virus. This infection often results in
the finding of atypical lymphocytes on a CBC. As she has splenomegaly,
she should be restricted from a sport, such as basketball, until her spleen is
no longer palpable. Mononucleosis is a self-limiting disease.

CLINICAL PEARLS

❖ The main concerns with pharyngitis are to rule out more serious conditions, such as epiglottitis or peritonsillar abscess, and to diagnose group A β-hemolytic streptococcal infections.

❖ Hepatosplenomegaly can be found in infectious mononucleosis infection.

❖ A tonsillopharyngeal exudate does not differentiate viral and bacterial causes.

❖ Tonsillopharyngeal/palatal petechiae are seen in GAS infections and infectious mononucleosis.

REFERENCES

Tierney LM, McPhee SJ, Papadakis MA. Current medical diagnosis and treatment. 42nd ed. New York: McGraw-Hill, 2003: 203–205, 1346–1347.

Gonzales R, Bartlett JG, Besser RE, et al. Principles of appropriate antibiotic use for treatment of uncomplicated acute bronchitis: background. Ann Intern Med 2001; 134(6):521–529.

Knutson D, Braun C. Diagnosis and management of acute bronchitis. Am Fam Physician 2002;65:2039–2044, 2046.

Ong S. Bronchitis. 2004. Available at: www.emedicine.com/emerg/topic69.htm.

Scheid DC, Hamm RM. Acute bacterial rhinosinusitis in adults: part I. Evaluation. Am Fam Physician 2004;70:1685–1692.

Scheid DC, Hamm RM. Acute bacterial rhinosinusitis in adults: part II. Treatment. Am Fam Physician 2004;70(9):1697–1704.

A 56-year-old male is brought to the emergency department complaining of chest discomfort for about 90 minutes. He has had occasional symptoms for a month, but it is worse today. Today's symptoms began while he was walking his dog and decreased slightly with rest, but have not resolved. He describes the feeling as a pressure sensation in the left substernal area of his chest associated with shortness of breath and mild diaphoresis. He does not have any radiation of the discomfort today, but has experienced radiation to the left upper extremity in the past. The patient denies any health problems, but his wife reports that he has not seen a physician in years. His wife made him come in because his younger brother had a heart attack 6 months ago. He is a vice president of a bank and lives with his wife and 3 daughters. He has smoked 1.5 packs of cigarettes per day for more than 30 years and denies drinking alcohol or any drug use.

On physical examination he is an anxious, obese gentleman who appears pale and has a moist brow. His temperature is 98.8°F, his pulse is 105 beats/min, his respirations is 18 breaths/min, his blood pressure is 190/95 mm Hg, his height is 74 inches, and his weight is 250 pounds. Cardiac examination reveals regular rhythm without murmur, but he has an S_4 gallop. Lungs are clear to auscultation. Neck is without carotid bruits or jugular venous distension. Abdomen is normal. He does have a right femoral bruit. Extremities reveal trace edema but no clubbing or cyanosis. He has 2+ pulses in radial and dorsal pedalis arteries. Rectal examination has no masses or tenderness with a normal prostate, and is guaiac negative.

◆ **What is your most likely diagnosis?**

◆ **What is your next diagnostic step?**

◆ **What is the next step in therapy?**

ANSWERS TO CASE 20: Chest Pain

Summary: A 56-year-old obese male presents to the emergency department with chest discomfort. He has a pressure sensation in the left substernal area of his chest associated with shortness of breath and diaphoresis. His symptoms began with minimal exertion. The patient is without prior medical care. He has a family history of coronary artery disease (CAD) and a history of tobacco abuse. He is hypertensive and tachycardic. He has a cardiac gallop. Lower extremities have trace edema and a femoral bruit.

◆ **Most likely diagnosis:** Unstable angina pectoris; must rule out myocardial infarction.

◆ **Next diagnostic step:** *Initial studies in the emergency room:* complete blood count (CBC), electrolytes, blood urea nitrogen (BUN), creatinine, prothrombin time (PT), partial thromboplastin time (PTT), international normalized ratio (INR), glucose, 12-lead electrocardiography (EKG) and chest x-ray (CXR); markers of myocardial damage including creatine kinase (CK) and MB isoenzyme (CK-MB), troponin T and troponin I to be done stat and every 6–10 hours for 3 cycles. Oxygen saturation must be monitored, as well.

Studies that can be performed later include: fasting lipids, liver function tests, magnesium, homocysteine level, urine drug screen, urinalysis, and myoglobin.

◆ **Next step in therapy:** *MONA* therapy: *M*orphine, *O*xygen, *N*itroglycerin, *A*spirin

> **Morphine** can achieve adequate analgesia which decreases levels of circulating catecholamines, thus reducing myocardial oxygen consumption. It must be initiated rapidly if nitroglycerin cannot alleviate the discomfort.
>
> **Oxygen** 2–4 L/min by nasal cannula; may be discontinued after 6 hours if oxygen saturation remains normal without other complications.
>
> **Nitroglycerin** must be given sublingually initially every 5 minutes for a total of 3 doses (in the absence of hypotension or contraindications such as sildenafil [Viagra] use), then advanced to IV or transdermal routes.
>
> **Aspirin** 325 mg should be chewed and swallowed (clopidogrel [Plavix] if allergy to aspirin exists).
>
> **β-Adrenergic antagonist** reduces myocardial damage and may limit infarct size.
>
> **Glycoprotein (GP) IIb/IIIa inhibitors** reduce end point of death or recurrent ischemia when given in addition to standard therapy for patients with high risk unstable angina or non-ST elevation myocardial infarction treated with percutaneous coronary intervention, or who are refractory to prior treatment.

Analysis

Objectives

1. Understand a diagnostic approach to chest pain and how to reduce potential damage to myocardium by implementing rapid evaluation.
2. Know the acute evaluation of chest pain and how to best implement the primary and secondary treatment of chest pain.
3. Identify the risks and the need to educate patients to reduce their risks.
4. Be familiar with the differential diagnosis of chest pain and how to best rule in and out the more life-threatening problems.

Considerations

This 56-year-old male has unstable angina with a variety of risk factors for CAD. All patients who present to primary care physicians with chest pain are immediate challenges. Most resources emphasize the life-threatening etiologies; however, the non–life-threatening etiologies are far more common in presentation. Physicians must master a cost-effective approach to diagnosing the various etiologies of chest pain, determining which patients warrant further evaluation, putting a large emphasis on thorough history and physical exam. The cause of this patient's symptoms must be determined as soon as possible. If the etiology is determined to be cardiac, there are medications and interventions that can dramatically reduce both morbidity and mortality. A complete history and physical exam can give information that can guide if and when other more expensive and invasive tests are necessary. The patient's most immediate problem is his acute symptoms. His anxiety will decrease slightly when he perceives that he is getting adequate care and information.

Nearly 1.5 million people in the United States experience a myocardial infarction each year. This is fatal approximately one-third of the time. However, there has been a continuous decline in the mortality rate over the past 3 decades because of a better understanding of the etiology and pathophysiology of myocardial infarction, and because of advances in therapeutic treatments.

The **first priority** is to obtain EKG and CXR, while giving medications to decrease the damage caused to his myocardium and simultaneously reducing his blood pressure. Nitroglycerin and β-adrenergic antagonists will begin achieving these goals. He will need constant monitoring and continuous telemetry. Oxygen needs to be continued as well. Before the EKG and CXR have been completed, aspirin, oxygen, nitroglycerin, morphine, and β-adrenergic antagonist should be given. The providers must assume cardiac etiology until it has been effectively ruled out to limit possible morbidity and mortality to the patient.

The labs previously listed need to be drawn, at which time IV access can be started in two places. The results of the tests will determine if the patient has other risk factors in addition to his known hypertension, family history of CAD, tobacco abuse, and obesity. If he routinely walks his dog, his lifestyle contains at least minimal physical activity.

The changes seen in an EKG that are indicative of angina include ST wave elevation or depression and/or T wave inversion. Myocardial infarctions include these changes plus elevated CK-MB and/or troponin levels. Pathologic Q waves may also indicate cardiac pathology, but typically represent myocardial tissue necrosis from a completed infarction. When Q waves are present, the benefits of thrombolytic therapy are uncertain. **Not all myocardial infarctions will have EKG changes.** A normal EKG reduces the likelihood of myocardial infarction but does not rule out cardiac pathology. Any person with symptoms of angina who has a left bundle-branch block (LBBB) on EKG must have serum cardiac enzymes drawn, because there is a high degree of correlation between LBBB and organic heart disease, especially CAD. LBBB can mask signs of myocardial pathology, as it can mimic both acute and chronic ischemic changes. All of the listed EKG changes each have a differential diagnosis that includes myocardial infarction. The clinical picture is of utmost importance, again demonstrating the need for complete history and physical examination.

APPROACH TO CHEST PAIN

Definitions

Angina pectoris: Severe pain around the heart caused by a relative deficiency of oxygen supply to the heart muscle.

Myocardial infarction (MI): Cardiac muscle death caused by partial or complete occlusion of one or more of the coronary arteries.

New York Heart Association Functional Classification of Angina:
Class I—Angina only with unusually strenuous activity
Class II—Angina with slightly more prolonged or slightly more vigorous activity than usual
Class III—Angina with usual daily activity
Class IV—Angina at rest

Unstable angina: Angina of new onset, angina at rest or with minimal exertion, or a crescendo pattern of angina with episodes of increasing frequency, severity, or duration.

Clinical Approach

Etiologies

Atherosclerosis leading to plaque rupture and then cascading to coronary artery thrombosis is the cause of an acute MI approximately 90% of the time, but **many different conditions can be the culprit for angina.** Coronary artery spasm, including cocaine-induced injury, can cause angina. Aortic dissection extending into a coronary artery will cause extensive damage. An embolus to a coronary artery can be caused by endocarditis, prosthetic heart valves, or myxoma. Embolism can also cause cerebral vascular accidents, increasing the extent of the initial evaluation that is warranted.

Chest pain or discomfort is one the most common complaints in both the outpatient and emergency setting. Determining the cause of such symptoms in a rapid fashion is of utmost importance. **If the patient is experiencing myocardial ischemia or infarction, time is myocardium.** Initial evaluation should be done within 10 minutes of presentation. Ischemic heart disease remains the leading cause of morbidity and mortality in the United States.

Treatment

Primary Treatment

All patients who rule in for myocardial infarction should receive aspirin and an antithrombotic treatment, if there are no contraindications. Aspirin and heparin reduce the risk of subsequent MI and cardiac death in patients with unstable angina. Studies present different recommendations for using clopidogrel in addition to aspirin and heparin. Current American College of Cardiology/American Heart Association recommendations advise withholding clopidogrel for 5–7 days before planned bypass surgery. It is reasonable to give clopidogrel 300 mg orally to patients with suspected acute coronary syndrome (ACS) (without EKG or cardiac marker changes) who are either allergic to or have gastrointestinal intolerance of aspirin.

Heparin usually should be continued for 48 hours or until angiography is performed. Patients suffering from unstable angina with EKG changes should also be given platelet glycoprotein IIb/IIIa receptor inhibitors because the composite risk of death, myocardial infarction, or recurrent ischemia is significantly reduced with these medications.

Nitroglycerin is best given IV initially because of the ability to achieve predictable blood levels rapidly. Once stabilized after 24 hours, the asymptomatic patient should be switched to a long-acting oral or transdermal nitrate. A β-adrenergic antagonist should also be given, unless contraindicated. The **combination of nitroglycerin and β-adrenergic antagonist reduces the risk of subsequent myocardial infarction.** β-Adrenergic antagonists decreased mortality and reduced infarct size in many clinical trials.

Angiotensin-converting enzyme (ACE) inhibitors reduce short-term mortality when started within 24 hours of acute myocardial infarction. Postinfarction ACE inhibitors prevent left ventricular remodeling and recurrent ischemic events. It is reasonable to recommend their indefinite use in the absence of any contraindications. All trials with oral ACE inhibitors have shown benefit from their early use, including those in which early entry criteria included clinical suspicion of acute infarctions. Magnesium sulfate if levels are low, as hypomagnesemia can increase the incidence of *torsade de pointes*-type ventricular tachycardia.

Despite the widespread use of calcium channel blockers both during and after myocardial ischemia, no evidence exists supporting any benefit when taking these medications. Rapid release, short-acting dihydropyridines (e.g., nifedipine) are contraindicated because they increased mortality in multiple trials.

Patients who are asymptomatic after 48 hours of drug therapy can perform a modified Bruce protocol stress test. Patients who have a markedly positive stress test should be referred for angiography. There is some debate concerning when angiography should be done. One approach shows that an early invasive approach with angiography within 24–48 hours is beneficial, whereas others recommend a more conservative approach, doing angiography only if recurrent ischemia is present or a positive stress test is done. There is no clear consensus as to which approach is superior.

All patients admitted for angina or myocardial infarction should receive a reduced saturated fat and cholesterol diet. These patients may benefit from nutrition counselors to help them develop healthy lifestyle changes.

Secondary Treatment

Primary prevention of CAD must be encouraged for all patients. **Risk factors for CAD include diabetes mellitus, dyslipidemia, age, hypertension, tobacco abuse, family history of premature CAD, male gender, postmenopausal status, left ventricular hypertrophy, and homocystinemia** (Table 20–1). Modification of these risk factors has a direct link to reduce morbidity and mortality. Patient education is particularly important.

Table 20–1
RISK FACTORS FOR CAUSES OF CHEST PAIN

RISK FACTOR	EVENT
Age/gender: male >40 years old	CAD
Hypertension	Risk for CAD and aortic dissection
Tobacco abuse	CAD, thromboembolism, aortic dissection, pneumothorax, and pneumonia
Diabetes mellitus	CAD
Cocaine use	MI
Hyperlipidemia Increasing TC, TG, LDL Decreasing HDL	MI
Left ventricular hypertrophy	MI
Family history of premature CAD	MI
Blunt trauma to chest	Pneumothorax, myocardial or pulmonary contusion, chest wall injury

Abbreviations: CAD, coronary artery disease; HDL, high-density lipoprotein; LDL, low-density lipoprotein; MI, myocardial infarction; TC, total cholesterol; TG, triglyceride.

Aspirin, nitrates, and β-adrenergic antagonist have proven benefits for both primary and secondary treatment. Prolonged treatment with aspirin reduces risks for both CAD and cerebrovascular disease. β-Adrenergic antagonist reduces first-year mortality. If no adverse affects are experienced, patients should continue β-adrenergic antagonist 2–3 years or longer. Long-acting nitrates can treat angina symptoms.

Beta-hydroxy-beta-methylglutaryl-coenzyme A (HMG-CoA) reductase inhibitors (statins) have documented a consistent decrease in the incidence of major adverse cardiovascular events when given within a few days after onset of ACS. There are few data on patients treated within 24 hours of the onset of symptoms. It is safe and feasible to start statin therapy early (within 24 hours) in patients; once started, continue statin therapy uninterrupted. The goal level for low-density lipoprotein (LDL) cholesterol in anyone with a history of CAD and high risk for future cardiac events is <70 mg/dL.

Hypertension must be treated using agents that reduce cardiac complications, as previously discussed. If further reduction is necessary, many medications treat hypertension and angina. Blood pressure and coronary pathology have a linear relationship; as blood pressure is reduced the risk, morbidity, and mortality of cardiac disease is also reduced. Agents used often depend on a patient's comorbid conditions.

Physical activity is an important component of lifestyle change. Recommendation of a minimum goal of 30 minutes of exercise on most days should be given to all patients. Weight management is also encouraged, but often requires numerous interventions. A minimum of a 5% reduction in weight will provide benefits to the patient. Body mass index needs to become part of the vital signs examined every visit.

Clinical Presentation

The history should focus on onset and evolution of the chest pain. The cardinal features of all chief complaints should be followed, paying attention to patient's description of the pain/discomfort, location, radiation of pain, quality of pain, quantity of pain, duration, associating factors, and aggravating and/or alleviating factors (Table 20–2). **Many people do not describe angina as chest pain.** It is more effective to ask the patient to describe the discomfort. Some describe it as pressure, squeezing, crushing, or smothering. Some may use a "Levine sign," a fist held firmly against the chest. The discomfort is usually central and substernal. It may radiate to the jaw, shoulder, arm, or hand; usually to the left side. Cardiogenic nausea and vomiting are associated with larger MIs.

The relationship of the symptoms to exertion is very important. Exertion, emotional stress, or other situations that either increase myocardial oxygen demand or decrease oxygen supply can increase symptoms. **Angina usually responds promptly to measures that reduce myocardial oxygen demand,** such as rest. Pain typically resolves in less than 5 minutes. If angina persists for longer than 20–30 minutes, a myocardial infarction is more likely. In this setting, hospitalization and further evaluation is warranted.

Table 20–2
DIFFERENTIAL DIAGNOSIS OF CHEST PAIN

DISORDER	SYMPTOMS/FINDINGS	STUDIES
Angina	Substernal pressure for duration <30 min Radiation to arm, neck, jaw ± dyspnea, N/V, diaphoresis ↑ with exertion; ↓ with rest and NTG	EKG, CXR, serum values
MI	Anginal symptoms but duration >30 min	EKG, CXR, serum values
Pericarditis	Sharp pain radiates to trapezius ↑ with respiration; ↓ with sitting forward	Friction rub, EKG, ± pericardial effusion
Aortic dissection	Sudden onset of tearing pain with radiation to back	CXR, widened mediastinum CT, TEE, MRI
Heart failure	Exertional chest pain and dyspnea (uncommon cause of angina, but often patients may also have CAD)	CXR, displaced apical impulse, edema (pulmonary, lower extremities), JVD, cardiac gallop, murmurs
Pneumonia	Dyspnea, fever, and cough; pleuritic pain	CXR, egophony, dullness to percussion
Pneumothorax	Unilateral sharp pleuritic pain of sudden onset, CXR findings	Unilateral ↓ breath sounds and/or hyperresonance
Pulmonary embolism	Sudden onset of pleuritic pain, tachycardia, tachypnea, hypoxemia	D-dimer, V/Q scan, CT chest, pulmonary angiogram
Gastroesophageal reflux	Burning epigastric/substernal pain, acid taste in mouth, ↑ with meals; ↓ with PPIs or antacids	Endoscopy, esophageal pH probe
Peptic ulcer disease	Epigastric pain ↓ with antacids and PPIs	Endoscopy *Helicobacter pylori* test
Pancreatitis	Severe epigastric and back pain	↑ amylase and lipase, abdominal CT

Table 20–2
DIFFERENTIAL DIAGNOSIS OF CHEST PAIN

DISORDER	SYMPTOMS/FINDINGS	STUDIES
Costochondritis	Localized pain that is easily reproducible, tender to palpation	Tenderness to palpation
Anxiety	"Tightness" sensation of chest, SOB, tachycardia	Ask screening questions for anxiety and panic
Herpes zoster	Pain often presents prior to rash	Unilateral pain in dermatomal distribution

Abbreviations: ↓, Decreasing; ↑, increasing; CAD, coronary artery disease; CT, computed tomography; CXR, chest x-ray; EKG, electrocardiogram; JVD, jugular venous distension; MI, myocardial infarction; MRI, magnetic resonance imaging; NTG, nitroglycerin; N/V, nausea and vomiting; PPI, proton pump inhibitor; SOB, shortness of breath; TEE, transesophageal echocardiogram.

The targeted history in patients with angina needs to ascertain whether the patient has had prior episodes of myocardial ischemia (stable or unstable angina, MI, interventions such as bypass surgery or angioplasty). Evaluation of the patient's complaints should focus on chest discomfort, associated symptoms, gender and age-related differences in presentation, hypertension, diabetes mellitus, possibility of aortic dissection, risk of bleeding, and clinical cerebrovascular disease (amaurosis fugax, face/limb weakness or clumsiness, face/limb numbness or sensory loss, ataxia, or vertigo).

The physical examination needs to concentrate on evidence that supports or disproves a diagnosis of cardiovascular disease. General appearance and vital signs can reveal much about the patient and the patient's stability. Hypertension, evidence of elevated lipids, changes consistent with diabetes mellitus, and signs of peripheral vascular disease all increase the risk of CAD.

Funduscopic examination can show signs of chronic hypertension or diabetes mellitus. All blood vessels must be auscultated for bruits, a direct sign of atherosclerotic disease. Diminished peripheral pulses are also a sign of atherosclerotic disease. Signs of heart failure include pulmonary edema, rales, jugular venous distension, and hepatojugular reflux. New gallops or murmurs can signal myocardial ischemia. Shallow, painful breathing suggests chest pain of with a pleural cause. Asymmetric expansion of the chest with unilateral hyperresonance to percussion and diminished breath sounds are indicative of a possible pneumothorax.

The cardiac examination requires careful evaluation. **Unequal carotid pulses or upper extremity pulses can indicate aortic dissection, but most patients with dissection will not have pulse deficit.** The murmur of aortic stenosis can be significant, as aortic stenosis can present with angina, which can then lead to syncope and heart failure.

The patient's chest wall should be palpated. If this examination reproduces the chest pain, costochondritis becomes more likely. **Musculoskeletal causes of chest pain are the most common etiology in an outpatient setting.** Abdominal examination is also important, as gastrointestinal etiology is the second most common culprit for chest pain in an outpatient setting. Careful examination of both upper quadrants and epigastric area must be done. The abdominal aorta warrants careful examination.

Comprehension Questions

[20.1] Which of the following medications would be contraindicated as a first-line agent for the treatment of angina pectoris?

    A. Labetalol
    B. Nitroglycerin
    C. Enalapril
    D. Nifedipine
    E. Aspirin

[20.2] Which of the following diagnostic studies is not necessary to be done on someone presenting with angina pectoris?

    A. EKG
    B. CXR
    C. Complete blood count
    D. Fasting lipids
    E. All should be done

[20.3] Which of the following EKG changes makes the determination of acute MI the most difficult?

    A. Q wave
    B. ST segment elevation
    C. Left bundle-branch block
    D. First-degree atrioventricular block
    E. T wave inversion

Answers

[20.1] **D.** Rapid release, short-acting dihydropyridines (nifedipine) are contraindicated because they increased mortality in multiple trials.

[20.2] **E.** All of the studies listed should be performed to fully evaluate patients presenting with angina pectoris.

[20.3] **C.** The changes of left bundle-branch block make the determination of an acute MI by an EKG extremely difficult. In these patients, it is particularly important to obtain serum markers of myocardial damage.

CLINICAL PEARLS

❖ Angina pectoris is the most frequent symptom of intermittent ischemia.
❖ Targeted history and physical exam of patients with angina is vital to
   expedite proper diagnosis and treatment of patients. The patient's
   description of their discomfort is key; history must be given attention because it is the most important diagnostic factor.
❖ Physical examination may be normal in many patients.
❖ Aspirin, nitrates, β-adrenergic antagonists, and statins are the backbone
   in treatment and prevention of myocardial pathology, having proven
   benefit for both primary and secondary treatment.
❖ Time is myocardium. Initial diagnosis and treatment must be done
   as soon as possible.
❖ Be mindful of polypharmacy, as many drugs have side effects that
   can exacerbate myocardial damage.

REFERENCES

Bosker G. Textbook of adult and pediatric emergency medicine. 2nd ed. Atlanta,
   GA: American Health Consultants, 2002.
Cayley W. Diagnosing the cause of chest pain. Am Fam Physician 2005;72:
   2012–2021.
Elliott A. ACC/AHA guidelines for the management of patients with ST-elevation
   myocardial infarction—executive summary. A report of the American College of
   Cardiology/American Heart Association Task Force on Practice Guidelines.
   Circulation 2004;110:588–636.
Lilly L. Pathophysiology of heart disease. 2nd ed. Baltimore: Williams & Wilkins,
   1998.
Marshall S. On call principles and protocols. 3rd ed. Philadelphia: WB Saunders,
   2000.
Meisel J. Diagnostic approach to chest pain in adults. UpToDate 2005. Available at:
   www.uptodate.com
Sabatine M. Pocket medicine. The Massachusetts General Hospital handbook of
   internal medicine. Baltimore: Lippincott Williams & Wilkins, 2000.
Shubhada A, Kellie F, Subramanian P. The Washington manual of medical thera-
   peutics. 30th ed. Baltimore: Lippincott Williams & Wilkins, 2001.
Simons M. Classification of unstable angina and non-ST elevation (non-Q wave)
   myocardial infarction. UpToDate 2005. Available at: www.uptodate.com
Tallia A. Swanson's family practice review. 4th ed. St. Louis: CV Mosby, 2001.
Thomas C. Taber's cyclopedic medical dictionary. 18th ed. Philadelphia: FA Davis,
   1997.
Wiviott S, Braunwald E. Myocardial infarction. Am Fam Physician 2004;70:535–538.
American Heart Association. 2005 International consensus conference on cardiopul-
   monary resuscitation and emergency cardiovascular care science with treatment
   recommendations. Dallas, Texas. January 23–30, 2005.

A 46-year-old female presents to the clinic for the first time, complaining of decreased urinary output for 5 months with a foamy appearance. She also complains of swelling in both legs and nonbloody, nonbilious emesis a few times a week. She was diagnosed with diabetes 10 years ago and has been taking insulin for 2 years. She does not check her sugars at home because she does not like to stick herself. When asked about her diet she states that she eats the best she can for what she can afford but often has very little appetite. The patient last saw her physician 8 months ago and insulin is her only medication. On examination, the patient is an obese female. Her temperature is 99°F, her heart rate is 108 beats/min, her blood pressure is 198/105 mmHg, her respiration is 19 breaths/min, and her oxygen saturation is 94% on room air. A head, ears, eyes, nose, and throat (HEENT) examination reveals periorbital edema. Her skin is hyperpigmented on both lower extremities. Her heart is tachycardic with an S_1, S_2, S_4 gallop auscultated with no murmur or rub. When palpating the heart's point of maximal impulse (PMI), it is lateral to the left midclavicular line. There are vesicular breath sounds in both lungs throughout. Her neck reveals no jugular venous distension and there are no carotid bruits. Her abdomen is nontender, with no bruits or masses palpated. The lower extremities reveal pitting pretibial edema with a pit recovery time less than 40 seconds. Laboratory studies in your office include a urinalysis showing hyaline casts, 3+ proteinuria and glucose, but negative for ketones. Her hemoglobin is 10.9 g/dL and her hematocrit is 32% with a mean corpuscular volume (MCV) of 82.3 g/dL.

◆ **What is the most likely diagnosis?**

◆ **What is your next diagnostic step?**

◆ **What is the next step in therapy?**

ANSWERS TO CASE 21: Chronic Renal Failure

Summary: This is a 46-year-old female with chronic renal failure (CRF). She has a history of uncontrolled diabetes and currently has uncontrolled hypertension. She presents with periorbital edema, long-standing lower-extremity edema, an S_4 and displaced PMI, and central obesity. The urinalysis shows hyaline casts, 3+ proteinuria and glucose, negative ketones, hemoglobin 10.9 g/dL with an MCV of 82.3 g/dL.

◆ **Most likely diagnosis:** Acute worsening of chronic renal failure.

◆ **Next diagnostic step:** Measurement of serum electrolytes, blood urea nitrogen (BUN), and creatinine; imaging of the kidneys.

◆ **Next step in therapy:** Further history to identify and remove any offending agents (such as nonsteroidal antiinflammatory drugs [NSAIDs]), and control of blood pressure and diabetes. May require dialysis if she develops complications such as pulmonary edema, severe hyperkalemia, or anuria.

Analysis

Objectives

1. Know the risks for developing CRF.
2. Learn to evaluate for CRF.
3. Be familiar with the management of CRF.
4. Recognize the complications associated with CRF.

Considerations

This 46-year-old patient presents with a concerning symptom of a decrease in urination with a change in the appearance of the urine. The most immediate concern is how often she is urinating and to what degree is she urinating less. A significant reduction requires immediate evaluation of creatinine function and volume status. Volume status is assessed by skin turgor, mucous membranes, specific gravity in the urinalysis, and orthostatic blood pressure, which also measures heart rate in the lying, sitting, and standing positions. A low volume status with an elevated creatinine requires that the patient be given IV fluids to see if there can be any recovery of kidney function. The patient's uncontrolled diabetes and hypertension predispose her to kidney damage. Another common offender is a patient with this history who is taking NSAIDs. This will increase the patient's already high risk of damage.

With chronic kidney failure, patients are often able to compensate for the metabolic imbalances that occur such as hyper- or hyponatremia, hyperkalemia, elevated uric acid levels, and metabolic acidosis. Patients also experience hyperparathyroidism. Significantly elevated potassium levels require treatment with sodium polystyrene sulfonate (Kayexalate), insulin with glucose, and retention enemas, depending on the degree of elevation. When the patient is no longer compensating, there are symptoms of pulmonary edema, which include shortness of breath, lower-extremity edema, jugular venous distension, and abnormal lung sounds (rales). This patient was compensating and mostly demonstrated the result of a hypoalbuminemic state from the loss of protein in the urine. She had lower-extremity edema with a long pit time that reflected her low albumin state. Her occasional emesis reflects high levels of urea and other toxins. Persistent emesis mandates treatment. Her normocytic anemia was the result of reduced erythropoietin from the kidneys. In this setting, treatment with exogenous erythropoietin improves prognosis for cardiovascular mortality. The hyaline casts reflect the long-standing damage to the kidneys.

Increasing the patient's chance of improved kidney function requires glucose and blood pressure control, removing offenders such as NSAIDs and diuretics (if allowable), maintaining normal volume status (which is difficult with a low albumin state), and adding agents that both treat blood pressure and improve kidney and cardiovascular function such as angiotensin-converting enzyme (ACE) inhibitors and angiotensin receptor blockers (ARBs). CRF itself is a cardiovascular risk factor. Patients are more likely to die from cardiovascular disease than to develop end-stage renal disease (ESRD) requiring dialysis. The patient's gross proteinuria of 3+ reflects her high risk for cardiovascular disease.

APPROACH TO CHRONIC RENAL FAILURE

Definitions

CRF: A pathophysiologic process that leads to a decrease in nephrons and function. There are several known causes. This can be detected by imaging studies and, or blood and urine analysis. It is also defined by a glomerular filtration rate (GFR) of <60 mL/min for 3 or more months.

ESRD: The irreversible loss of kidney function such that the patient is permanently dependent on renal replacement therapy (dialysis or transplantation). Also defined as a GFR of <15 mL/min.

Clinical Approach

Etiologies

Chronic renal failure is becoming more common in the United States. **The most common etiologies are diabetes, hypertension, and glomerulonephritis**. Diabetic kidney disease occurs in 30–40% of type I diabetics, in 25% of type II diabetics, and in 24% of hypertensive patients. Within the diabetic patient population, 20–60% have hypertension. Many patients present at a later stage of CRF and it is then difficult to determine the etiology.

Evaluation

The Kidney Disease Outcomes Quality Initiative (KDOQI) from the National Kidney Foundation (NKF) recommends both a serum creatinine (CR) to estimate GFR and random urinalysis for albuminuria in those groups at risk for CRF. The stage of CRF is based on GFR, which can be estimated with a random CR level calculated with one of two commonly used equations:

Modification of Diet in Renal Disease (MDRD) equation:

$$\text{GFR (mL per min per 1.73 m}^2) = 186 \times (\text{Scr})^{-1.54} \times (\text{age})^{-0.203}$$
$$\times (0.742, \text{if female}) \times (1.210, \text{if black})$$

Cockcroft-Gault equation:

$$\text{Ccr (mL per min)} = ((140 - \text{age}) \times \text{weight}/72 \times \text{Scr}) \times (0.85, \text{if female})$$

(Scr = serum creatinine concentration; Ccr = creatinine clearance).

A normal GFR for a woman is between 100 and 120 mL/min. Stage 1 of CRF correlates with a GFR >90 mL/min; stage 2 correlates with a GFR of 60–89 mL/min; stage 3 correlates with a GFR of 30–59 mL/min; stage 4 correlates with a GFR of 15–29 mL/min; and stage 5 correlates with a GFR <15 mL/min or dialysis. The Cockcroft-Gault equation is preferred for older patients. A 24-hour urine collection is recommended for persons with extremes of age and weight, malnutrition, skeletal muscle disease, paraplegia or quadriplegia, or a vegetarian diet.

The evaluation in all patients with CRF includes renal imaging and microscopic evaluation of urine. Treatment may be more successful in patients with normal-size kidneys. Small kidneys show irreversible disease. Asymmetry suggests renovascular disease. Evidence of proteinuria or microalbuminuria should be evaluated in all patients with CRF. If the urine dipstick does not reveal gross proteinuria, a sample should be sent to evaluate for microalbumin. A test is positive if there is >30 mg of microalbumin per gram CR. It is recommended in the case of <200 mg of protein per gram CR that the test be repeated yearly. Any patient with >200 mg of protein per gram CR will need diagnostic evaluation and treatment. The protein-to-creatinine ratio in an early morning random urine sample may be used instead of a 24-hour urine protein excretion.

Underlying causes may be ascertained through clinical presentation, symptomatology, and past medical and family history. Some common lab studies include C3, C4, hepatitis panel, HIV test, protein and urine electrophoresis for those patients older than age 40, hemoglobin A_{1c}, fasting blood sugar, and analysis of urine sediment. Renal biopsy is indicated in patients with unknown etiology after history and lab evaluation, if parenchymal disease is suspected, or if treatment or prognosis will be based on the biopsy.

Management

Managing CRF includes treatment of reversible causes. Hypovolemia, hypotension, infection leading to sepsis, and drugs that lower the GFR all reduce renal perfusion. History and physical examination allow for this diagnosis, and a trial of fluids may improve kidney function. Drugs such as NSAIDs, aminoglycosides at full strength, and radiographic contrast material can affect kidney function. Urinary tract obstruction, commonly caused by prostate enlargement in elderly males, is a potentially reversible cause.

Goals of treatment include a blood pressure <130/80 mmHg and a reduction of protein excretion to less than 500–1000 mg/d (or at least 60% of the baseline value). KDOQI guidelines recommend starting with an ACE inhibitor or an ARB, followed by a diuretic if the blood pressure goal is not achieved. Additional medications are diltiazem, verapamil, or a β-blocker. If the proteinuria goal continues to be unmet after achieving blood pressure control, add either the ACE inhibitor or an ARB. Combining both an ACE inhibitor and an ARB requires reevaluating the potassium and CR 3–5 days after initiation, because of its potential for worsening function. Nonproteinuric renal disease strictly requires blood pressure control.

Other treatments may be beneficial in CRF. Dietary protein restrictions of 0.8–1.0 mg/kg/d may be beneficial. Hyperlipidemia should be treated with a goal low-density lipoprotein (LDL) of <100 mg/dL, and some say the goal should be <70 mg/dL because CRF is a cardiovascular equivalent. The volume overload associated with CRF responds well to sodium restriction and loop diuretics. This lowers the intraglomerular pressure. Hyperkalemia may be prevented by a low-potassium diet and avoiding drugs such as NSAIDs and, sometimes, ACE inhibitors. Metabolic acidosis may be treated with sodium bicarbonate, with a goal to maintain a concentration of 22 mEq/L. Dietary phosphate restriction may limit the development of secondary hyperparathyroidism in these patients.

When the GFR is below 25–30 mL/min, oral phosphate binders are usually required. Caution is used when treating hyperphosphatemia in stages 3 to 5 CRF. It is suggested that calcium intake not exceed 2000 mg/d, as this may contribute to cardiovascular disease.

The KDOQI guidelines suggest evaluation of anemia with a hemoglobin <11 g/dL in premenopausal females and prepubertal patients, and <12 g/dL in adult males and postmenopausal females. This should include evaluation for nonrenal causes of anemia. Treating patients with CRF with erythropoietin before they develop ESRD may reduce symptoms of anemia, show cardiovascular improvement, and possibly decrease mortality. Ultimately, the patient that is going toward ESRD must be identified and adequately prepared for renal replacement therapy. It is recommended that patients with a creatinine >1.2 mg/dL in women and >1.5 mg/dL in men be referred to a nephrologist for evaluation and recommendations.

Comprehension Questions

[21.1] A 56-year-old man with known CRF presents with a 3-day history of shortness of breath and rapid weight gain. On examination you are able to auscultate an S_3, hear crackles at the bases, and see moderate jugular venous distension (JVD). What is your next step in evaluation?

    A. Perform an echocardiogram
    B. Do a chest x-ray
    C. Measure a CR to calculate GFR
    D. Check for cardiac enzymes

[21.2] Which conditions do you want to modify to stop the worsening of renal function?

    A. Blood pressure control
    B. Cholesterol
    C. Hyperparathyroid disease
    D. Metabolic acidosis
    E. Volume depletion
    F. A, B, D, and E

[21.3] A 72-year-old male, with a long history of hypertension, presents to the emergency department complaining of a 2-day history of emesis and 36 hours of no urination. On examination, the abdomen is firm and tender, and the prostate is enlarged. His CR analysis is 3.4 mg/dL. What is the next step?

    A. Give him IV fluids and see if he begins to make urine
    B. Perform a renal ultrasound in the emergency department
    C. Maintain tight control of his blood pressure
    D. Place an indwelling Foley catheter

[21.4] A 38-year-old female with type I diabetes presents to the clinic with decreased vision in the left eye for 1 year, 1+ proteinuria, a baseline CR of 1.6 mg/dL, an LDL of 135 mg/dL, blood pressure of 145/92 mm Hg, and occasional chest pressure for 2 months. What are her cardiovascular risk factors?

    A. CRF
    B. Uncontrolled hypertension
    C. Hyperlipidemia
    D. Diabetes
    E. All of the above

Answers

[21.1] **B.** The patient has CRF with volume overload as evidenced by symptoms and physical examination. A simple first step is to do a chest x-ray to confirm what you already suspect—pulmonary edema. After initiating furosemide (Lasix), the chest x-ray may be repeated to see to what degree the diuresis has improved the overload. Cardiac work-up is also indicated but would not be the first test done.

[21.2] **F.** High blood pressure, acidosis, volume depletion, and cholesterol all worsen kidney function when left untreated. Treating secondary hyperparathyroidism prevents complications such as renal osteodystrophy.

[21.3] **D.** The patient has an enlarged prostate that has caused urinary obstruction and potentially reversible renal failure, depending on at which point the obstruction is resolved. Placing the Foley catheter will usually allow for significant reversal of an elevated CR. Following catheter placement, the urine output needs to be carefully monitored and the CR repeated later. Another clue is the tense lower abdomen that is caused by a very enlarged bladder. It is especially important to rely on clinical examination skills in elderly patients who have less-than-optimal communication skills as a consequence of dementia or who have a history of stroke when evaluating for a cause.

[21.4] **E.** Both diabetes and CRF are known to be cardiovascular equivalents. Other factors, such as uncontrolled blood pressure and cholesterol, add to the patient's high risk, which is why it is so important for all diabetics and CRF patients to improve all modifiable risk factors. The goals become much more stringent when looking at these two groups of patients.

REFERENCES

Craig JC, Craig M, Strippoli GFM. Antihypertensive agents for preventing diabetic kidney disease [review]. The Cochrane Database Syst Reviews 2005;4:1–2, 8.

Goljan E. Pathology. Philadelphia: WB Saunders, 1998:376–377.

Orient J. Sapira's art and science of bedside diagnosis. 2nd ed. Philadelphia: Williams & Wilkins, 2000:323–324, 491–492.

Post T, Rose B. Overview of the management of chronic kidney disease in adults. UpToDate 2005:1–15.

Skorecki K, Green J, Brenner B. Chronic renal failure In Braunwald E, Fauci A, Kasper D, et al (eds). Harrison's principles of internal medicine. 15th ed. New York: McGraw-Hill, 2001: 1551–1559.

Snyder S, Pendergraph B. Detection and evaluation of chronic kidney disease. Am Fam Physician 2005:1723–1731.

A 25-year-old woman presents to the office with a 1-week history of vaginal discharge. She describes the discharge as being green-yellow in color with a bad odor. She has never had this type of discharge in the past. She complains of increased vaginal soreness and discharge after she has intercourse. She denies any itching, abdominal pain, nausea, vomiting, fever, chills, or sweats. She is currently sexually active and is using an intrauterine device (IUD) as her contraceptive method. She has been with a one male partner for the past 3 months and he has no symptoms. She does state that she first had intercourse at age 15 and has had multiple sexual partners. She had a chlamydial infection 2 years ago that was treated with oral antibiotics. Her last menstrual period was 2 weeks ago and was normal. She also denies any recent antibiotic treatment. On examination, she is afebrile, has normal vital signs, and appears to be in no acute distress. Her general physical examination is normal. On pelvic examination, she has normal external genitalia. She has a small amount of frothy, homogenous green-gray discharge at the introitus. The cervix has a "strawberry"-red appearance with a slight amount of discharge noted in the os. The IUD string is in place. Chlamydia and gonorrhea specimens are obtained from the os and a sample of the vaginal discharge is collected for microscopic evaluation. Bimanual examination shows no cervical motion tenderness, and a normal uterus and adnexa.

◆ **What organism is the most likely cause of her symptoms?**

◆ **What would you expect to see on microscopic examination of the vaginal discharge?**

◆ **What is the recommended treatment for this infection?**

ANSWERS TO CASE 22: Vaginitis

Summary: A 25-year-old woman presents with a foul-smelling vaginal discharge. She has a greenish, frothy discharge and a "strawberry cervix" noted on examination.

◆ **Organism most likely to cause this infection:** *Trichomonas vaginalis*

◆ **Expected microscopic examination findings:** Motile, flagellated trichomonads, and many white blood cells

◆ **Recommended treatment:** Metronidazole 2 g by mouth in a single dose for both the patient and her sexual partner. Metronidazole 500 mg twice a day for a week is an alternate regimen.

Analysis

Objectives

1. Be able to differentiate among common presentations of vaginitis on the basis of clinical information and laboratory testing.
2. Know the current guidelines for treatment of the various etiologies of vaginitis.

Considerations

Women with vaginitis may present with a variety of symptoms, including vaginal discharge, itching, odor, and dysuria. There are many potential causes of vaginitis, including sexually transmitted pathogens and overgrowth of organisms found in the normal vaginal flora. Common among the causes of vaginitis are *Candida albicans, Trichomonas vaginalis,* and *Gardnerella vaginalis.*

Certain historical information may lead a clinician to suspect a specific cause of vaginitis in a given patient. For example, a history of recent antibiotic use may predispose to a *Candida* vaginitis, as the antibiotic may alter the normal vaginal flora and allow the overgrowth of a fungal organism. Women with diabetes mellitus are also more predisposed to developing yeast infections. A history of multiple sexual partners may raise the likelihood of a sexually transmitted infection, such as trichomoniasis.

The patient's symptoms and signs may also suggest a specific organism as the cause of her vaginitis. Fungal infections tend to have thick discharge and cause significant pruritus. The discharge of bacterial vaginosis is often thinner and patients complain of a "fishy" odor. *Trichomonas* produces a discharge that is usually frothy and the patient's cervix is frequently very erythematous.

The key test to determining the cause of vaginal discharge, which guides the specific treatment, is microscopic examination of the discharge. A sample of the discharge is examined both as a "wet mount" (i.e., mixed with a small amount of normal saline) and as a "KOH prep" (i.e., mixed with a small amount of 10% potassium hydroxide). On wet mount, the examiner can evaluate the normal epithelial cells and look for white blood cells, red blood cells, clue cells, and motile trichomonads. The hyphae or pseudohyphae of *Candida* are best seen on KOH prep.

Etiologies

Vulvovaginal Candidiasis

This infection is typically caused by *C. albicans*, although other species are occasionally identified. **More than 75% of women have at least one episode during their lifetime.** The presenting symptom is a thick, whitish discharge that has no odor and the patient complains of significant pruritus of the external and internal genitalia. On physical examination, the vaginal area can be edematous with erythema present. The discharge has a pH between 4.0 and 5.0. The diagnosis is confirmed by wet mount or KOH preparation showing budding yeast or pseudohyphae. **Fungal cultures are not needed to confirm the diagnosis,** but they are useful if the infection recurs or is unresponsive to treatment. Numerous treatment options are available for patients with vulvovaginal candidiasis, including over-the-counter and prescription medications. Uncomplicated candidiasis can be treated effectively with short-term intravaginal preparations (creams or vaginal suppositories) or single-dose oral therapies (fluconazole 150 mg). Treatment of complicated or recurrent infection should begin with an intensive regimen for 10–14 days followed by 6 months of maintenance therapy to reduce the likelihood of recurrence. Treatment of sexual partners is not indicated unless symptomatic (e.g., male partners with balanitis).

Trichomoniasis

This infection is caused by the protozoan *T. vaginalis* and is classified as a sexually transmitted disease. The incubation period is 3–21 days after exposure. **Certain factors predispose to infection, such as multiple sexual partners, pregnancy, and menopause.** The presenting complaint is copious amounts of a thin, frothy, green-yellow or gray malodorous vaginal discharge. Women can also have vaginal soreness or dyspareunia. Symptoms may start or be exacerbated during the time of their menses. Vaginal examination may reveal that the **cervix has a "strawberry" appearance** (red and inflamed with punctuations) or that redness of the vagina and perineum is present. Microscopically, the **wet mount preparation can demonstrate motile trichomonads,** although cultures may be necessary because of the significant number of false-negative results. The recommended treatment for trichomoniasis is oral metronidazole, given in a single, 2-g oral dose or 1-week regimen of 500 mg BID to both the patient and her sexual partner. **It is important to screen for other sexually transmitted diseases (STDs) and to remember to treat the partner to ensure better cure rates.**

Bacterial Vaginosis

Bacterial vaginosis (BV) arises when normal vaginal bacteria are replaced with an **overgrowth of anaerobic bacteria and *G. vaginalis*.** Although not an STD, it is associated with having multiple sexual partners. **Diagnosis can be based on the presence of three of four clinical criteria:** (a) a thin, homogenous vaginal discharge; (b) a vaginal pH >4.5; (c) a positive KOH "whiff" test (a fishy odor present after the addition of 10% KOH to a sample of the discharge); and (d) the presence of clue cells in a wet mount preparation (Fig. 22–1). Culture is generally not needed. Treatment options include both oral and topical vaginal preparations of metronidazole or clindamycin. There are no advantages to any of these regimens with regard to cure rates or recurrence, although patients do

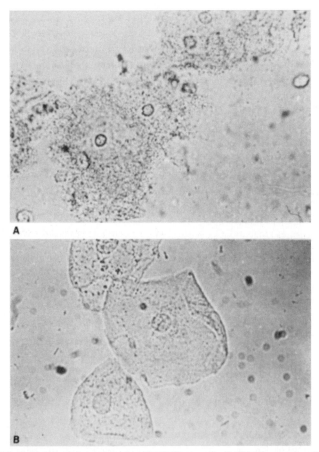

Figure 22–1. Bacterial vaginosis. (A) "Clue cells." (B) Normal epithelium.
(*Reproduced with permission from Kasper DL, Braunwauld E, Fauci A, et al. Harrison's principles of internal medicine. 16th ed. New York: McGraw-Hill, 2005:767.*)

report more satisfaction with the vaginal preparations. **Treatment of BV in asymptomatic pregnant women may reduce the incidence of preterm delivery.** Treatment of sexual partners is not necessary and does not reduce the risk of recurrent infection.

Mucopurulent Cervicitis

This infection is characterized by purulent or mucopurulent discharge from the endocervix, which may be associated with vaginal discharge and/or cervical bleeding. The diagnostic evaluation should include testing for *Chlamydia trachomatis* and *Neisseria gonorrhoeae,* although the etiologic agent is not always found. Absence of symptoms should not prevent additional evaluation and treatment, as **approximately 50% of gonococcal infections and 70% of chlamydial infections are asymptomatic in women.** The gold standard for establishing the diagnosis is a culture of the cervical discharge. **Empiric treatment should be considered in areas of high prevalence of infection or if follow-up is unlikely.** The treatment recommendation for gonorrhea is ceftriaxone 125 mg intramuscularly; alternative therapies are ciprofloxacin 500 mg or ofloxacin 400 mg in a single oral dose. The recommended treatment for *Chlamydia* infections is doxycycline 100 mg orally twice daily for 7 days or azithromycin in a single 1-g oral dose when compliance is a concern. Typical treatment regimens will cover for both gonorrhea and chlamydia and the treatment of sexual partners is advised.

Pelvic Inflammatory Disease

Pelvic inflammatory disease (PID) is defined as inflammation of the upper genital tract, including pelvic peritonitis, endometritis, salpingitis, and tuboovarian abscess caused by infection with gonorrhea, *Chlamydia*, or vaginal and bowel flora. **Lower abdominal tenderness with both adnexal and cervical motion tenderness without other explanation of illness is enough to diagnose PID.** Other criteria that enhance the specificity of the diagnosis include temperature >101°F, abnormal cervical or vaginal discharge, elevated sedimentation rate, elevated C-reactive protein, and cervical infection with gonorrhea or *Chlamydia*. Definitive diagnosis rests on techniques that are not generally used or readily available to make the diagnosis, such as laparoscopic findings consistent with PID, endometrial biopsy showing endometritis, and ultrasound examination findings showing thickened fluid-filled tubes with or without free pelvic fluid or tuboovarian complex. **Because of the clinical similarity between PID and ectopic pregnancy, a serum pregnancy test should be performed on all patients suspected of having PID.**

Determination of appropriate treatment should consider pregnancy status, severity of illness, and compliance. **Less-severe disease can generally be treated on an outpatient basis. Women who are pregnant, have HIV, or have severe disease generally require inpatient therapy and treatment with parenteral antibiotics.** Table 22–1 lists PID treatment regimens.

Table 22–1
TREATMENT REGIMENS FOR PID

Oral
  Ofloxacin 400 mg PO BID for 14 days *or*
  Levofloxacin 500 mg PO BID for 14 days
    With or without metronidazole 500 mg PO BID for 14 days
  Ceftriaxone 250 mg IM single dose *or*
  Cefoxitin 2 g IM and probenecid 1 g PO given concurrently *plus* doxycycline
  100 mg PO BID for 14 days
    With or without metronidazole 500 mg PO BID for 14 days
Parenteral
  Cefotetan 2 g IV of 12 h *or*
  Cefoxitin 2 g IV of 12 h *plus* doxycycline 100 mg PO *or* IV of 12 h
  Clindamycin 900 mg IV of 8 h *plus* gentamicin 2 mg/kg loading dose followed by
  1.5 mg/kg IV of 8 h
  Ofloxacin 400 mg IV of 12 h *or* levofloxacin 500 mg IV daily
    With or without metronidazole 500 mg IV of 8 h
  Ampicillin/sulbactam 3 g IV of 6 h *plus* doxycycline 100 mg PO *or* IV of 2 h

Patients who have PID need to be aware of potential complications, including the potential for recurrence of disease, the development of tuboovarian abscess, chronic abdominal pain, infertility, and the increased risk of ectopic pregnancy. It is important to discuss these potential problems with patients who are given a diagnosis of PID. All patients with STDs or who are at risk for developing STDs should be counseled on safer sexual practices, including abstinence, monogamy, and the use of latex condoms.

Comprehension Questions

[22.1] Which of the following vaginitis infections does not require treatment in the sexual partner to prevent recurrence of infection in the patient?

    A. Vaginal candidiasis
    B. Bacterial vaginosis
    C. Gonococcal cervicitis
    D. Trichomoniasis

[22.2] Which of the following factors predisposes females to vulvovaginal candidiasis infections?

    A. Recent antibiotic use
    B. Hypothyroidism
    C. Condom use
    D. Menopause

[22.3] Which of the following treatments regimens for PID is correct?

A. Ceftriaxone 125 mg IM plus azithromycin 1 g PO
B. Cefoxitin 2 g IV q 12 h plus doxycycline 100 mg PO BID
C. Ceftriaxone 250 mg IM plus doxycycline 100 mg PO BID for 7 days
D. Ciprofloxacin 500 mg PO single dose plus doxycycline 100 mg PO BID for 7 days

Answers

[22.1] **B.** Partner treatment is not necessary for bacterial vaginosis. In most cases, it is not necessary in candida vaginitis, unless the partner has a symptomatic infection such as balanitis. Partner treatment is necessary for any sexually transmitted disease.

[22.2] **A.** Recent antibiotic use is a risk factor for developing a candidal infection. Other risk factors include diabetes mellitus, pregnancy, and oral contraceptive use.

[22.3] **B.** Option B is an appropriate regimen for the in-patient management of PID. The other regimens listed are appropriate for the treatment of cervicitis but not PID.

CLINICAL PEARLS

❖ Remember to treat sexual partners when you diagnose a sexually transmitted infection and consider testing for infections that may initially be asymptomatic, such as HIV and syphilis.

❖ Single-dose therapy is available for many types of infections, including *Trichomonas,* gonococcal and chlamydial cervicitis, candida vaginitis. Providing single-dose therapy in your office will improve your patient's compliance, as well as rates of successful treatment.

REFERENCES

Newkirk GR. Pelvic inflammatory disease: a contemporary approach. Am Fam Physician 1996;53:1127–1135.

Rakel RE. Essentials of family practice. Philadelphia: WB Saunders, 1993.

South-Paul JE, Matheny SC., Lewis EL (eds.). Current diagnosis and treatment in family medicine. New York: McGraw-Hill, 2004.

Workowski KA, Levine WC. Sexually transmitted diseases treatment guidelines. MMWR 2002;51(RR06):1–80.

A 62-year-old male presents to your office for a routine evaluation. His only complaint is of fatigue over the past 2–3 months despite no changes in diet or lifestyle. On questioning, the patient reports that he has never smoked and admits to an increase in his consumption of alcohol upon retiring, to about 2–3 beers per day. He has occasional headaches on the day after a night of heavier drinking, which are easily relieved by the use of over-the-counter nonsteroidal anti-inflammatory drug (NSAID) preparations. While talking to the patient and examining his chart you note no distress and proceed with your examination. You note a 4 lb weight loss since his last visit 6 months ago and a relative increase in his pulse with a blood pressure of 129/81 mmHg. Remarkable to this visit is the paleness of his conjunctivae, but the rest of his general examination is unchanged from the previous examination. You perform a digital rectal exam and find a smooth, normal-size prostate and some soft, reducible protrusions within the internal sphincter, along with guaiac-positive stools. You decide on a more direct approach and delve into his drinking, bowel habits, and NSAID use. His only addition is the occasional production of bloody stools accompanied by some diffuse abdominal discomfort.

◆ **What is the most likely diagnosis?**

◆ **What is your next diagnostic step?**

◆ **What is the next step in therapy?**

ANSWERS TO CASE 23: Lower Gastrointestinal Bleeding

Summary: A 62-year-old male presents to your office for a routine checkup. He reports having occasional bloody stools and you discover guaiac-positive stools. He is a bit pale, but hemodynamically stable at the moment. You decide that further evaluation of this bleeding is necessary, but most of it can be carried out on an outpatient basis with close follow-up.

◆ **Most likely diagnosis:** Hemorrhoids

◆ **Next diagnostic step:** Complete blood count (CBC) and colonoscopy

◆ **Next step in therapy:** Discontinue NSAID use and decrease alcohol consumption

Objectives

1. Know how to recognize the subtle signs and symptoms of lower GI bleeding.
2. Understand the etiologies of lower GI bleeding.
3. Understand how to correctly evaluate and treat patients with lower GI bleeding in outpatient settings.

Considerations

This 62-year-old male presented to your office for a routine examination but was found to have some type of lower gastrointestinal bleeding that needs further evaluation. During his office visit there are no signs of hemodynamic instability or active bleeding that require immediate referral to an emergency room or inpatient treatment, so you decide on close outpatient follow-up during his work-up. His immediate identifiable and modifiable risk factors for GI bleeding include the regular consumption of alcohol and NSAIDs. You counsel him on both these matters and send him to the lab for a CBC, chemistry panel, liver function tests, and coagulation profile prior to his discharge home from your office. Barring any abnormal lab values that require emergent management, you schedule him for an outpatient colonoscopy later in the week. Your differential diagnosis at this time is wide but you start to consider the most frequent offenders in his age group, which include diverticular disease, hemorrhoids, tumors, and ulcerative colitis. For the time being, you modify those factors that may contribute to any of these etiologies and await the results of his laboratory tests.

APPROACH TO LOWER GI BLEEDING

Definitions

Hematochezia: Bright red blood visible in the stool.
Lower GI bleeding: Bleeding that comes from a source distal to the ligament of Treitz.

Clinical Presentation

The manifestations of GI bleeding depend on the source, rate of bleeding, and underlying or coexisting disease. An older patient, or someone with significant comorbidities, such as coronary artery disease, would be at a higher risk of presenting in shock. A younger, healthier individual may present with symptoms such as fatigue or dyspnea on exertion, or may complain directly of seeing blood in the stool. Signs and symptoms of anemia are common and include weakness, easy fatigability, pallor of the conjunctivae or skin, chest pain, dizziness, tachycardia, hypotension, and orthostasis.

A history of blood in the stool or finding guaiac-positive stool on examination should prompt further evaluation to determine the source of the bleeding. Depending on a patient's history and hemodynamic status, more immediate and invasive measures may be necessary once GI bleeding is identified. For example, **hematochezia is usually pathognomonic of lower GI bleeding, but can also be found in patients with heavy upper GI bleeding.** In this setting, a nasogastric aspirate may help differentiate this small subset of patients.

Evaluation of the "ABCs" (airway, breathing, and circulation) is critical in unstable patients who present with GI bleeding. ICU admission should not be delayed in those with severe bleeding and a team approach, consisting of a gastroenterologist, a surgeon with expertise in GI surgery, and skilled nursing, should always be anticipated. Major causes of morbidity and mortality in patients with GI bleeding include blood aspiration and shock. To prevent these complications, endotracheal intubation should always be considered to protect the airway of patients with altered mental status. Most lower GI bleeding does not warrant emergency therapy, but be prepared for decompensation in the elderly and in those with borderline normal hemodynamic parameters.

Diagnosis

The test of choice for the determination of the source of lower GI bleeding is colonoscopy. Adequate bowel preparation with an oral sulfate purge to clear the bowel of blood, clots, and stool increases the yield in diagnosing colonic bleeding sites. Angiography and technetium-labeled colloid or red blood cell scans may be of value if colonoscopy cannot be performed or if heavy bleeding prevents adequate visualization of the colon. However, the magnitude of bleeding required to show the bleeding site limits their usefulness. Sigmoidoscopy with air-contrast barium enema x-rays may be an alternative when colonoscopy is unavailable or if the patient refuses colonoscopy. If the initial sigmoidoscopy is negative, a colonoscopy must be performed. If both of these studies are negative, panendoscopy should be carried out.

Always consider the possibility of upper GI bleeding as a source of hematochezia. An aspirate from a nasogastric tube can help to make this determination. An aspirate that shows bile but not blood will help to confirm that the bleeding is from a lower GI source.

Etiologies

Hemorrhoids

Hemorrhoids are dilated veins in the hemorrhoidal plexus of the anus. They are defined as "internal" if they arise above the dentate line and "external" if they arise below the dentate line; both can be the cause of hematochezia. Chronic constipation, straining for bowel movements, pregnancy, and prolonged sitting (e.g., truck drivers) are risk factors. Along with bleeding, external hemorrhoids can cause pain, irritation, and a palpable lump. Internal hemorrhoids can cause bleeding and can prolapse through the anus. Conservative treatment with a high-fiber diet, stool softeners, and precautions against prolonged straining are usually successful. When necessary, various surgical procedures can be performed for definitive treatment.

Diverticular Disease

Diverticula are outpouchings of the colonic mucosa through weakened areas of the colon wall. They occur most often where blood vessels penetrate through the muscles of the colon. They are **most often asymptomatic and found on endoscopy or bowel imaging studies.** They can cause symptomatic, and occasionally massive, bleeding that is usually painless. Diverticular bleeding usually stops spontaneously. When the bleeding is extremely heavy or fails to stop, surgical resection of the affected portion of the colon may be necessary. Asymptomatic diverticulosis is managed with dietary modification, primarily a high-fiber diet.

Diverticulitis is a painful inflammation and infection of a diverticulum. Diverticulitis frequently causes left lower quadrant abdominal pain along with fever, nausea, diarrhea, and constipation. Perforation of a diverticulum resulting in peritonitis or intraabdominal abscess formation can be a complication. Diverticulitis is typically treated with bowel rest and antibiotics effective against gut flora. A combination of a quinolone and an agent for anaerobic organisms, such as metronidazole, is one commonly used regimen. In severe cases, or when perforation occurs, surgery may be indicated.

Inflammatory Bowel Disease

Ulcerative colitis and Crohn disease are the two primary diagnoses considered in the category of inflammatory bowel disease (IBD). **Ulcerative colitis causes**

continuous inflammation of the large bowel, starting from the rectum and extending proximally. Severe disease can cause pancolitis, affecting the entire colon. **Crohn disease causes areas of focal inflammation, but can occur anywhere in the gastrointestinal tract.** Both diseases can cause recurrent episodes of abdominal pain, diarrhea, weight loss, rectal bleeding, fistulas, and abscesses. The definitive etiology of IBD is not known, but these are autoimmune syndromes and a family history of IBD is a major risk factor. Along with GI symptoms, **numerous extraintestinal manifestations may occur, most frequently arthritis.** Other extraintestinal manifestations include sclerosing cholangitis, cirrhosis, fatty liver, pyoderma gangrenosum, and erythema nodosum. Ulcerative colitis is a significant risk factor for the development of colon cancer. Patients with ulcerative colitis require frequent surveillance colonoscopic examinations. IBD can be managed with symptomatic therapy, such as antidiarrheal medications, along with antiinflammatory medications (aminosalicylates, corticosteroids) given orally or as enemas, and immunosuppressive medications. Ulcerative colitis can be definitively treated with a total colectomy, which is usually reserved for severe pancolitis, failure to respond to medical therapy, or because of the risk of colon cancer.

Colon Neoplasms

Polyps are benign neoplasms of the colon. Hyperplastic polyps tend to be small, smooth growths found incidentally during endoscopy and are of no prognostic significance. Adenomatous polyps are benign growths that have a potential to become malignant. Listed in order of potential for becoming cancerous (from least to most), the three types of adenomas are tubular adenomas, tubulovillous adenomas, and villous adenomas. Larger polyps have a higher risk of causing bleeding and becoming malignant than smaller polyps. Polyps can be identified and removed during a colonoscopy.

Colon cancer is the second leading cause of cancer death in men and women. The risk of colon cancer increases with age, with a history of colon polyps, a family history of colon cancer or a personal history of ulcerative colitis. **Any patient older than age 50 years who has lower GI bleeding must be evaluated for the presence of colon cancer.** Because of the presence of premalignant lesions (polyps) that can be identified and removed in asymptomatic patients, colon cancer screening is recommended for all adults older than age 50, and at younger ages for those with increased risks. The treatment and prognosis of colon cancer depends upon the stage in which it is found. The Dukes System stages colon cancer from A to D, depending on the penetration through the bowel wall layer, the presence of lymph node spread, and distant metastases. Dukes A colon cancer has an excellent prognosis with surgical resection; Dukes D cancer is usually not curable and is treated with combinations of surgery, chemotherapy and radiation.

Diverticular bleeding occurs in 10–20% of cases of lower GI bleeding, with most cases being increased by NSAID or aspirin use. In diverticular disease, bleeding is often self-limited and ceases approximately 75% of the time, while recurring at a rate of approximately 38%. More common causes include hemorrhoids (59%), colorectal polyps (38–52%), diverticulosis (34–51%), colorectal cancer (8%), ulcerative colitis, arteriovenous malformations and colonic strictures. These percentages vary amongst age groups and most serious causes are expected in the elderly.

Comprehension Questions

Match the following pathology with their most frequent clinical presentation:

      A. Hypertrophic polyps
      B. Hemorrhoids
      C. Adenomatous colon polyps
      D. Colon cancer
      E. Ulcerative colitis
      F. Diverticular disease

[23.1] Premalignant colon neoplasm

[23.2] Left lower quadrant pain accompanied by alternating bouts of constipation and diarrhea

[23.3] Small growth in colon with no prognostic significance

[23.4] Prognosis depends on depth of invasion

[23.5] Chronic, painful, loose stooling with blood and joint pain

[23.6] Blood-tinged sanitary paper upon wiping after a bowel movement

Answers

[23.1] **C.** Adenomatous colon polyps are premalignant lesions. The risk of becoming malignant increases as the polyp grows larger. Villous adenomas have the highest risk of malignant transformation, tubular adenomas have the lowest risk, and tubulovillous are intermediate.

[23.2] **F.** Left lower quadrant abdominal pain with constipation, diarrhea, or alternating bouts is consistent with diverticulitis.

[23.3] **A.** Hyperplastic polyps are commonly seen during colonoscopy and are of no prognostic significance.

[23.4] **D.** Colon cancer is the second most common cause of cancer death in the United States. Its prognosis is related to the depth of invasion at the time of diagnosis.

[23.5] **E.** Chronic, recurrent, painful, loose stooling, often with blood, is consistent with ulcerative colitis. Arthritis can also occur with this disease.

[23.6] **B.** Blood with wiping, a palpable anal lump, itching, or irritation are common presentations of hemorrhoids.

CLINICAL PEARLS

❖ Lower GI bleeding is usually suspected in lesions or pathology that is distal to the angle of Treitz. Simple measures like nasogastric lavage can aid in ruling out upper GI bleeding as a cause of hematochezia.

❖ In a patient with acute bleeding, avoid performing a test that will not give an adequate diagnostic yield, such as a flexible sigmoidoscopy or barium enema.

❖ Any patient older than age 50 years with blood in the stool must be evaluated for colon cancer.

REFERENCES

Anthony T, Penta P, Todd RD, et al. Rebleeding and survival after acute lower gastrointestinal bleeding. Am J Surg 2004;188:485–490.

Bassford T. Treatment of common anorectal disorders. Am Fam Physician 1992;45:1787–1794.

Manning-Dimmitt LL, Dimmitt SG, Wilson GR. Diagnosis of gastrointestinal bleeding in adults. Am Fam Physician 2005;71:1339–1346.

Salzman H, Lillie D. Diverticular disease: diagnosis and treatment. Am Fam Physician 2005;72:1229–1234.

Stenson WF, Goldman L, Ausiello D. Inflammatory bowel disease. In: Cecil textbook of medicine. 22nd ed. Philadelphia: WB Saunders, 2004:861–869.

Zuber TJ. Hemorrhoidectomy for thrombosed external hemorrhoids. Am Fam Physician 2002;65:1629–1639.

A 61-year-old female presents to the emergency room complaining of cough for 2 weeks. The cough is productive of green sputum and is associated with sweating, shaking chills, and fever up to 102°F. She was exposed to her grand-children who were told that they had upper respiratory infections 2 weeks ago but now are fine. Her past medical history is significant for diabetes for 10 years, which is under good control using oral hypoglycemics. She denies tobacco, alcohol, or drug use. On examination, she looks ill and in distress, with continuous coughing and chills. Her blood pressure is 100/80 mm Hg, her pulse is 110 beats/min, her temperature is 101°F, her respirations are 24 breaths/min, and her oxygen saturation is 97% on room air. Examination of the head and neck is unremarkable. Her lungs have rhonchi and decreased breath sounds, with dullness to percussion in bilateral bases. Her heart is tachycardic but reg-ular. Her extremities are without signs of cyanosis or edema. The remainder of her examination is normal. A complete blood count (CBC) shows a high white blood cell (WBC) count of 17,000 cells/mm^3, with a differential of 85% neu-trophils and 20% lymphocytes. Her blood sugar is 120 mg/dL.

◆ **What is the most likely diagnosis?**

◆ **What is your next diagnostic step?**

◆ **What is the next step in therapy?**

◆ **What are potential complications of this diagnosis?**

ANSWERS TO CASE 24: Pneumonia

Summary: This is a 61-year-old female with fever, chills, and productive cough. She has an abnormal pulmonary examination and is found to have a high white cell count. Her significant medical history is diabetes mellitus.

◆ **Most likely diagnosis:** Community-acquired pneumonia

◆ **Next diagnostic step:** Chest x-ray, sputum Gram stain and culture, and blood cultures

◆ **Next therapeutic step:** Determine whether patient requires in-patient or out-patient therapy and start antibiotics.

◆ **Potential complications:** Bacteremia, sepsis, parapneumonic pleural effusion, empyema

Analysis

Objectives

1. Recognize the differential diagnosis of pneumonia.
2. Be familiar with widely accepted decision-making strategies for the diagnosis and management of different kinds of pneumonia.
3. Learn about the treatment and follow-up of pneumonia.
4. Recognize the effects of comorbid conditions.

Considerations

This 61-year-old patient presents with a common diagnostic dilemma: productive cough with green sputum and fever. The first priority for the physician is to assess whether the patient is more ill than the complaint would indicate. Helpful clues to the patient's overall condition include a toxic appearance, using accessory muscles to breathe, and low oxygen saturation. Tachycardia, hypotension, and altered mentation are signs of more critical illness. **Airway, breathing, and circulation must always be addressed.**

Fortunately, this patient does not have those alarming symptoms. If a patient has respiratory distress, the physician may need to check arterial blood gases. If the patient has low oxygen saturation, give oxygen by nasal cannula and then proceed to your history and physical examination.

The most common etiology of cough is an upper respiratory tract infection. This patient has several features that make pneumonia more likely, including her **age, cough with green sputum, fever with chills, and exposure to close contacts with respiratory infections.** The gold standard for diagnosis of pneumonia is the presence of an infiltrate on chest x-ray, although normal x-ray does not exclude the diagnosis. X-rays may be normal early in the course of disease and a patient who is dehydrated may not demonstrate an infiltrate until the patient is adequately rehydrated.

APPROACH TO PNEUMONIA

Bronchitis and pneumonia represent a continuum of lower respiratory infection. The extent of involvement of adjacent lung parenchyma determines whether there is an infiltrate on x-ray. **Pneumonia is defined as infection of lung parenchyma** caused by agents that include bacteria, viruses, fungi, and parasites. It should be distinguished from pneumonitis, which is an inflammation of the lungs from a variety of noninfectious causes such as chemicals, blood, radiation, and autoimmune processes. The occurrence and severity of pneumonia depends on both the state of the body's defense mechanism against infection and the characteristics of the infectious agent. The **most common mechanism triggering pneumonia is upper airway colonization** by potentially pathogenic organisms that are subsequently aspirated. The type of organism involved depends, in part, on host characteristics.

Community-Acquired Pneumonia

Pneumonia that occurs in persons who are not hospital in-patients or residents of long-term care facilities is defined as community acquired. The most common bacterial cause of community-acquired pneumonia is *Streptococcus pneumoniae* (pneumonococcus). Other common bacterial etiologies are *Haemophilus influenzae* and *Moraxella catarrhalis.* Pneumococcal pneumonia classically causes an illness of acute onset with cough productive of rust-colored sputum, fever, shaking chills, and a lobar infiltrate on chest x-ray. *H. influenzae* is often seen in patients with underlying chronic obstructive pulmonary disease.

   Mycoplasma pneumoniae, Chlamydia pneumoniae, and *Legionella pneumophila* are bacteria that cause what is classified as "atypical" pneumonia. Atypical pneumonia is also caused by several different viruses. The **typical pneumonia organisms are more common in the very young and in the older patient.** Atypical pneumonias occur more commonly in adolescent or young adult patients. Atypical organisms tend to cause bilateral, diffuse infiltrates, rather than focal, lobar infiltrates, on x-ray.

Hospital-Acquired Pneumonia

Hospital-acquired pneumonia is a major source of morbidity, mortality, and prolonged hospitalization. **Risk factors include intubation, nasogastric tube feeding, preexisting lung disease, and multisystem failure.** The organisms involved include the pathogens involved in community-acquired pneumonia as well as aerobic Gram-negative bacteria (*Pseudomonas, Klebsiella, Acinetobacter*) and Gram-positive cocci such as *Staphylococcus aureus.* The incidence of drug-resistant organisms, such as methicillin-resistant *Staphylococcus aureus,* is increasing. Avoiding intubation when possible, using oropharyngeal intubation as opposed to nasopharyngeal intubation, keeping the head of the patient's bed elevated during tube feedings, and infection control techniques, such as careful handwashing and use of alcohol-based hand disinfectants, can reduce risks.

Diagnosis

Patient history in pneumonia commonly includes the symptoms of productive cough, fever, pleuritic chest pain, and dyspnea. The symptoms can be very nonspecific in the very old and very young. In young children, rapid breathing is commonly seen; in the elderly, pneumonia may present as altered mental status.

Sometimes the history may lead to assistance in determining the specific organism involved. An abrupt onset or abruptly worsening illness is seen frequently in pneumococcal pneumonia. *Legionella* often causes diarrhea along with pneumonia. *S. aureus* is a common cause of postinfluenza pneumonia.

Physical examination findings can include fever, tachycardia, tachypnea, hypotension, and reduced oxygen saturation. Auscultation of the lungs may reveal rhonchi or rales. Egophony (E to A change) can be a sign of focal lung consolidation and dullness to percussion may be the result of a pulmonary effusion.

All patients with suspected pneumonia should have a chest x-ray. The presence of an infiltrate can confirm the diagnosis. Absence of an infiltrate does not rule out pneumonia as a diagnosis. A chest x-ray can also identify a pleural effusion, which may be a complication of pneumonia (parapneumonic effusion).

Specific x-ray findings may also lead to consideration of certain etiologic agents or types of pneumonia. As noted previously, lobar infiltrates are more common with typical infections and diffuse infiltrates are more likely with atypical infections. A bilateral, "ground glass"-appearing infiltrate is associated with *Pneumocystis carinii* infections, which are seen most often in patients with AIDS. Apical consolidation may be seen with tuberculosis. Pneumonia caused by the aspiration of gastrointestinal contents commonly is seen in the right lower lobe because of the branching of the bronchial tree.

Other testing indicated in patients with pneumonia includes a complete blood count (CBC) and a chemistry panel. Specific microbiologic diagnosis is possible with blood or sputum cultures. **Cultures have a low sensitivity** (many false negatives), but a positive culture can help to guide treatment. Direct fluorescent antibody testing on sputum can be used to identify *Legionella* and *Mycoplasma; Legionella* can also be identified by urinary antigen testing.

Treatment

When pneumonia is diagnosed, the initial decision to be made is can the patient be treated safely as an outpatient or is hospitalization required. One method of making this determination is to use the **Pneumonia Severity Index, which assigns patients to a risk category based on their age, comorbid illnesses, specific examination, and laboratory findings.** High-risk comorbidities include neoplastic disease, liver disease, renal disease, congestive heart failure, and diabetes. Physical examination findings taken into consideration are tachypnea, fever, hypotension, tachycardia, and altered mental status. Laboratory findings include a low pH, low serum sodium, low hematocrit, low oxygen saturation, high glucose, high blood urea nitrogen (BUN), and pleural effusion on x-ray. Based on the patient's demographics and individual findings, a risk class and mortality risk is assigned. Low-risk classes (classes 1 and 2) can be safely treated as an outpatient; higher-risk classes (classes 3, 4, and 5) should be hospitalized.

The emergence of drug-resistant pneumococci and the development of new antimicrobials have changed the empiric treatment of community acquired pneumonia. Newer fluoroquinolones with activity against *S. pneumoniae* offer alternatives in the treatment of drug-resistant *S. pneumoniae* infection. Macrolides, such as azithromycin and clarithromycin, may be preferable to erythromycin because of better GI tolerance. For outpatient therapy, a macrolide or an oral β-lactam (e.g., cefuroxime, amoxicillin, or amoxicillin-clavulanate) is recommended by the CDC. An oral fluoroquinolone with activity against *S. pneumoniae* can be substituted if the patient is allergic to macrolides or β-lactam antibiotics.

For hospitalized patients with community-acquired pneumonia, an intravenous β-lactam (e.g., cefuroxime, cefotaxime, ceftriaxone, or ampicillin-sulbactam) and an intravenous macrolide (erythromycin or azithromycin) are recommended. An IV fluoroquinolone with activity against *S. pneumoniae* can be substituted.

The follow-up visit to the office 3–4 days later will help to assess response to therapy. Early follow-up chest x-rays are mandatory in those who fail to show clinical improvement by 5–7 days, because bronchogenic carcinoma can present with the picture of a typical pneumonitis.

Hospital-acquired pneumonias require broader antibiotic coverage of the likely pathogens, many of which have developed multiple-drug resistance. One regimen includes a β-lactam plus an antipseudomonal fluoroquinolone or aminoglycoside. Methicillin-resistant *S. aureus* may require treatment with vancomycin.

The duration of the treatment is influenced by the severity of illness, the etiologic agent, response to therapy, the presence of other medical problems, and complications. Therapy until the patient is afebrile for at least 72 hours is usually sufficient for pneumonia caused by *S. pneumoniae*. A minimum of 2 weeks of therapy is appropriate for pneumonia caused by *S. aureus, Pseudomonas aeruginosa, Klebsiella*, anaerobes, *Mycoplasma pneumoniae, Chlamydia pneumoniae*, or *Legionella* species.

Complications

Bacteremia occurs in approximately 25–30% of patients with pneumococcal pneumonia. Mortality rates range for patients with bacteremia from 20–30%, but can be as high as 60% in the elderly. Parapneumonic pleural effusion develops in 40% of hospitalized patients with pneumococcal pneumonia. Fewer than 5% of cases progress to empyema. If more than a minimal amount of fluid is present, as evidenced by significant blunting of the costophrenic angle on x-ray, it may be necessary to perform a thoracentesis with Gram stain and culture of the pleural fluid. The presence of an empyema usually requires drainage with a chest tube or surgical procedure.

Prevention

Pneumococcal vaccine is recommended for all persons age 65 years and older, all adults with chronic cardiopulmonary diseases, and all immunocompromised persons. Consider revaccination every 5 years in patients known to have a rapid decline in antibody titers, such as those with nephritic syndrome or renal failure. Also consider repeating pneumococcal vaccination in asplenic patients. Revaccination has minimal side effects; the most common is a localized reaction at the site of injection.

Influenza vaccination is recommended in the late fall and winter months for populations at risk for infection, complications, or transmission of the influenza virus. The association between influenza virus infection and pneumonia is well recognized. The number of cases of invasive pneumococcal disease peaks in midwinter, when influenza is prevalent. Influenza virus infection can facilitate bacterial colonization and impair host defense mechanism. A prospective study of patients 65 years of age and older demonstrated the effectiveness of influenza and pneumococcal vaccination at reducing hospitalizations for pneumonia and at preventing invasive pneumococcal disease.

Comprehension Questions

[24.1] In which of the following settings are you most likely to find a bilateral, diffuse infiltrate on x-ray?

A. Pneumonia caused by *S. pneumoniae*
B. Pneumonia caused by *H. influenzae*
C. Pneumonia caused by aspiration of GI contents
D. Pneumonia caused by *M. pneumoniae*

[24.2] Which of the following tests should be ordered on any patient with a suspected pneumonia?

A. Chest x-ray
B. Blood cultures
C. HIV test
D. Urine for *Legionella* antigen

[24.3] Which of the following is most likely to reduce the risk of pneumonia in hospitalized patients?

A. Nasotracheal intubation
B. Placing the patient flat during tube feedings
C. Use of alcohol-based antimicrobial gel by healthcare workers
D. Changing the patient from face-mask oxygen to mechanical ventilation

Answers

[24.1] **D.** Bilateral, diffuse infiltrates are more likely to be seen in patients with pneumonia caused by atypical agents, such as *Mycoplasma*, than in patients with typical pneumonia or aspiration pneumonia.

[24.2] **A.** All patients with suspected pneumonia should have a chest x-ray. The other tests listed may be indicated depending on the clinical situation.

[24.3] **C.** The use of alcohol-based hand gels and strict handwashing techniques can reduce the risk of nosocomial pneumonia. All of the other listed options will increase the likelihood of pneumonia developing.

CLINICAL PEARLS

❖ Elderly patients often have fewer or less-severe symptoms or atypical presentations of pneumonia. Consider pneumonia in the differential diagnosis of altered mental status in the elderly.

❖ Appropriate use of influenza and pneumococcal vaccination reduces the risk of pneumonia in susceptible populations.

❖ Consider the diagnosis of empyema in patients with pneumonia and a pleural effusion, especially if the patients continue to have fever despite appropriate antibiotic therapy.

REFERENCES

American Thoracic Society and Infectious Diseases Society of America. Guidelines for the management of adults with hospital-acquired, ventilator-associated and healthcare-associated pneumonia. Am J Respir Crit Care Med 2005;171:388–416.

Bartlett JG. Diagnostic approach to community acquired pneumonia in adults. Up to Date 13.3. Available at: www.uptodate.com

Lutfiyya MN, Henley E, Chang LF. Diagnosis and treatment of community-acquired pneumonia. Am Fam Physician 2006;73:442–450.

Patel N, Criner G. Community acquired pneumonia in the elderly: Update on treatment strategies. Consultant 2003;43(6):689–701.

Tierney LM, McPhee SJ, Papadakis MA. Current medical diagnosis and treatment. New York: McGraw-Hill, 2004.

A 38-year-old female presents to the office with complaints of weight loss, fatigue, and insomnia of 3 months' duration. She reports that she has been feeling gradually more tired and staying up late at night because she can't sleep. She does not feel that she is doing as well in her occupation as a secretary and states that she has trouble remembering things. She does not go outdoors as much as she used to and cannot recall the last time she went out with friends or enjoyed a social gathering. She feels tired most of the week and states she feels that she wants to go to sleep and frequently does not want to get out of bed. She denies any recent medication, illicit drug, or alcohol use. She feels intense guilt regarding past failed relationships because she perceives them as faults. She states she has never thought of suicide, but has begun to feel increasingly worthless.

Her vital signs and general physical examination are normal, although she becomes tearful while talking. Her mental status examination is significant for depressed mood, psychomotor retardation, and difficulty attending to questions. Laboratory studies reveal a normal metabolic panel, normal complete blood count, and normal thyroid functions.

◆ **What is the most likely diagnosis?**

◆ **What is your next step?**

◆ **What are important considerations and potential complications of management?**

ANSWERS TO CASE 25: Major Depression

Summary: This is a 38-year-old female with depression. She meets at least five of the *Diagnostic and Statistical Manual of Mental Disorders, 4th Edition* (DSM-IV) diagnostic criteria during a 2-week period that represents a change from her previous level of functioning. At least one of the symptoms must be either depressed mood or loss of interest or pleasure.

◆ **Most likely diagnosis:** Major depression

◆ **Next step:** Evaluate the patient for suicidal risk, begin pharmacologic and psychotherapeutic management.

◆ **Important considerations and potential complications:** Rule out other medical diagnoses such as hypothyroidism, anemia, and infectious processes that could mimic some symptoms of depression; verify that no substance abuse or use is taking place; screen for bipolar disorder and inquire about a family history of mood disorders; investigate and address suicidal ideations; review any recent medication changes for agents that may contribute to these symptoms (e.g., β-blockers, steroids, sedatives, chemotherapy agents).

Analysis

Objectives

1. Recognize the common presenting signs and symptoms of depression.
2. Understand the multifactorial pathogenesis of depression.
3. Learn about the treatment of depression and the sequelae of this condition.
4. Be familiar with the appropriate follow-up of this condition.
5. Recognize the importance of assessing for suicidal risk.

APPROACH TO DEPRESSION

Background

Depression has a lifetime prevalence of 15–25%, with a **greater incidence in women and the elderly.** Symptoms for depression must include at least 5 of the 9 following symptoms, must occur during the same 2-week time period, must represent a change from previous functioning and must include either depressed mood or loss of interest or pleasure:

A.
    1. Depressed mood
    2. Diminished interest or pleasure
    3. Significant weight loss or weight gain
    4. Insomnia or hypersomnia
    5. Psychomotor agitation or retardation

6. Fatigue or loss of energy
7. Fatigue of worthlessness
8. Diminished ability to think or concentrate; indecisiveness
9. Recurrent thoughts of death, suicidal ideation, suicide attempt, or specific plan

B. Symptoms do not meet criteria for a mixed episode (both mania and depressive episode)
C. Symptoms cause clinically significant distress or impairment of functioning
D. Symptoms are not a result of the direct physiologic effects of a substance or a generalized medical condition
E. Symptoms are not accounted for by bereavement

A patient with depression commonly presents to the physician with various somatic complaints and decreased energy level rather than a complaint of depression. Patients often complain of sadness, sometimes of irritability or mood swings. Difficulty concentrating or loss of energy and motivation are common. Their thinking is often negative, frequently with feelings of worthlessness, hopelessness, or helplessness. Poor memory or concentration may be a complaint in others. The elderly may present with confusion or a general decline in functioning. **The diagnosis of depression needs to be considered in scenarios where a patient presents with multiple unrelated physical symptoms.**

The differential diagnosis of depression includes many other psychiatric and medical disorders. The psychiatric disorders include dysthymic disorder, bereavement, and bipolar disorder. **Numerous medical conditions can cause depressive symptoms.** Common among these are hypothyroidism and anemia. The role of pharmacologic agents and substance use, abuse, or dependence also should be investigated, as these can cause significant mood changes. This is especially true of alcohol, sedatives, narcotics, and cocaine.

Pathophysiology

The etiology of depression is thought to be multifactorial, involving a complex interaction of genetic, psychosocial, and neurobiologic factors. Multiple neurotransmitter systems are implicated, including the serotoninergic, noradrenergic, and dopaminergic systems. Evidence of the effects of neurotransmitters on mood disorders is supported by the knowledge of the mechanism of action of antidepressant medications. All currently available antidepressant agents appear to work by increasing the amount of neurotransmitter available to the postsynaptic nerve. They accomplish this by (a) enhancing neurotransmitter release, (b) reducing neurotransmitter breakdown, or (c) inhibiting the reuptake of the neurotransmitter by the presynaptic neuron.

Morbidity and Mortality

Depression causes significant morbidity and mortality in numerous ways. Depression is frequently reported in persons with underlying medical conditions.

It is a common occurrence following myocardial infarctions and cerebrovascular accidents. Persons with depression and preexisting cardiovascular disease have a 3.5-times greater risk of dying of a heart attack than do nondepressed patients. Studies also show that **persons with depression have a greater chance of developing or dying from cardiovascular disease,** even after controlling for traditional risk factors such as smoking, blood pressure, and lipid levels. Depression also contributes the disruption of interpersonal relationships, the development of substance abuse, and absenteeism from work and school.

All depressed patients should be screened for suicidal and homicidal/violent ideations. A history of suicide attempts or violence is a significant risk factor for future attempts. Major depression plays a role in more than half of all suicide attempts. Women, especially those younger than age 30 years, attempt suicide more frequently than men, but men are more likely to complete suicide. Firearms are the most commonly used method in completed suicides. Table 25–1 lists the risk factors for suicide attempts and completion.

Physical Findings

Most patients with depression have no significant physical abnormalities on examination. Those who have more severe symptoms may reveal decline in

Table 25–1
RISK FACTORS FOR SUICIDE ATTEMPTS
AND COMPLETED SUICIDES

ATTEMPT	COMPLETED
Female sex	Male sex
Age <30 years	Age >55 years
Living alone	Concurrent chronic medical illness
Current psychosocial stressors (loss of job, relationship, etc.)	Social isolation (divorced, widowed)
Substance abuse	History of suicide attempt
Personality disorder	Family history of suicide
Depression	Substance abuse
	Depression and family history of depression

Data from, American Psychiatric Association: Diagnostic and Statistical Manual of Mental Disorders. 4th ed. Washington, DC: American Psychiatric Association Press; 1994; and Guck TP, et al. Assessment and Treatment of Depression following Myocardial Infarction. *Am Fam Physician* 2001;64:641–8,651–2.

grooming or hygiene along with significant weight changes. Speech may be normal, slow, monotonic, or lacking in content. Pressured speech is suggestive of mania, whereas disorganized speech suggests the need to evaluate for psychosis. The thought content of patients with depression includes feelings of inadequacy, helplessness, or hopelessness. Sometimes patients complain of being overwhelmed. Psychomotor retardation can manifest as slowing of movements or reactions, especially in the elderly.

Treatment

Initial pharmacotherapy should be based on physician familiarity with medication, anticipated safety and tolerability, anticipation of adverse effects, and history of prior treatments. Pharmacotherapy with psychotherapy is more effective than either pharmacotherapy or psychotherapy alone. Treatment should be geared toward doing both to improve chances of successful therapy. **Treatment failures typically result from medication noncompliance, inadequate duration of therapy, or inadequate dosing.** No class of medication has been proven to be more effective than other classes. Patients treated for a first episode of major depression should be treated for at least 6–9 months; recurrent depression needs to be treated for longer periods of time. The need for lifelong therapy is higher with increasing number of episodes of depression.

Classes of Medications

Table 25–2 lists the medications used in the treatment of depression.

Table 25–2
MEDICATIONS USED IN THE TREATMENT OF DEPRESSION

SSRI	SNRI	TCA	ATYPICAL	MAOI
Fluoxetine (Prozac)	Venlafaxine (Effexor)	Amitriptyline (Elavil)	Bupropion (Wellbutrin)	Phenelzine (Nardil)
Paroxetine (Paxil)	Duloxetine (Cymbalta)	Nortriptyline (Pamelor)	Mirtazapine (Remeron)	Tranylcypromine (Parnate)
Sertraline (Zoloft)		Desipramine (Norpramin)	Trazodone (Desyrel)	
Fluvoxamine (Luvox)		Clomipramine (Anafranil)		
Citalopram (Celexa)		Doxepin (Sinequan)		
Escitalopram (Lexapro)		Imipramine (Tofranil)		

Selective Serotonin Reuptake Inhibitors

Selective serotonin reuptake inhibitors (SSRIs) increase the amount of the neurotransmitter serotonin (5-hydroxytryptamine) available to the postsynaptic neuron by blocking the presynaptic neuron's ability to reuptake serotonin. Because it can take 3–6 weeks of therapy before significant improvement in mood occurs, dosage adjustments of these medications should occur no more often than monthly. These agents are have a low risk of toxicity if taken as an overdose (either accidentally or intentionally), making them very safe to use. Common side effects include sexual dysfunction, weight gain, gastrointestinal disturbance, fatigue, and agitation. Because of their efficacy and safety, SSRIs are frequently used as first-line agents for the treatment of depression.

Serotonin-Norepinephrine Reuptake Inhibitors

Serotonin-norepinephrine reuptake inhibitors (SNRIs) affect both the serotonergic and noradrenergic systems. They act primarily on the serotonergic system at lower dosages and on the noradrenergic system at higher dosages. Their side effects are similar to SSRIs. They can be used as first-line treatment for depression and, because of their effects on two neurotransmitter systems, may be used as second-line agents in SSRI failure.

Tricyclic Antidepressants

Tricyclic antidepressants (TCAs) are older agents that affect, to varying degrees, the reuptake of norepinephrine and serotonin. They are effective for the treatment of depression and, because they have been in use for many years, are inexpensive. However, they have numerous side effects, including sedation, dry mouth, dry eyes, urinary retention, weight gain, and sexual disturbance. They also carry the risk that they are highly toxic and potentially fatal in overdose. Because of the side effects and risks, TCAs have largely been replaced by SSRIs as the first-line treatment of depression.

Monamine Oxidase Inhibitors

Monoamine oxidase inhibitors (MAOIs) cause increased amounts of serotonin and norepinephrine to be released during nerve stimulation. Patients taking MAOIs must be on a tyramine-restricted diet to reduce the risk of severe, and sometimes fatal, hypertensive crisis. MAOIs also interact with numerous other medications, including SSRIs and meperidine (Demerol). These interactions can also be fatal. Because of the risks, MAOIs should only be used by experienced practitioners and only when the benefits outweigh the risks.

Atypical Agents

The different atypical agents may act similarly to SSRIs, TCAs, and MAOIs, in varying degrees. Their primary benefit is a lower incidence of sexual disturbance as a side effect. Bupropion is associated with a risk of seizure at higher doses and is contraindicated in patients with a history of seizure disorders.

Trazodone carries the risk, although rare, of causing priapism. It is also highly sedating and is frequently used as a sleep aid.

Inpatient Management

Inpatient management is indicated when the patient presents a significant risk to self (suicide, inability to care for self) or others (risk of violence), or the symptoms are sufficiently severe to initiate treatment in controlled settings. Involvement of a psychiatrist is warranted in the care of patients in whom more severe symptoms require more intensive care (suicidal ideations, psychosis, mania, and severe decline in physical health).

Other Mood Disorders

Anxiety Disorders

Anxiety disorders is a classification of mood disorders that are common in the population such as **panic disorder, obsessive-compulsive disorder** (OCD), **generalized anxiety disorder, posttraumatic stress disorder** (PTSD), **and phobia.** Patients with generalized anxiety disorder have excessive and difficult-to-control worry and anxiety that causes physical symptoms, including restlessness, irritability, sleep disturbance, and difficulty concentrating. Panic disorder is characterized by recurrent panic attacks, which are defined as periods of intense fear of abrupt onset. OCD manifests as either obsessions (recurrent, intrusive, and inappropriate thoughts) or compulsions (repetitive behaviors) that are unreasonable, excessive, and cause much distress to the patient. PTSD is a response to a severe traumatic event in which the patient suffers fear, helplessness, or horror. A phobia is an irrational fear that causes a conscious avoidance of a situation, subject, or activity. **Patients with anxiety disorders are at high risk for developing comorbid depression.**

Bereavement

Bereavement is defined as symptoms of a major depressive episode that occur after the loss of a loved one. If the symptoms last longer than 2 months and involve suicidal ideations, morbid preoccupations, or psychosis, then a diagnosis of major depression is made.

Bipolar Disorder (Manic-Depression)

This mood disorder affects genders equally but often presents in young people. Symptoms include the abrupt onset of increased energy, decreased need for sleep, pressured speech, decreased attention span, hypersexuality, spending large amounts of money, and engaging in outrageous activities. Concomitant substance abuse should always be investigated. Episodes must last longer than 1 week and should be abrupt, not continuous. Continuous behavior of this type suggests personality disorders or schizophrenia. A single episode of mania is sufficient for the diagnosis of bipolar disorder. **All patients diagnosed with depression should be questioned about mania,** as the treatments are different. Bipolar disorder is typically treated with mood stabilizers, which include valproate, carbamazepine, and lithium. The use of antidepressant agents in bipolar disorder may precipitate acute manic behaviors.

Dysthymic Disorder

This mood disorder presents with continuous low mood as the primary symptom. Typically 2 years of low mood is used for diagnosis. Dysthymia is less acute but longer in duration than major depression. If a major depressive episode takes place during the 2 years of dysthymia, then, by definition, it is major depression rather than dysthymia.

Comprehension Questions

Which of the following best explains each situation?

    A. Bipolar disorder
    B. Generalized anxiety
    C. Panic attacks
    D. Major depression
    E. Bereavement

[25.1] A 26-year-old male is brought to the emergency room by police after he was found shouting at staff at a busy hotel where he claimed that "I am owner of the hotel." He had checked into the hotel 10 days ago with the intention of "buying all hotels in the area." Since checking in, he has been noticed to be up all night working on paperwork. Additionally, when approached by the staff concerning his stay, he replies by going on tangents without answering the question and always seems to be in a hurry because he speaks quickly.

[25.2] A 74-year-old male is brought to your office by his family for his annual examination. While conducting the examination, you notice that he is less social than usual. The patient tells you that his wife passed away 6 weeks ago and he has been unhappy most of the time. His daughter tells you he doesn't garden anymore and frequently cries around the house.

[25.3] A 25-year-old female states that she has been feeling more irritable and worries constantly about her children, who recently started school. She also worries about her father, who recently was diagnosed with high blood pressure. She is concerned that her husband might leave her because they have been fighting more often than usual. She appears restless and fidgets frequently, wringing her hands while speaking. She adds that she has been on edge for at least the past 8 months and that she is having problems doing her job, which is another of her worries.

Answers

[25.1] **A.** The decreased need for sleep, pressured speech, and outrageous behavior are consistent with an acute manic event and consistent with the diagnosis of bipolar disorder.

[25.2] **E.** Symptoms of depression that occur following the death of a loved one are suggestive of bereavement. If the symptoms become prolonged or involve suicidal thoughts or psychoses, a diagnosis of depression may be made.

[25.3] **B.** Excessive worry associated with physical manifestations, such as nervousness and restlessness, are consistent with the diagnosis of generalized anxiety disorder.

CLINICAL PEARLS

❖ Rule out other medical diagnoses such as hypothyroidism, anemia, or infectious processes that could mimic some symptoms of depression.

❖ Always investigate the use of alcohol and drugs when evaluating for mood disorders.

❖ Suicidal ideations should always be investigated and appropriately addressed when diagnosing depression.

❖ Any recent medication addition should be investigated to ensure it is not contributing to the patient's symptoms.

REFERENCES

American Psychiatric Association. Diagnostic and Statistical Manual of Mental Disorders. 4th ed. Washington, DC: American Psychiatric Association Press, 1994.

Aronson SC. Depression. Available at: http://www.emedicine.com/MED/topic532.htm. Last accessed March 29, 2005.

Bhatia SC, Bhatia SK. Depression in women: diagnostic and treatment considerations. Am Fam Physician 1999;60:225–240.

Guck TP, Kavan MG, Elsasser GN, et al. Assessment and treatment of depression following myocardial infarction. Am Fam Physician 2001;64:641–648, 651–652.

Tierney LM, McPhee SJ, Papadakis, MA. Current Medical Diagnosis and Treatment 2003. 42nd ed. New York: Lange Medical Books, 2003:1034–1047.

A 26-year-old gravida$_1$ para$_{1001}$ woman presents for a routine postpartum visit 6 weeks following the vaginal delivery of a 7-lb baby girl. She had an uncomplicated prenatal course. She went into labor spontaneously at 39 2/7 weeks' gestation. Her labor was augmented with oxytocin (Pitocin). The first stage of labor lasted for 9 hours, the second stage for 45 minutes, and the third stage for 15 minutes. She had a second-degree episiotomy that was repaired without difficulty. She started breast-feeding her baby immediately after delivery. Her postpartum course was uncomplicated and she was discharged from the hospital on the second postpartum day. She is exclusively breast-feeding her baby and reports that it is going well. She says that she felt "stressed, sad, and overwhelmed" during her first week at home, but that those feelings resolved after a week or so. She is now in excellent spirits and has strong support at home from her husband and her mother. She had some light vaginal bleeding that stopped about a week after delivery. She had a mild, white discharge for a couple of weeks that has also stopped and has had no vaginal discharge since. On examination, she appears well and has normal vital signs. Her general physical examination is normal. A pelvic examination shows a well-healed episiotomy, no cervical or vaginal discharge, and no cervical motion tenderness. Her uterus is normal size, firm, and nontender, and there are no adnexal masses.

◆ **What are the maternal benefits of breast-feeding?**

◆ **The patient had been using a diaphragm for contraception prior to her pregnancy and wishes to use one again. What counseling should be given?**

◆ **She desires hormonal contraception. Which type is most recommended for a patient like her?**

ANSWERS TO CASE 26: Postpartum Care

Summary: A 26-year-old first-time mother presents for a routine, 6-week postpartum examination. She is breast-feeding her baby. Her examination is normal. She had a brief period in which she felt sad and overwhelmed, but this has resolved. She requests counseling about contraception.

◆ **Maternal benefits of breast-feeding:** Along with benefits to the baby, the maternal benefits include (but are not limited to) a more rapid return of uterine tone with reduced bleeding and a quicker return to nonpregnant size; a more rapid return to prepregnant body weight; a reduced incidence of ovarian and breast cancer; the convenience of always having a readily available feeding supply for baby; and lower cost (no need to purchase formula).

◆ **Counseling regarding use of diaphragm:** There is no contraindication to using a diaphragm but she should have a new fitting.

◆ **Recommended hormonal contraception:** In breast-feeding women, the progestin-only "minipill" is recommended, as combined hormonal contraceptives can interfere with milk supply.

Analysis

Objectives

1. Know the normal changes that occur in the postpartum period.
2. Be familiar with the diagnosis and management of common postpartum complications.
3. Be able to counsel patients on common postpartum issues such as contraception, breast-feeding, and postpartum depression.

Considerations

The postpartum period is defined as the time starting after the delivery of the placenta and lasting for 6–12 weeks. The postpartum period is a time of great change for the woman and the family. There are numerous normal physiologic changes that occur during the change from the pregnant to the nonpregnant state. Just as important are the many personal, social, and family changes that occur, which can be magnified for first-time parents or when there are unforeseen complications.

The immediate postpartum period, while still in the delivery suite, is usually focused on the medical conditions of both the neonate and the mother. The delivery attendant examines the mother, repairs any lacerations or episiotomy, and monitors for complications, such as postpartum hemorrhage. Simultaneous to this, the neonate is assessed and cared for during her initial transition to extrauterine life. The baby is often quite alert during this time, making it an ideal time to start breast-feeding efforts.

A typical postdelivery hospital stay is 24–48 hours for an uncomplicated vaginal delivery and 72–96 hours for a cesarean delivery. This time allows for recovery from the delivery or surgery, allows further monitoring for both maternal and neonatal problems, and can be used to provide education and support for the new mother and family. Typical maternal problems that occur during this time frame include pain, bleeding, lactation problems, and urinary difficulties (infections, incontinence, retention). Postpartum fever is most often a sign of endometritis (infection of the uterus), but can also be caused by urinary tract or wound infections, thromboembolic disease, and mastitis.

The time following discharge from the hospital and for the subsequent 6–12 weeks usually represents the period of greatest adjustment. There are normal changes that occur, along with many potential medical and emotional complications. Future family planning and contraceptive issues often need to be addressed as well. A 6-week postpartum examination is usually scheduled, but many of the issues that can occur during this time frame should be addressed prior to discharge from the hospital.

APPROACH TO POSTPARTUM CARE

Definitions

Endometritis: A polymicrobial infection of the endometrium of the uterus, usually caused by ascending infection from the vagina.

Lochia: Yellow-white discharge, consisting of blood cells, decidual cells, and fibrinous products, that occurs following delivery.

Normal Changes

Immediately following delivery, the uterus begins the process of involution, the return to its nonpregnant size. Contraction of the uterine musculature promotes hemostasis by compressing the uterine blood vessels. An IV infusion of oxytocin (Pitocin) given during or immediately after the third stage of labor will aid in producing increased uterine tone. Early breast-feeding also leads to uterine contraction, further promoting involution. In most cases, the uterus has returned to normal size by the time of the 6-week follow-up visit.

Vaginal bleeding is usually heaviest in the hours following delivery, then decreases significantly. Brown or blood-tinged lochia occurs for about the next week. This is followed by white or yellow lochia, which continues for approximately 3–6 more weeks. **In women who are not breast-feeding, menstruation usually restarts by the third postpartum month.** In women who are breast-feeding, ovulation and menstruation can be suppressed for much longer. Anovulation will persist for longer periods of time in women who exclusively breast-feed their babies.

Breast engorgement, signaling increased milk production, typically occurs 1–4 days after delivery. In breast-feeding women, this is best managed by increased frequency of feedings. In women who are not breast-feeding, the use of ice packs, supportive bras, and nonsteroidal antiinflammatory drugs (NSAIDs) can reduce discomfort.

Medical Complications

Hemorrhage

Postpartum hemorrhage is categorized as "early" or "late," depending on when the hemorrhage began. Early postpartum hemorrhage occurs within 24 hours of delivery, most often immediately postpartum; late postpartum hemorrhage occurs between 24 hours and 6 weeks after delivery. The causes of most cases of postpartum hemorrhage can be remembered with the mnemonic "The Four Ts" (Table 26–1). Careful examination focused on the likely causes should be performed promptly to identify the source of the bleeding.

As with all emergency situations, the **first priority in this setting is assessment of the ABCs—airway, breathing, and circulation.** It is important to ensure that adequate IV access is available, preferably 2 large-bore IV catheters. Fluid resuscitation with a crystalloid solution (normal saline, lactated Ringer solution) should be given as necessary and massive hemorrhage may require transfusion with packed red blood cells.

Uterine atony is the most common cause of postpartum hemorrhage. Failure of the uterus to contract adequately results in continued bleeding from uterine vasculature. Risks include prolonged labor, prolonged use of oxytocin during labor, a large baby, and grand multipara (5 or more previous children). **Initial management of uterine atony includes the IV administration of oxytocin and initiation of bimanual uterine massage.** When these fail to control the bleeding, methylergonovine (Methergine) may be given intramuscularly. **Methylergonovine is contraindicated in patients with hypertension,** as it may cause an abrupt increase in blood pressure. If the bleeding continues following this, or if the patient is hypertensive, prostaglandin $F_{2\alpha}$ (Hemabate) can be injected intramuscularly or intramyometrially. Prostaglandin $F_{2\alpha}$ is contraindicated in women with asthma.

Table 26–1
THE FOUR TS OF POSTPARTUM HEMORRHAGE

Tone	Uterine atony
Trauma	Cervical, vaginal, or perineal lacerations; uterine inversion
Tissue	Retained placenta or membranes
Thrombin	Coagulopathies

Fever

Postpartum fever, especially if associated with uterine tenderness and foul-smelling lochia, is often a sign of endometritis. Endometritis complicates approximately 10% of cesarean and 1–2% of vaginal deliveries. Antibiotics given prophylactically during a cesarean delivery can reduce the risk of this complication. When it does occur, endometritis should be treated with broad-spectrum antibiotics that cover vaginal and gastrointestinal flora.

Urinary tract infections (UTI) are another common cause of fever after both vaginal and cesarean deliveries. Urinary frequency, urgency, and burning are typical presenting symptoms. Catheterization of the urinary bladder, which occurs routinely during a cesarean delivery and frequently during vaginal deliveries, raises the risk of introducing bacteria into the normally sterile environment of the bladder.

Other causes of fever in the postpartum period, especially in women delivered by cesarean, are identical to causes of fever in other postsurgical patients. These include atelectasis, wound infections, and venous thromboembolic disease.

Mood Disorders

Up to three-fourths of women develop some type of psychological reaction following the delivery of a child. In most cases, the symptoms are mild and self-limited. However, a smaller but significant percentage can have a reaction of such severity as to require medical or psychiatric intervention.

Approximately 30–70% of women develop a temporary state known as the **"maternity blues"** or "baby blues." This condition **develops within the first week after delivery and typically resolves by the 10th postpartum day.** Symptoms include tearfulness, sadness, and emotional lability. The etiology is not entirely clear, but may be multifactorial and include both hormonal changes following delivery along with components of stress, sleep deprivation, and adjustment to the new role of mother. Postpartum depression occurs following 10–20% of pregnancies and can occur following gestations of any length—term, preterm, miscarriages, or abortions. The onset is defined as occurring within 4 weeks postpartum, but it has been seen up to a year later. **The symptoms of postpartum depression are the same as in major depression.** The severity can vary from mild to severe and suicidal. There is a **high recurrence rate in subsequent pregnancies** and an increased risk in women with a history of depression unrelated to pregnancy. Untreated, postpartum depression can last for 6 months or more and can be a significant cause of morbidity. All women should be screened for a history of psychiatric disorders during their prenatal care and should be questioned about symptoms of depression during postpartum visits. The **treatment is similar to the treatment of nonpregnancy-related depression.** Women who are a risk to themselves, or to others, or who are unable to care for themselves should be admitted to the hospital. Selective serotonin reuptake inhibitors (SSRIs) are first-line therapy because of their efficacy and safety. They also are considered safe in breast-feeding. Counseling and general supportive measures at home are also important adjuncts to treatment.

Postpartum psychosis is a rare, but potentially devastating, complication following pregnancy. Manic or frankly delusional behaviors may present within a few days to a few weeks of delivery in up to 1 in 1000 postpartum patients. All women with postpartum psychosis should be hospitalized and managed, as well as treated by a psychiatrist. Without proper treatment, there is a high risk of suicide and infanticide associated with this diagnosis.

Breast-Feeding

Counseling and encouragement regarding both the maternal and infant benefits of breast-feeding should start during the prenatal period. Neonatal benefits include ideal nutrition, increased resistance to infection, and a reduced risk of gastrointestinal difficulties. Maternal benefits include improved mother–child bonding, more rapid uterine involution, quicker return to prepregnant body weight, convenience, decreased costs, and long-term reduced risks of ovarian and breast cancer. Breast-feeding promotion and education can increase the rate of breast-feeding and the duration for which women breast-feed their babies.

Women should be allowed to nurse their newborns as soon as possible following delivery. During this time, the newborns are often very alert and have strong rooting and sucking reflexes, which promote latching on to the nipple. Initial feedings provide colostrum, an antibody-rich clear/yellow nourishment for the newborn. Breast engorgement and milk letdown commonly occurs between the second and fourth postpartum days.

There are few contraindications to breast-feeding. HIV infection is a contraindication, as vertical transmission can occur through infected breast milk. Most mothers with hepatitis B and C can safely breast-feed, although women with acute, active hepatitis B infection should not breast-feed. Women who have had breast-reduction surgery with nipple transplantation will be unable to breast-feed.

Common maternal complications of breast-feeding include sore or cracked nipples and mastitis. Sore nipples can be managed with frequent position changes, alternating breasts during feedings, and applications of lanolin. Mastitis, an obstruction of milk glands sometimes secondarily infected with bacteria, is treated by increased nursing or breast pumping and oral antibiotics, such as cephalexin or dicloxacillin. Mastitis should not result in discontinuation of nursing.

Family Planning

Most women resume sexual activity by 3 months postpartum. Numerous options are available to women for contraception and family planning. Discussion of these options ideally should occur in the prenatal period and again before discharge from the hospital.

Oral contraceptive pills (OCPs) are the most widely used reversible form of contraception. Available OCPs contain either combined estrogen and progestin or are progestin only. **In breast-feeding women, the progestin-only pills are**

preferred because the combination OCPs might reduce lactation. Both the American College of Obstetricians and Gynecologists and the World Health Organization recommend waiting for 6 weeks postpartum to start oral contraceptives in breast-feeding women. Injectable long-acting depot medroxyprogesterone (Depo-Provera) may also be used in breast-feeding women and should also be given at least 6 weeks postpartum. **Non–breast-feeding women should wait 3 weeks after delivery to start combined OCPs,** as the risk of thromboembolic disease is higher in those who start at earlier times.

Barrier methods of contraception may also be used regardless of breast-feeding status. An intrauterine device (IUD) may be placed at the 6-week postpartum visit; earlier placement is associated with an increased rate of expulsion of the device. **Diaphragms and cervical caps can be used, but should be refitted at the 6-week visit** to ensure an appropriate fit.

Lactation-induced amenorrhea provides a high level of natural contraception in the first 6 months postpartum. Women who breast-feed exclusively and who are amenorrheic have a 98% contraceptive protection for 6 months. After 6 months, if menses restart, or if breast-feeding is reduced, the risk of pregnancy increases and alternate forms of contraception should be used.

Comprehension Questions

[26.1] You are called by the postpartum nurse to see a 20-year-old woman who delivered an 8 lb 9 oz baby boy approximately 6 hours ago. The nurse noted that the patient is continuing to bleed more than expected. The patient is awake and talking, but feels dizzy. Her blood pressure is 90/40 mm Hg and her pulse is 110 beats/min. You see that her perineal pad is soaked with blood. Which of the following is your most appropriate initial intervention?

    A. Add 20 units of oxytocin (Pitocin) to the IV of 0.45% saline that is currently running at 125 mL/hr

    B. Perform bimanual uterine massage

    C. Place a large-bore IV and give a 1 liter bolus of 0.9% saline

    D. Give an IM injection of methylergonovine (Methergine)

[26.2] A 29-year-old first-time mother comes to you for her routine 6-week postpartum visit. Her husband, who accompanied her to the visit, reports that his wife is tearful much of the time. She has not been sleeping well, has little energy, and a reduced appetite. She denies any suicidal thoughts, hallucinations, or feelings that she wants to harm her baby. Which of the following is the most likely diagnosis?

    A. Maternal blues

    B. Postpartum psychosis

    C. Postpartum depression

    D. Normal response to the overwhelming new responsibilities of motherhood

[26.3] You see a 30-year-old woman for an acute visit 16 days postpartum. She has been nursing her baby daughter but has developed a very sore left breast. On examination, the patient is afebrile. The breast is diffusely tender but primarily in the upper inner quadrant. The skin overlying the area of most tenderness is erythematous and warm. The remainder of the examination is normal. Which of the following statements is correct?

A. This condition is self-limited but she should stop nursing the baby until this condition resolves.
B. She may nurse from the unaffected breast but should pump and discard the milk from the painful breast.
C. She will require oral antibiotics but may not breast-feed while taking them.
D. Oral antibiotics and increased nursing are recommended.

Answers

[26.1] **C.** This patient is symptomatically hypovolemic, with dizziness, hypotension, and tachycardia. Fluid resuscitation must be your first intervention—remember the ABCs first! Once you have started the management of this critical issue, you should turn your attention to identifying and correcting the source of the bleeding.

[26.2] **C.** This is a picture of postpartum depression. The symptoms are identical to those of a major depressive episode. The maternity blues is a self-limited condition that starts in the first postpartum week and resolves in the second. Fortunately, this patient doesn't have signs of postpartum psychosis—mania, hallucinations, and delusions. Appropriate management includes the use of an SSRI, counseling, and close follow-up.

[26.3] **D.** Mastitis is a common complication of breast-feeding. It is caused by gland obstruction and sometimes, as in this case, there also are signs of infection. Treatment is directed at relieving the obstruction, so increased breast-feeding or pumping is helpful. The antibiotics typically used for this complication are considered safe to use while nursing.

CLINICAL PEARLS

❖ Many of the important postpartum issues—mood problems, contraception, and breast-feeding—are best managed by addressing them in the prenatal course first, and then readdressing or reinforcing them in the postpartum period.

❖ Most causes of postpartum hemorrhage can be remembered with the four Ts: Tone, Trauma, Tissue, and Thrombin.

REFERENCES

Anderson J, Etches D, Smith D. Postpartum hemorrhage: third stage emergency. In: Atwood L, Deutchman M, Bailey E, et al. (eds). Advanced life support in obstetrics manual. 4th ed. Leawood, KS: American Academy of Family Physicians, 2003.

Blenning CE, Paladine H. An approach to the postpartum office visit. Am Fam Physician 2005;72:2491–2498.

Bowes WA, Katz VL. Postpartum care. In: Gabbe SG, Niebyl JR, Simpson JL (eds). Obstetrics: normal and problem pregnancies. 4th ed. Philadelphia: Churchill Livingstone, 2002:701–722.

A 66-year-old woman presents to your office complaining of shortness of breath and bilateral leg edema that have been worsening for 3 months. She emphatically tells you, "I get out of breath when I do housework and I can't even walk to the corner." She has also noticed difficulty sleeping secondary to a dry cough that wakes her up at night and further exacerbation of her shortness of breath while lying flat. This has forced her to use 3 pillows for a good night's sleep. She denies any chest pain, wheezing, or febrile illness. She has no past illnesses and takes no medications. She's never smoked and drinks socially. On examination, her blood pressure is 187/90 mm Hg; her pulse is 97 beats/min; her respiratory rate is 16 breaths/min; her temperature is 98°F; and her oxygen saturation is 93% on room air by pulse oximetry. She has a pronounced jugular vein. Cardiac exam reveals a pansystolic murmur. Examination of her lung bases produces dullness bilaterally. You find 2+ pitting edema of both ankles. An EKG shows a normal sinus rhythm and a chest x-ray demonstrates mild cardiomegaly with bilateral pleural effusions. You decide she needs further work-up, so you call the hospital where you have admitting privileges and arrange for a telemetry bed.

◆ **What is the most likely diagnosis?**

◆ **What is the next diagnostic step?**

◆ **What is the next step in therapy?**

ANSWERS TO CASE 27: Congestive Heart Failure

Summary: A 66-year-old female presents to your office with worsening short-ness of breath, bilateral leg edema and 3-pillow orthopnea. She is not known to be hypertensive, but her blood pressure is 187/90 mm Hg and she is only saturating 93% on room air. Her examination reveals jugular venous distension (JVD), a murmur, and decreased breath sounds at both lung bases. On a chest x-ray you find bilateral pleural effusions and decide you must admit her for further work-up.

◆ **Most likely diagnosis:** New-onset congestive heart failure

◆ **Next diagnostic step:** Echocardiogram, serial cardiac enzymes, and EKG analysis

◆ **Next step in therapy:** Telemetry monitoring, IV diuretics, and oxygen

Objectives

1. Know how to clinically recognize congestive heart failure (CHF).
2. Understand the classification of CHF.
3. Understand the mechanism of action of the drugs used in the treatment of acute and chronic CHF.
4. Understand the underlying pathophysiology that occurs in CHF and the rationale for treatment options.
5. Be familiar with the outpatient management of CHF and the impor-tance of patient education.

Considerations

This 66-year-old female presented with congestive heart failure. Her most immediate problem is oxygenation and volume overload on her weakened heart. The **first priority is optimizing oxygen exchange** by administering oxygen via nasal cannula, dilating pulmonary vasculature and decreasing car-diac preload and afterload. Most cases of CHF are caused by either coronary artery disease or hypertension, so it's imperative to admit these patients for serial cardiac enzymes and further assessment of heart function. The over-loading of fluid in the lungs is a common cause of anxiety and distress in patients with acute CHF because of the continuous struggle to oxygenate ade-quately. This anxiety activates sympathetic pathways and mounts catecholamine-induced responses, which produce further worsening of acute heart failure by causing tachycardia and increasing peripheral vascular resistance, leading to greater stress on the heart and worsening of symptoms. These triggers can, in part, be suppressed by the use of an agent such as morphine sulfate, which acts as both an anxiolytic and a vasodilator. Furosemide (Lasix) is the diuretic of choice, not only for its diuretic effect but also for its immediate vasodilatory action on bronchial vasculature. Admitting these patients to the hospital allows for closer maintenance of homeostasis in their fluid balances and evaluation of any underlying condition that may have precipitated the CHF. Other medications, including angiotensin-converting enzyme (ACE) inhibitors and β-blockers, help to control heart failure symptoms by decreasing preload and afterload, and reducing cardiac remodeling.

APPROACH TO CONGESTIVE HEART FAILURE

Definitions

Congestive heart failure: Imbalance in pump function where the heart fails to maintain the circulation of blood adequately.

Framingham Heart Study: Large, prospective cohort study of the epidemiologic factors associated with cardiovascular diseases.

Clinical Presentation

CHF is divided into two main categories: systolic and diastolic dysfunction. Systolic dysfunction exists when there is a dilated left ventricle with impaired contractility. Diastolic dysfunction occurs in a normal or intact left ventricle that has an impaired ability to relax, fill, and eject blood. Table 27–1 lists the findings frequently associated with CHF.

Dyspnea on exertion is the most sensitive symptom for the diagnosis of CHF, but its specificity is much lower. Other symptoms, which are common but less sensitive for the diagnosis, include dyspnea at rest, anxiety, orthopnea, paroxysmal nocturnal dyspnea, and cough productive of pink, frothy sputum. Nonspecific symptoms sometimes reported are weakness, lightheadedness, abdominal pain, malaise, wheezing, and nausea. Patients may have a medical history of hypertension, coronary artery disease, or other heart diseases (cardiomyopathy, valvular disease). Histories of cigarette smoking and alcohol abuse may also be found.

Etiologies

The symptoms and signs that occur are unique and characteristic of the alterations to the normal physiologic function. Symptoms of right-sided heart failure include venous congestion, nausea/vomiting, distension/bloating, constipation, abdominal pain, and decreased appetite. Common signs of right-sided heart failure are fluid retention, weight gain, peripheral edema, JVD, hepatojugular reflux, hepatic ascites, and splenomegaly.

Left-sided heart failure manifests with pulmonary congestion, resulting in the symptoms of dyspnea on exertion, paroxysmal nocturnal dyspnea, orthopnea, wheezing, tachypnea, and cough. The signs of pulmonary congestion are

Table 27–1
ETIOLOGIES OF HEART FAILURE

FINDING	COMMON CAUSES
Cardiac rhythm disorders	Complete heart block Supraventricular tachycardia Ventricular tachycardia Sinus node dysfunction
Volume overload	Structural heart disease (ventricular septal defect; patent ductus arteriosis; aortic or mitral regurgitation, complex cardiac lesions) Anemia Sepsis
Pressure overload	Structural heart disease (aortic or pulmonary stenosis; aortic coarctation) Hypertension
Systolic ventricular dysfunction or failure	Myocarditis Dilated cardiomyopathy Malnutrition Ischemia
Diastolic ventricular dysfunction or failure	Hypertrophic cardiomyopathy Restrictive cardiomyopathy

bilateral pulmonary rales, S_3 gallop rhythm, Cheyne-Stokes respiration, pleural effusion, and pulmonary edema. Pulmonary edema is often the first manifestation of congestive heart failure, but it can also be caused by a variety of non-cardiac conditions (Table 27–2).

Signs common to both left- and right-heart failure are tachycardia, cardiomegaly, cyanosis, oliguria, nocturia, and peripheral edema. Symptoms common to both include weakness, fatigue, confusion (delirium), decreased mental status, insomnia, decreased exercise tolerance, headache, stupor, coma, paroxysmal nocturnal dyspnea, and declining functional status.

After the Framingham Heart Study was reviewed, criteria were devised to help diagnose CHF by both signs and symptoms. Two major criteria or one major and two minor criteria can lead to a presumptive diagnosis of CHF. The major signs are paroxysmal nocturnal dyspnea; JVD; rales; cardiomegaly; pulmonary edema; S_3 gallop; central venous pressure >16 cm H_2O; circulation time of 25 seconds; hepatojugular reflex; and weight loss of 4.5 kg over 5 days of treatment. Minor criteria include bilateral ankle edema; nocturnal cough; dyspnea on exertion; hepatomegaly; pleural effusions; decreased vital capacity by one-third of maximum; and tachycardia.

Table 27–2
NONCARDIAC CAUSES OF PULMONARY EDEMA

Altered capillary permeability	Acute respiratory distress syndrome (ARDS) Inhaled or circulating toxins Vasoactive substances Dissminated intravascular coagulation (DIC) Aspirations (including near-drowning) Uremia
Increased pulmonary capillary pressure (noncardiac causes)	Pulmonary vein thrombosis Pulmonary vein stenosis Volume overload
Decreased oncotic pressure	Hypoalbuminemia
Lymphatic insufficiency	
Large negative pleural pressure	
Mixed or unknown mechanism	High altitude Neurogenic Drug overdoses Pulmonary embolism Eclampsia Postanesthesia Postcardiac bypass Postcardioversion Postextubation

Modified with permission from Ingram RH, Braunwald E. Dyspnea and pulmonary edema. In: Braunwald E, Fauci AS, Kasper DL, et al. (eds). Harrision principles of internal medicine. 15th ed. New York: McGraw-Hill, 2001:202.

Epidemiology

Of the general population between the ages of 50 and 59 years, 1–2% will have CHF, but that number increases to 10% in persons older than age 75. Approximately 30–40% of patients with CHF are hospitalized every year; **it is the leading diagnosis-related group (DRG) among hospitalized patients older than age 65 years.** The 5-year mortality rate remained essentially unchanged from 1971 to 1991, at 60% in men and 45% in women. Data from the Framingham Heart Study shows a **median survival of 3.2 years for males and 5.4 years for females with CHF.** The most common cause of death is progressive heart failure, but sudden death may account for up to 45% of all deaths. African-Americans are 1.5 times more likely to die of CHF than are Whites. Nevertheless, African-American patients appear to have similar or lower in-hospital mortality rates than White patients. The prevalence is greater in males than in females for patients ages 40–75 years; after the age of 75, however, there is no difference.

Evaluation

After an initial assessment of the "ABCs"—airway, breathing, and circulation— patients presenting with dyspnea suggestive of heart failure should be evaluated with a history, physical examination, and focused testing. The testing should be designed to confirm CHF (or lead to an alternate diagnosis), identify a cause, and assess the severity of the disease. These initial tests should include blood tests, radiographic studies, electrocardiography, and echocardiography.

Initial blood tests should generally include a complete blood count (CBC), serum electrolytes, renal function tests, hepatic function tests, and cardiac enzymes. A high white blood cell count can help to identify the presence of an underlying infection, a common triggering event of CHF. Anemia is another common trigger of CHF. In an anemic patient, the oxygen-carrying ability of the blood is reduced. The cardiac output must increase to compensate for this. If the anemia is mild, or if the heart is normal, this compensation may occur without producing symptoms; if the anemia is severe or if there is underlying cardiac abnormality (from previous ischemia, hypertension, valvular abnormality, etc.), heart failure may occur.

Electrolyte abnormalities are common in the presence of CHF. Neurohumoral responses to a failing heart result in water and sodium retention and potassium excretion. Severe heart failure can result in a dilutional hyponatremia. Medications used by patients with chronic heart disease (diuretics, ACE inhibitors, others) also can lead to electrolyte abnormalities. Increased vascular congestion can lead to passive congestion of the liver, resulting in increases in serum transaminases. Severe CHF can lead to jaundice as a consequence of impaired hepatic function caused by congestion. Serial measurement of cardiac enzymes is necessary to evaluate for the presence of acute myocardial infarction as the inciting event.

One of the neurohumoral responses to the presence of a failing ventricle is release of brain natriuretic peptide (BNP). The "Breathing Not Properly" study, published in 2004, showed that elevated levels of BNP and its prohormone (pro-BNP) can be used to assist in the diagnosis of CHF as a cause of acute dyspnea. Elevated levels of BNP and pro-BNP are a sensitive and specific marker for the diagnosis of CHF. In a dyspneic patient, a level of BNP <100 pg/mL suggests that the symptoms are unlikely to be caused by CHF; a BNP level >500 pg/mL is consistent with the diagnosis of CHF.

EKG findings in CHF are variable. An EKG is useful to evaluate for evidence of acute ischemia or arrhythmia as cause of the CHF and can also reveal the presence of ventricular hypertrophy, often seen in chronic hypertension. Chest x-ray can also show cardiomegaly and cardiac chamber enlargement. Typically, the cardiothoracic ratio is greater than 50%. One of the earliest chest x-ray findings in CHF is cephalization of the pulmonary vasculature. As the failure progresses, interstitial pulmonary edema can be seen as perihilar infiltrates, often in a butterfly pattern. Pleural effusions can also be found. Effusions are usually bilateral but, if unilateral, are more often seen on the right hemithorax than the left.

Echocardiography is the gold-standard diagnostic modality in the presence of CHF. It may help to identify regional or global wall motion abnormalities, cardiomyopathy, ventricular or septal hypertrophy, and cardiac ejection fraction. It also can find cardiac tamponade, pericardial constriction, and pulmonary embolus. Echocardiography also is useful in identifying valvular stenosis or regurgitation, either of which can lead to heart failure. These findings aid in the determination of whether the heart failure is a systolic or diastolic dysfunction, an important distinction in the decision of appropriate treatment.

Classification of CHF

CHF severity is characterized by the symptoms a patient has and the degree that the symptoms limit a patient's lifestyle. There are several classification systems in use; two of the most widely used are the New York Heart Association (NYHA) and the American Heart Association (AHA) classifications. Table 27–3 summarizes these systems. The classification of CHF is important in determining the appropriate treatment and prognosis for the patient.

Table 27–3

CLASSIFICATION OF SEVERITY OF CONGESTIVE
HEART FAILURE

AMERICAN HEART ASSOCIATION	NEW YORK HEART ASSOCIATION	LIMITATIONS	SYMPTOMS
A	—	None	Risk factors
B	I	None with normal activities	Left ventricular dysfunction
B	II	Mild	Fatigue, dyspnea with normal activities
C	III	Moderate	Activities of daily living
D	IV	Severe	At rest

Management of Heart Failure

In all cases of acute CHF, **the initial management imperative is the "ABCs"**—airway, breathing, and circulation. Supplemental oxygen, initially 100% via non-rebreather face mask, should be administered. If necessary, ventilation can be assisted with continuous positive airway pressure (CPAP), bilevel positive airway pressure (BiPAP), or mechanical ventilation. Cardiac and continuous pulse oximetry monitors should be placed and IV access obtained.

When acute pulmonary edema caused by CHF is diagnosed, the next step in management is the administration of a loop diuretic. Furosemide is generally the treatment of choice, both for its potent diuretic effect and for its rapid bronchial vasculature vasodilation. Nitrates, particularly nitroglycerin when given IV, reduce myocardial oxygen demand by reducing preload and afterload. Nitroglycerin also can rapidly reduce blood pressure and is the treatment of choice in a patient who has CHF and whose blood pressure is elevated. It should be used with caution or avoided in a hypotensive patient. IV morphine sulphate can be an effective adjunct to therapy. Along with its analgesic and anxiolytic properties, morphine is a venodilator (primary effect) and arterial dilator, resulting in a reduction in preload and an increase in cardiac output.

Most patients who present to the emergency department with symptomatic CHF will require admission to a telemetry unit for treatment and monitoring. Discharge criteria from the emergency department includes the gradual onset of symptoms, rapid resolution of symptoms with treatment, oxygen saturation of >90% on room air, and exclusion of an acute coronary syndrome as the cause of the CHF.

Outpatient Management of CHF

Patient education is an important aspect of the care for all patients with CHF. All patients should be advised about the importance of dietary sodium and fluid restriction. A normal American diet contains 6–10 g sodium chloride a day; initial restriction in patients with CHF should be to 2–4 g per day. Stricter restrictions may be necessary in those with more severe disease. Overweight and obese patients should be counseled on appropriate caloric restrictions and encouraged to exercise to reduce weight. The importance of strict management of blood pressure and modification of other cardiac risk factors should be emphasized as well.

ACE inhibitors should be considered first-line therapy in patients with CHF and reduced left ventricular function. ACE inhibitors reduce preload, afterload, improve cardiac output, and inhibit tissue rennin–angiotensin systems. The result of this is an improvement in symptoms and a reduction in mortality. ACE inhibitors can also delay the development of symptomatic CHF in asymptomatic patients with a reduced cardiac ejection fraction. Angiotensin receptor blockers (ARBs) can be used in place of an ACE inhibitor in a patient who does not tolerate an ACE inhibitor because of side effects (e.g., cough).

ACE inhibitors are contraindicated in pregnancy, hypotension, hyperkalemia, and bilateral renal artery stenosis, and should be used with caution in patients with renal insufficiency.

For many years, the teaching was to avoid the use of β-blockers in the setting of CHF. However, more recent data support the use of β-blockers for both systolic and diastolic heart failure. **The administration of β-blockers, especially in high doses, in the setting of acute CHF, can worsen symptoms;** consequently, initial doses should be low and titrated up over several weeks. β-Blockers can reduce the sympathetic tone and the cardiac muscle remodeling associated with chronic heart failure. β-Blockers reduce mortality in patients with an ejection fraction of less than 35% and are primarily indicated in patients with NYHA class II or III heart failure, or in patients with coronary artery disease.

Diuretics should be used to reduce fluid overload in both the acute and chronic settings. Loop diuretics (furosemide, bumetanide, torsemide, ethacrynic acid) can be used in all stages of CHF and are useful in pulmonary edema and refractory heart failure. Thiazide diuretics (hydrochlorothiazide, chlorthalidone, others) are used in mild heart failure and may be used in combination with other diuretics in more severe CHF. Diuretic doses can be adjusted based on daily weight measurements by the patient.

The aldosterone antagonist spironolactone reduces mortality in advanced heart failure. It also functions as a diuretic and should be considered in NYHA classes III and IV heart failure. Patients on this medication must be closely monitored for the development of hyperkalemia, which can become profound and lead to arrhythmia.

Calcium channel blockers, in general, are contraindicated in systolic heart failure, because they increase mortality. The exception to this is the dihydropyridine calcium channel blocker amlodipine (Norvasc), which did not increase or decrease mortality. Nondihydropyridine calcium channel blockers (diltiazem, verapamil) are useful in heart failure because of diastolic dysfunction, as they promote increased cardiac output by lowering heart rate, which allows for more ventricular filling time.

Comprehension Questions

Match the following class of drugs with their mechanism of action:

[27.1] β-Blockers

[27.2] ACE inhibitor

[27.3] Loop diuretics

[27.4] Morphine sulfate

[27.5] Nitroglycerin

    A. Anxiolytic and vasodilator

    B. Decrease preload and afterload

    C. Decrease sympathetic tone and prevent cardiac remodeling

    D. Bronchial smooth muscle relaxation and decrease preload

    E. Reduce oxygen demand in heart by vasodilation

Answers

[27.1] **C.** β-Blockers decrease mortality, especially with an ejection fraction of <35%.

[27.2] **B.** ACE inhibitors decrease mortality when there is an ejection fraction of <35% and should be considered first-line therapy for the management of CHF.

[27.3] **D.** Loop diuretics are a first-line agent in CHF exacerbation with pulmonary edema.

[27.4] **A.** Morphine sulfate reduces preload and acts as an arterial dilating agent, which reduces systemic vascular resistance and increases cardiac output.

[27.5] **E.** Nitroglycerin is a potent venodilator that aids in reducing afterload.

CLINICAL PEARLS

❖ The initial hour in the management of a patient with either new-onset CHF or an acute exacerbation is crucial to their outcome.

❖ Simple measures, such as decreasing cardiac preload by sitting the patient up with their legs on the ground and their arms by their side, maintaining an airway and giving oxygen, and giving sublingual nitroglycerin, can alleviate CHF immediately.

REFERENCES

Abraham WT. Switching between beta blockers in heart failure patients: rationale and practical considerations. Congest Heart Fail 2003;9:251–258.

Braunwald E. Heart Failure. In: Braunwald E, Fauci AS, Kasper DL, et al (eds). Harrison's principles of internal medicine. 15th ed. New York: McGraw-Hill, 2001:1318–1326.

Dosh SA. Diagnosis of heart failure in adults. Am Fam Physician 2004;70: 2145–2152.

Hoyt R, Bowling SL. Reducing readmissions for congestive heart failure. Am Fam Physician 2001;63:8.

Mueller C, Scholer A, Laule-Kilian K, et al. Use of B-type natriuretic peptide in the evaluation and management of acute dyspnea. N Engl J Med 2004;350(7):647–654.

Peacock WF, Emerman CL. Safety and efficacy of nesiritide in the treatment of decompensated heart failure in observation patients: the PROACTION trial (abstract). J Am Coll Cardiol 2003;4(Suppl A):336A.

Schocken DD, Arrieta PM, Leaverton PE, Ross EA. Prevalence and mortality rate of congestive heart failure in the United States. J Am Coll Cardiol 1992;20:301–306.

A 38-year-old gravida$_3$ para$_3$, divorced executive presents to your clinic for contraceptive advice. She is currently in a monogamous relationship and has been in it for several months. She denies any allergy. She occasionally drinks alcohol and smokes half a pack of cigarettes a day. She mentions that she used to take birth control pills without any problems. All of her three children were born via vaginal delivery without complication. She and her boyfriend are sexually transmitted disease (STD) free based on their recent checkups. She reports that she is tired of using over-the-counter contraceptives because they are inconvenient. She said that her life is very busy because of work. She fears any form of surgery and hasn't excluded having another child. Her lab workup is normal. Her physical examination is normal. She is looking for the "best contraceptive method" for her situation.

◆ **What contraceptive options are available to this woman?**

◆ **Which contraceptives are contraindicated for her?**

ANSWERS TO CASE 28: Family Planning—Contraceptives

Summary: A 38-year-old parous woman presents for counseling regarding her contraceptive options. She is in a monogamous relationship. She reports that she is dissatisfied with using over-the-counter options and that she is not ready for permanent sterilization. She smokes a half-pack of cigarettes daily.

 Available contraceptive options: Barrier contraceptives, intrauterine device, natural family planning

 Contraindicated contraceptive options: Oral contraceptive pills

Analysis

Objectives

1. To know the available methods of contraception.
2. To be aware of contraindications for and the side effects of contraceptives.

Considerations

Choosing a method of contraception is a personal decision, based on individual preferences, medical history, and lifestyle. Each method of contraception has a number of risks and benefits of which the patient should be aware. In the United States, approximately 50% of pregnancies are unintended and approximately 50% of these pregnancies end in abortion. Each method of contraceptive has a failure rate, which is an inability to prevent pregnancy over a 1-year period. Sometimes the failure rate is a result of the method and sometimes it is a result of human error. Each method has possible side effects. Some methods require lifestyle modifications. Patients with certain medical conditions cannot use certain types of contraceptives.

There are numerous contraceptive options available and recommendations regarding contraceptive use must be individualized. In the case given, there are several important factors that must be considered. Hormonal contraceptives are contraindicated in women older than age 35 years who smoke cigarettes. Given the patient's fear of surgery and because she is not certain whether she wants to have more children in the future, surgical sterilization via tubal ligation is not a choice. Barrier methods are too much of an inconvenience to the patient's busy lifestyle. A vasectomy might not be welcomed by the boyfriend. Given that both the patient and her boyfriend have no history of STDs and are in a long-term relationship, the best method of contraception for them may be an intrauterine device (IUD). A copper-T IUD can last up to 10 years before replacement, does not require the woman's busy lifestyle to be inconvenienced, and, in appropriately selected cases, is safe, effective, and well tolerated. Figure 28–1 is an algorithm that can be used as a guide to approaching family planning options.

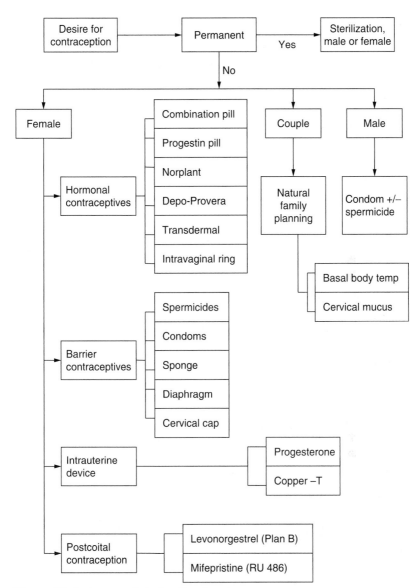

Figure 28–1. Approach to family planning.

Hormonal Contraception

Hormonal contraception involves ways of delivering estrogen and progesterone. Hormones interact with the body and have the potential for serious side effects, although this is rare. When properly used, hormonal methods are extremely effective. Hormonal methods are available only by prescription.

Oral Contraceptives

There are **two types of oral contraceptive pills (OCPs):** combination pills, which contain both estrogen and a progestin (a natural or synthetic progesterone), and "minipills," which contain only progestin. The combination pill suppresses ovulation through inhibition of the hypothalamic–pituitary–ovarian axis, alters the cervical mucus, retards sperm entry, and discourages implantation into an unfavorable endometrium. **Combination oral contraceptives offer significant protection against ovarian cancer, endometrial cancer, iron-deficiency anemia, pelvic inflammatory disease (PID), and fibrocystic breast disease.** Women who take combination pills have a lower risk of functional ovarian cysts. The minipill reduces cervical mucus and causes it to thicken. The mucus thickening prevents the sperm from reaching the egg and keeps the uterine lining from thickening, which prevents the fertilized egg from implanting in the uterus. When taken as directed, the failure rate for the minipill is 1–3%; the failure rate of the combination pill is 1–2%.

Smokers and women with certain medical conditions should not take the OCP. Table 28–1 lists the absolute and relative contraindications to taking the OCP. Minor side effects, which usually subside after a few months of usage, include nausea, headaches, breast swelling, fluid retention, weight gain, irregular bleeding, and depression.

When starting an OCP, patients should take the first pill the first day after the start of menses. Many women choose to start on the Sunday after the start of

Table 28–1
CONTRAINDICATIONS TO HORMONAL CONTRACEPTION

ABSOLUTE CONTRAINDICATIONS	RELATIVE CONTRAINDICATIONS
Thrombophlebitis, thromboembolic disease	Severe vascular headache (migraine, cluster)
Cerebral vascular disease	Severe hypertension (if younger
Coronary occlusion	than 35–40 years of age and in good
Impaired liver function	medical control, can elect OCP)
Known or suspected breast cancer	Diabetes mellitus (prevention of pregnancy outweighs the risk of complicating vascular
Undiagnosed abnormal vaginal bleeding	disease in diabetic who is younger than age 35–40 years)
Known or suspected pregnancy	Gallbladder disease (may exacerbate
Smokers older than the age of 35 years	emergence of symptoms when gallstones are present)
Congenital hyperlipidemia	Obstructive jaundice in pregnancy
	Epilepsy (antiepileptic drugs may decrease effectiveness of OCPs)
	Morbid obesity

their menses for convenience. Postpartum, non–breast-feeding women should start the OCP during the fourth week after delivery. OCPs can be started the day after an induced or spontaneous abortion. **If a pill is missed, it should be taken as soon as possible and the next dose should be taken as usual.** If two pills are missed, take 2 pills together on 2 consecutive days to catch up and alternative contraception should be used for 7 days.

The effectiveness of OCPs may be reduced by a few other medications, including some antibiotics, barbiturates, and antifungal medications. On the other hand, OCPs may prolong the effects of theophylline, benzodiazepine, and caffeine.

Medroxyprogesterone (Depo-Provera)

Medroxyprogesterone (Depo-Provera) is an injectable form of a progestin. Depo-Provera has a failure rate of only 1%. **Each injection provides contraceptive protection for 14 weeks.** It is injected every 3 months into a muscle in the buttocks or arm. Its side effects include irregular menses, weight gain, and facial/body hair growth. In addition, there may be irregular bleeding and spotting during the first months followed by periods of amenorrhea. About half of women develop amenorrhea after a year of Depo-Provera use.

Transdermal Contraceptive

A transdermal contraceptive patch (Ortho Evra) is available. It is a combined hormone patch containing norelgestromin (the active metabolite of norgestimate) and ethinyl estradiol. The treatment regimen for each cycle is three consecutive 7-day patches followed by one patch-free week, so that withdrawal bleeding can occur. **The patch's efficacy and side effects are comparable to that of combined OCPs.**

Intravaginal Ring Contraceptive

NuvaRing is a flexible, transparent ring made of ethylene vinylacetate copolymers that delivers etonogestrel and ethinyl estradiol. **A woman inserts the NuvaRing herself, wears it for 3 weeks, then removes and discards the device.** After one ring-free week, during which withdrawal bleeding occurs, a new ring is inserted. The side effects of NuvaRing are similar to those of combined OCPs, with the main adverse effect being disrupted bleeding.

Spermicides Used Alone

Spermicides come in many forms (foams, jellies, gels, and suppositories) and work by forming a physical and chemical barrier to sperm. They should be inserted into the vagina within an hour before intercourse. If intercourse is repeated, more spermicide should be inserted. The active ingredient in most spermicides is the chemical nonoxynol-9. The failure rate for spermicides in preventing pregnancy when used alone is 20–30%. Spermicides are available without a prescription. When **spermicides are used with a condom, the failure rate is comparable to that of oral contraceptives** and is much better than for either spermicides or condoms used alone.

Barrier Methods

There are **five barrier methods of contraception:** male condoms, female condoms, diaphragm, sponge, and cervical cap. In each, the method works by keeping the sperm and egg apart. The main possible side effect is an allergic reaction either to the material of the barrier or the spermicides that should be used with them. Using the methods correctly for each and every sexual intercourse gives the best protection.

Male Condom

Condoms on the market are made of either latex rubber or natural skin (from sheep intestines). Of these two types, **only latex condoms are highly effective preventing STDs.** Latex provides a good barrier to viruses such as HIV and hepatitis B. Each condom can only be used once. Condoms have a birth control failure rate of approximately 15%, with most of the failures a result of improper use. Some condoms have spermicide added, which may give some additional contraceptive protection. Vaginal spermicides may also be added before sexual intercourse.

Female Condom

The Reality Female Condom consists of a lubricated polyurethane sheath with a flexible polyurethane ring on each end. One ring is inserted into the vagina much like a diaphragm, while the other remains outside, partially covering the labia. The female condom may offer some protection against STDs; however, for highly effective protection, male latex condoms must be used. The estimated yearly failure rate ranges from 21–26%.

Sponge

The contraceptive sponge is made of white polyurethane foam. The sponge, shaped like a small doughnut, contains the spermicide nonoxynol-9. It is inserted into the vagina to cover the cervix during and after intercourse. It does not require fitting by a health professional and is available without prescription. It is to be used only once and then discarded. The failure rate is between 18% and 28%. An extremely rare side effect is toxic shock syndrome (TSS).

Diaphragm

The diaphragm is a flexible rubber disk with a rigid rim ranging in size from 2–4 inches in diameter. It is designed to cover the cervix during and after intercourse, so that sperm cannot reach the uterus. Spermicidal jelly or cream must be placed inside the diaphragm for it to be effective. The diaphragm must be fitted by a health professional and the correct size prescribed to ensure a snug seal with the vaginal wall. If intercourse is repeated, additional spermicide should be added with the diaphragm still in place. The **diaphragm should be left in place for at least 6 hours after intercourse.** The diaphragm used with spermicide has a failure rate of from 6–18%.

Cervical Cap

The cervical cap is a dome-shaped rubber cap in various sizes that fits snugly over the cervix. Like the diaphragm, it is used with a spermicide and must be fitted by a health professional. It is more difficult to insert than the diaphragm, but may be left in place for up to 48 hours. There also appears to be an increased incidence of irregular Papanicolaou (Pap) tests in the first 6 months of using the cap, and TSS is an extremely rare side effect. The cap has a failure rate of about 18%.

Intrauterine Devices

IUDs are small, plastic, flexible devices that are inserted into the uterus through the cervix by a trained physician. **Only two IUDs are presently marketed in the United States:** ParaGard T380A, a T-shaped device partially covered by copper and effective for 10 years, and Progestasert, which is also T-shaped but contains a progestin released over a 1-year period. Both IUDs have a 4–5% failure rate. An IUD alters the uterine and tubal fluids, particularly in the case of copper-bearing IUDs, inhibiting the transport of sperm through the cervical mucus and uterus. The risk of PID with IUD use is highest in those women with multiple sex partners or who have a history of previous PID. Consequently, the **IUD is recommended primarily for women in mutually monogamous relationships.**

Absolute contraindications for IUD include current, recent (within 3 months), or recurrent endometritis, PID, or STD; pregnancy; anatomically distorted uterine cavity; and known or suspected HIV infection. Relative contraindications include any history of gonorrhea or chlamydia; multiple sexual partners or a partner with multiple other partners; undiagnosed abnormal vaginal bleeding; known or suspected uterine or cervical malignancy; and previous problems with an IUD (pregnancy, expulsion, perforation, pain, heavy bleeding). In addition to PID, other complications include perforation of the uterus, septic abortion, and ectopic pregnancy. Women may also experience some short-term side effects such as cramping and dizziness at the time of insertion; bleeding, cramps, and backache that may continue for a few days after the insertion; spotting between periods; and longer and heavier menstruation during the first few periods after insertion. The patient should check that the string is palpable each month after her menses. Between 2% and 10% of women expel their IUD within the first year. The absolute rate of ectopic pregnancy is reduced with the IUD because of its high contraceptive efficacy. However, when accidental pregnancy does occur, there is an increased proportion of ectopics, highest with the Progestasert. Adolescence and nulliparity are not contraindications in properly selected young women in monogamous relationships.

Natural Family Planning

Periodic abstinence (natural family planning or rhythm method) entails not having sexual intercourse during the woman's fertile period. Using periodic abstinence is dependent on the ability to identify the approximately 10 days in each menstrual cycle that a woman is fertile. Periodic abstinence has a failure rate of 14–47%. Women with irregular cycles have the highest failure rates. The basal body temperature method is based on the knowledge that just before ovulation a woman's basal body temperature drops several tenths of a degree and after ovulation it returns to normal. The method requires that the woman take her temperature each morning before she gets out of bed. There are now electronic thermometers with memories and electrical resistance meters that can more accurately pinpoint a woman's fertile period. The cervical mucus method, also called the Billings method, depends on a woman recognizing the changes in cervical mucus that indicate ovulation is occurring or has occurred.

Surgical Sterilization

Tubal ligation seals a woman's fallopian tubes so that an egg cannot travel to the uterus. Vasectomy involves closing off a man's vas deferens so that sperm will not be carried to the penis. Vasectomy is a minor surgical procedure, most often performed in a doctor's office under local anesthesia. Tubal ligation is an operating room procedure performed under general anesthesia. Major complications, which are rare in female sterilization, include infection, hemorrhage, and problems associated with the use of general anesthesia. The failure rate is less than 1%. Although there has been some success in reopening the fallopian tubes and the vas deferens, the success rate is low, and **sterilization should be considered irreversible.**

Emergency Contraception

All female patients of reproductive age should be made aware of postcoital contraception. This knowledge does not increase the likelihood of high-risk behavior. The **Yuzpe method consists of taking combined OCPs for emergency contraception.** High doses of oral contraceptives, begun within 72 hours of unprotected intercourse, decrease the risk of pregnancy by 74%. Only RU-486 (mifepristone) is effective after 72 hours. Consider prescribing an antiemetic, as nausea and vomiting are common side effects. Two oral doses of levonorgestrel (Plan B) 0.75 mg, with 12 hours between doses, is an effective and well-tolerated regimen. Preven, a convenient emergency contraception kit, includes two doses of medication and a pregnancy test. Mifepristone (RU-486) 600 mg in a single dose is the most effective emergency contraceptive and has the fewest side effects.

Levonorgestrel Implants

Levonorgestrel in silastic capsules (Norplant) was the first contraceptive implant. In a minor surgical procedure, 6 matchstick-size rubber capsules containing progestin were placed just underneath the skin of the upper arm. The implant was effective within 24 hours and provided progestin for up to 5 years. The failure rate for Norplant was less than 1% for women who weighed less than 150 pounds. The potential side effects of the implant included irregular menstrual bleeding, headaches, nervousness, depression, nausea, dizziness, skin rash, acne, change of appetite, breast tenderness, weight gain, enlargement of the ovaries or fallopian tubes, and excessive growth of body and facial hair. Norplant is no longer manufactured.

Comprehension Questions

[28.1] Which of the following is a contraindication to IUD placement?

    A. Any history of STD

    B. Nulliparity

    C. Desire for future fertility

    D. HIV infection

[28.2] A patient reported having intercourse with her boyfriend 20 hours ago. She was concerned because the condom broke. She used no other form of contraception. The patient reported a history of regular periods. What is her risk of pregnancy?

    A. >40%

    B. ~30%

    C. ~15%

    D. ~8%

    E. <1%

[28.3] A 32-year-old woman reports that she and her acquaintance had consensual intercourse but the condom broke. She is midcycle. She has had chlamydial cervicitis in the past. Her pregnancy test is negative. She desires something to prevent pregnancy. Which of the following is the most appropriate method of "emergency contraception"?

    A. Yuzpe method

    B. Plan B method

    C. Insertion of an IUD

    D. Intramuscular methotrexate

[28.4] A combination oral contraceptive agent is being considered for a patient who wishes contraception. Which of the following is the most important contraindication to prescribing a combination OCP?

    A. Patient is older than age 35 years and smokes cigarettes.

    B. Patient is less than 2 weeks postpartum.

    C. Patient has hirsutism and irregular cycles,

    D. Patient is breast-feeding her 2-month-old daughter.

Answers

[28.1] **D.** Known or suspected HIV infection is a contraindication to IUD placement. IUDs can be used in selected nulliparous women and in women who desire future fertility. A history of an STD is a relative, but not an absolute, contraindication to IUD use.

[28.2] **D.** Approximately 8% of women will become pregnant after a single act of coitus.

[28.3] **B.** Emergency contraception may include combination hormonal therapy at time zero and at 72 hours; many OCPs are effective if used in the right doses and within 72 hours. Plan B is levonorgestrel and is more effective than the combined OCPs for postcoital contraception. In addition, it does not have the prominent side effect of nausea. The IUD is relatively contraindicated in this patient because of her history of *Chlamydia* infection.

[28.4] **A.** The most important contraindications to combination oral contraceptives are current cardiovascular disease, smoking, and older than age 35 years. Oral contraceptives can help in women with polycystic ovarian syndrome and hirsutism. Low-dose oral contraceptives are not contraindicated in breast-feeding patients, especially after the milk has come in.

CLINICAL PEARLS

❖ The male latex condom remains the best shield against AIDS and other STDs.

❖ Barrier methods, which work by keeping the sperm and egg apart, usually have only minor side effects.

❖ Combination oral contraceptives offer significant protection against ovarian cancer, endometrial cancer, iron-deficiency anemia, PID, and fibrocystic breast disease.

❖ Methods of hormonal contraception, when used properly, are extremely effective.

❖ Surgical sterilization must be considered permanent. Vasectomy is considered safer than tubal ligation.

❖ Noncontraceptive benefits of combination oral contraceptives include decreased incidence of benign breast disease, relief from menstrual disorders (dysmenorrhea and menorrhagia), reduced risk of uterine leiomyomata, protection against ovarian cysts, reduction of acne, improvement of bone mineral density, and a reduced risk of colorectal cancer.

REFERENCES

Beckmann CR, Ling FW, Laube DW, et al. Obstetrics and gynecology. 4th ed. Philadelphia, PA: Lippincott, Williams and Wilkins, 2002:327, 347.

Burkman RT. Oral contraceptives: current status. Clin Obstet Gynecol 2001;44:62.

Brunsell SC. Contraception. In: South-Paul JE, Matheny SC, Lewis EL (eds). Current diagnosis and treatment in family medicine. New York: McGraw-Hill, 2004:211.

Greydanus DE, Patel DR, Rimsza ME. Contraception in the adolescent: an update. Pediatrics 2001;107:562.

Jensen JT, Speroff L. Health benefits of oral contraceptives. Obstet Gynecol Clin North Am 2000;27:705.

A 16-year-old female presents for a routine well examination. She is a junior in high school and has no significant medical history. She plays on the school softball team and has a preparticipation clearance form for you to complete. She is accompanied by her mother who wants to know if her daughter should start having routine gynecologic examinations as part of her routine checkup. She states that the patient's last tetanus shot was at the age of 5 years. She received all of the routine childhood immunizations, including a complete hepatitis B series, and had chickenpox when she was 6 years old. The mother reports that there are no medical problems in the immediate family, but that one of the patient's cousins died at the age of 21 years of a sudden cardiac death. When interviewed without the mother in the room, the patient reports to you that she is generally happy, she gets As and Bs in school, and has an active social life. She denies ever being involved in sexual activity, or tobacco or drug use. She says that she will have a "drink or two" at a party with her friends. On examination, her vital signs are normal. Examination of her head and neck, lungs, abdomen, skin, and musculoskeletal and nervous systems are normal. On cardiac auscultation, you hear a 2/6 systolic murmur that gets louder when you have her Valsalva. Peripheral pulses are strong and symmetric, there is good capillary refill and no sign of cyanosis.

◆ **What immunizations should be recommended at this visit?**

◆ **At what age is it recommended to start routine Papanicolaou (Pap) smear screening?**

◆ **What is the most common cause of sudden cardiac death in young athletes?**

ANSWERS TO CASE 29: Adolescent Health Maintenance

Summary: A healthy 16-year-old female presents for a routine checkup and sports preparticipation examination. She is noted incidentally to have a heart murmur.

◆ **Recommended immunization:** Tetanus-diphtheria booster and meningococcal vaccination

◆ **Recommended age to start routine Pap smears:** Within 3 years of the start of sexual activity or age 21, whichever comes first

◆ **Most common cause of sudden cardiac death in young athletes:** Hypertrophic cardiomyopathy

Analysis

Objectives

1. Be familiar with the recommendations of the Guidelines for Adolescent Preventive Services (GAPS) for screening examinations and counseling in adolescents.
2. Know the immunizations routinely recommended for adolescents and teenagers.
3. Know the components of and the rationale for performing sports preparticipation examinations

Considerations

Adolescence is a time of physical, emotional, and psychosocial changes. It is also a time of experimentation and, frequently, risk taking. Fortunately, adolescence is also a time of relatively good health for most. However, the choices made during adolescence can affect both the short- and long-term health of the patient. Addressing the unique healthcare needs of adolescents can be difficult, as they may be more likely to present to the physician for acute illness than for health maintenance. For this reason, physicians should take the opportunity to consider age-appropriate health maintenance at each encounter with an adolescent and young adult.

Numerous issues can serve as barriers to providing effective care to adolescent patients; one of these is confidentiality. Many adolescents believe that physicians share any information provided with the parent. Consequently, they may not volunteer information, such as sexual activity or use of tobacco, alcohol, and drugs. One commonly used technique to address this is to take a history with the parent in the room, to allow the parent to present any concerns, then interview the patient alone, to allow the patient to speak confidentially with the doctor. **Physicians who treat adolescent patients should have policies in**

place to ensure doctor–patient confidentiality while balancing the parent's right to be involved with the child's care. These policies should be discussed with and agreed to by the patient and parent in advance, so as to promote an honest, trusting, and therapeutic relationship.

The American Medical Association has published *Guidelines for Adolescent Preventive Services (GAPS),* a series of recommendations regarding the delivery of health services, promotion of well-being, screening for common conditions, and provision of immunizations for adolescents and young adults between the ages of 11 and 21 years. These services are intended to be delivered as part of a series of annual healthcare visits that address biomedical and psychosocial aspects of health and emphasize preventive services. These visits should include at least 3 complete physical examinations, one in early adolescence (age 11–14), one in middle adolescence (age 15–17), and one in late adolescence (age 18–21).

The **GAPS guidelines recommend counseling for both parents and adolescents.** It recommends that physicians provide guidance to parents on normal physical, sexual, and emotional development, signs of physical and emotional problems, parenting behaviors to promote health, and methods to help their child to avoid harmful behaviors. The adolescent patient should receive counseling annually on their growth and development, injury prevention, healthy diet, exercise, and avoidance of harmful substances (alcohol, tobacco, drugs, anabolic steroids). Guidance should also emphasize responsible sexual behaviors, including abstinence and contraception, to reduce the risks of sexually transmitted diseases (STDs) and pregnancy.

GAPS recommends the routine screening for several medical, behavioral, and emotional conditions. All adolescents should be screened annually for hypertension, with further evaluation and treatment for those whose blood pressure is above the 90th percentile for their gender and age. All should be screened annually for eating disorders and obesity. All should also be screened for the use of tobacco (both cigarettes and smokeless tobacco), alcohol, and other abusable substances. Routine toxicology screening, however, is not recommended. Lipid screening is recommended for those at above average risk based on a personal history of comorbid conditions or a family history of hyperlipidemia, coronary artery disease, or other vascular diseases. Tuberculosis (TB) skin testing should be performed in those at high risk. These risks include having lived (or living) in a homeless shelter or in an area with a high prevalence of TB, having been (or being) incarcerated, having been exposed to active TB, and working in a healthcare setting.

All adolescents should be asked about sexual behaviors, including sexual orientation, use of contraception, number of sexual partners, and history of pregnancy or STDs. **Sexually active females should be screened for gonorrhea and *Chlamydia* by cervical sampling.** Cervical cancer screening should also be performed in sexually active females. The United States Preventive Services Task Force (USPSTF), in a 2003 guideline, states that screening for cervical cancer with Pap smears should begin within 3 years of onset of sexual activity or age 21 years, whichever comes first. **Sexually active males can** be screened for presumptive gonorrhea and *Chlamydia* infections by urine test for leukocyte esterase. Males and females at risk for HIV should be offered confidential testing.

Other recommendations include screening all adolescents annually for depression and risk of suicide, with appropriate management or referral of those in need. All should also be questioned annually about emotional, physical, or sexual abuse. Every state mandates the reporting of suspected abuse of minors to the designated child welfare agency or child protective service. Difficulties at school or with learning should also be evaluated annually, with subsequent management to be coordinated with the school and parent/guardian.

The adolescent health visit is also a time to ensure that the patient is appropriately immunized against preventable infections. In those who have received the recommended primary series, a tetanus-diphtheria (Td) booster is recommended at ages 11–12 years and then every 10 years thereafter. Varicella vaccine should be offered to those who have not been vaccinated and who do not have a history of chickenpox. A measles-mumps-rubella (MMR) booster should be given if the patient did not receive a booster at ages 4–6 years. The hepatitis B series should be given to any adolescent who has not been previously immunized. Hepatitis A vaccine can be offered to those who live in areas with high infection rates, travel to high risk areas, have chronic liver disease, or inject IV drugs, and to males who have sex with males.

In 2005, the Centers for Disease Control and Prevention's (CDC) Advisory Committee on Immunization Practices added a new recommendation for routine meningococcal vaccination using a tetravalent polysaccharide-protein conjugate vaccine (MCV4). Routine vaccination is recommended at ages 11–12 years. If not previously vaccinated, vaccination before high school is advised. Vaccination is also recommended for college freshmen living in dormitories and for others at increased risk, such as military recruits, travelers to endemic areas, or the functionally/anatomically asplenic.

Sports Preparticipation Examination

A common reason for healthy adolescents to present to primary care physicians is for a preparticipation examination as a requirement to play a sport in school. The goal of these examinations is to attempt to identify conditions that may place a young athlete at risk during athletic participation. These conditions are primarily cardiac and orthopedic, but are not limited to these systems. A preparticipation examination allows the physician to provide the comprehensive health maintenance, including counseling, anticipatory guidance, screening, and vaccination, recommended in the GAPS guidelines. These encounters also serve to meet legal and insurance requirements of the school or school system.

The rate of sudden cardiac death in athletes is very low. Congenital cardiac anomalies are the most common etiology, with hypertrophic cardiomyopathy accounting for about one-third and anomalous coronary arteries for about one-fifth of cardiac anomalies. The **history is the most important tool in screening for these abnormalities.** All adolescents and their parents should be asked about personal history of exertional chest pain, dyspnea, syncope, history of heart murmurs, and family history of hypertrophic cardiomyopathy other congenital cardiac abnormalities or premature cardiac deaths. Other important historical information includes history of asthma or other pulmonary disorders, orthopedic injuries, heat-related illness, and absence of one of a paired organ (e.g., single kidney, testicle, ovary, etc).

It is important to screen for eating disorders, as well as for a desire to change body weight, either for body image or for athletic purposes (e.g., "weight cutting" for wrestlers). Eating disorders are more common in female than male athletes. Females should be questioned about menstrual irregularities, as amenorrhea could signal anorexia and amenorrheic female athletes could be at risk for osteoporosis.

The examination should be thorough, but several aspects should be emphasized. Blood pressure should be measured and compared with age- and gender-appropriate norms. General appearance, specifically looking for signs of Marfan syndrome, should be noted. These signs, which include arachnodactyly, an arm span greater than height, pectus excavatum, tall-thin habitus, high arched palate, and ocular lens subluxations, should prompt further evaluation, as persons with Marfan can have aortic abnormalities that predispose to rupture during sports. Auscultation of the heart should be performed, at minimum, in both the lying and standing positions. **The murmur of hypertrophic cardiomyopathy, while not always present, is best heard along the left sternal border and accentuates with activities that decrease cardiac preload and end diastolic volume of the left ventricle.** Therefore, standing or straining with a Valsalva maneuver would increase the murmur; conversely, squatting would be expected to decrease the murmur. **Any adolescent with stigmata of Marfan syndrome, a murmur suggestive of hypertrophic cardiomyopathy, with a grade 3/6 or louder systolic murmur, or any diastolic murmur should be evaluated by a cardiologist prior to clearance for athletic participation.**

No specific tests are recommended for universal screening of all athletes, although specific tests may be indicated based upon history or physical examination findings. Echocardiography is the study of choice for the diagnosis of hypertrophic cardiomyopathy.

Participation in athletics or exercise should be encouraged. **Absolute contraindications to all athletic participation are rare;** more commonly, clearance to participate may be delayed for further evaluation of a suspected condition, rehabilitation of an injury, or recovery from an acute illness. In almost all cases, an adolescent should be able to find some athletic pursuit in which the adolescent may participate.

Comprehension Questions

[29.1] Which of the following should prompt a referral to a cardiologist prior to clearance to participate in high school sports?

    A. A 2/6 systolic murmur in an asymptomatic 16-year-old

    B. A 1/6 diastolic murmur heard at the apex in a 17-year-old

    C. A 2/6 systolic murmur heard while lying down that gets softer when standing

    D. An asymptomatic 16-year-old whose grandfather died of a heart attack at age 72

[29.2] Which of the following is recommended routinely in the Guidelines for Adolescent Preventive Services?

    A. Annual complete physical examinations between the ages of 11 and 21 years

    B. Periodic screening for drug use with a urine toxicology test

    C. Cholesterol testing for all teenagers

    D. Annual screening for hypertension for all adolescents

[29.3] A 17-year-old male reports that he has been sexually active with 2 female partners in the past year. He has used condoms "sometimes, but not always." He is asymptomatic for anything and has a normal physical examination. Which of the following tests would be recommended to screen him for gonorrhea and *Chlamydia*?

    A. Urethral swab

    B. Serum antibodies to *Neisseria gonorrhoeae* and *Chlamydia trachomatis*

    C. Urine for leukocyte esterase

    D. No screening is recommended

Answers

[29.1] **B.** Any patient with a diastolic murmur, grade 3/6 or louder systolic murmur, murmur suggestive of hypertrophic cardiomyopathy, or signs of Marfan syndrome should be evaluated by a cardiologist prior to clearance to participate in athletics. The murmur of hypertrophic cardiomyopathy typically gets louder with maneuvers that reduce preload, such as standing or Valsalva.

[29.2] **D.** GAPS recommends annual screening for hypertension by blood pressure measurement in all adolescents. Complete physical examinations are advised routinely, once during early adolescence, once in midadolescence, and once in late adolescence, as well as more often when indicated. Lipid screening should be targeted to those who are at high risk based on personal or family history. Routine toxicology screening is not recommended.

[29.3] **C.** Urine for leukocyte esterase is recommended as screening for presumptive gonorrhea or *Chlamydia* in sexually active males. A urethral swab is more appropriate for diagnostic testing in a male who has a urethral discharge.

CLINICAL PEARLS

❖ Adolescents tend to see physicians irregularly. Take the time at each visit, no matter what the chief complaint is, to review health maintenance issues.

❖ True contraindications to participation in all sports are rare. Almost everyone should be able to participate in some form of athletic activity.

❖ Universal adolescent vaccination with meningococcal vaccine became a recommendation in 2005; unvaccinated adolescents and teens should be offered vaccination routinely.

REFERENCES

American Medical Association. Guidelines for adolescent preventive services (GAPS): recommendations monograph. Chicago: American Medical Association, 1997.

Centers for Disease Control and Prevention. Prevention and control of meningococcal disease: recommendations of the Advisory Committee on Immunization Practices (ACIP). MMWR 2005;54(No. RR-7):1–28.

Kurowski K, Chandran S. The preparticipation athletic evaluation. Am Fam Physician 2000;61:2683–2690, 2696–268.

McKeag DB, Sallis RE. Factors at play in the athletic preparticipation examination [editorial]. Am Fam Physician 2000;61:2617.

United States Preventive Services Task Force. Screening for cervical cancer. Available at: www.ahrq.gov/clinic/uspstf/uspscerv.htm.

A 47-year-old male presents to your office for a follow-up visit. He was seen 3 weeks ago for an upper respiratory infection and noted incidentally to have a blood pressure of 164/98 mm Hg. He vaguely remembered being told in the past that his blood pressure was "borderline" in the past. He feels fine, has no complaints, and his review of systems is entirely negative. He does not smoke cigarettes, drinks "a couple of beers on the weekends," and does not exercise regularly. He has a sedentary job. His father died of a stroke at the age of 69 years. His mother is alive and in good health at the age of 72 years. He has two siblings and isn't aware of any chronic medical issues that they have. In the office today, his blood pressure is 156/96 mm Hg in his left arm and 152/98 mm Hg in the right arm. He is afebrile, his pulse is 78 beats/min, respiratory rate 14 breaths/min, he is 70 inches tall, and weighs 210 lb. A general physical examination is normal.

◆ **What diagnosis (or diagnoses) can you make today?**

◆ **What further evaluation needs to be performed?**

◆ **What nonpharmacologic intervention(s) may be beneficial?**

◆ **What is the recommended initial medication management?**

ANSWERS TO CASE 30: Hypertension

Summary: A 47-year-old male is found to have an elevated blood pressure reading when seen for an unrelated problem visit. On follow-up, his blood pressure remains elevated. He is obese and leads a sedentary lifestyle but does not have other high risks based on his personal or family history.

◆ **Diagnoses from today's visit:** Stage 1 hypertension and obesity

◆ **Necessary further evaluation:** Blood glucose; serum potassium, creatinine, and calcium levels; hematocrit; urinalysis; electrocardiogram (EKG)

◆ **Nonpharmacologic interventions:** DASH (Dietary Approaches to Stop Hypertension) diet; alcohol limitation to no more than 2 drinks per day; increased physical activity; weight reduction

◆ **Recommended initial medication:** Thiazide diuretic

Analysis

Objectives

1. Know the diagnostic criteria for hypertension.
2. Learn the recommended initial evaluation of persons found with an elevated blood pressure.
3. Know the medication and lifestyle modifications that can help to control blood pressure.
4. Learn the complications and risks of uncontrolled hypertension.

Considerations

The patient presented here is typical of one seen everyday in primary care offices and represents the most common presentation of hypertension. Most hypertensive patients do not have any symptoms of their disease. They are typically seen for another reason and noted to have a high blood pressure reading. Untreated hypertension significantly raises an individual's risk of myocardial infarction, cerebrovascular accidents, and renal failure, among other conditions. **The risk of cardiovascular disease doubles with each increase in blood pressure of 20/10 mm Hg above 115/75 mm Hg.** Because of the high prevalence of the problem, the lack of symptoms and the demonstrated efficacy of treatment in reducing the risk of complications, the United States Preventive Services Task Force recommends screening every adult patient for hypertension by measuring their blood pressure. The appropriate screening interval is not clearly defined, but most practitioners will check the blood pressure of every adult patient at every office visit.

APPROACH TO HYPERTENSION

Definition

JNC 7: The 7th report of the Joint National Committee on Prevention, Detection, Evaluation and Treatment of High Blood Pressure. A comprehensive, evidence-based, expert review of the diagnosis, evaluation, and management of hypertension (available at: www.nhlbi.nih.gov/guidelines/hypertension/ express.pdf).

Scope of Problem and Risks

Hypertension is the most common primary diagnosis at physician office visits in the United States each year. **Approximately 50 million Americans have hypertension and approximately 30% are unaware of their problem.** The prevalence is higher in African-Americans and in older patients. National Health and Nutritional Examination Surveys (NHANES) data suggest that hypertension is responsible for approximately one-third of heart attacks, one-half of heart failure, and one-fourth of premature deaths. Most patients with end-stage kidney disease are hypertensive. Hypertensive nephrosclerosis is responsible for approximately one-fourth of end-stage kidney disease. **The risk of complications is directly related to the elevation of the blood pressure—the higher the blood pressure, the higher the risk.**

Elevated systolic blood pressure is a greater risk for cardiovascular disease complications than elevated diastolic pressure. Control of systolic blood pressure tends to be more difficult to achieve, and when it is achieved, the diastolic blood pressure usually comes under control as well. The goal of treatment is to get the blood pressure to <140/90 mm Hg. For persons with diabetes or kidney disease, the goal is to achieve a blood pressure of <130/80 mm Hg.

Diagnosis and Work-Up

The diagnosis of hypertension relies on accurate measurement of blood pressure. The appropriate technique is to allow the patient to sit quietly in a chair (not on the examination table) with a supported back and feet on the floor for 5 minutes prior to making the measurement. The blood pressure should be measured at least twice, using a calibrated sphygmomanometer and an appropriately sized cuff for the patient. The blood pressure cuff should encircle at least 80% of the patient's arm; a cuff that is too small can result in a falsely elevated reading.

The diagnosis of hypertension is made based on the average of two properly taken blood pressure measurements at two or more office visits. JNC 7 places blood pressure readings into one of four categories: Normal, prehypertension, stage 1 hypertension, and stage 2 hypertension (Table 30–1). The prehypertension category was a new addition in JNC 7, in recognition of the fact that people with blood pressure in this range have twice the risk of progression to overt hypertension as those with normal blood pressure.

Table 30–1
CLASSIFICATION OF BLOOD PRESSURE

CLASSIFICATION	SYSTOLIC BLOOD PRESSURE (mm Hg)	DIASTOLIC BLOOD PRESSURE (mm Hg)
Normal	<120	and <80
Prehypertension	120–139	or 80–89
Stage 1 hypertension	140–159	or 90–99
Stage 2 hypertension	≥160	or ≥100

When hypertension is diagnosed, an **evaluation consisting of a history, physical examination, and focused diagnostic studies should be performed, with the goals of assessing overall cardiovascular risks, identification of possibly secondary causes of hypertension, and determination of the presence of any end-organ damage.** Historical information should include personal and family medical histories, an assessment of diet and activity levels, and specific questioning regarding tobacco, alcohol, recreational drug and medication (both prescription and nonprescription) use. Patients should be questioned about cardiovascular, cerebrovascular, and peripheral arterial disease symptoms.

Along with blood pressure, examination should include all other vital signs and a measurement of body mass index. Other specific components of the examination should include a funduscopic examination for signs of retinopathy, auscultation for carotid, femoral, and renal bruits, palpation of peripheral pulses, abdominal palpation for signs of organomegaly or aortic aneurysm, and a complete cardiopulmonary examination.

Initial testing should include measurement of serum potassium, creatinine (with glomerular filtration rate calculation) and calcium, blood glucose, and hematocrit. A urinalysis should be done to look for proteinuria or cellular components suggestive of renal disease. An EKG should be performed to evaluate for changes consistent with coronary artery disease and to screen for left ventricular hypertrophy (LVH).

Nonpharmacologic Management

Once the diagnosis of hypertension, or prehypertension, is made, patients should be advised of specific lifestyle modifications that can both reduce their blood pressure and reduce their overall cardiac risk factors. These should include efforts to lose weight if overweight or obese, an increase in physical activity, and reduced consumption of alcohol. Men should consume no more than two alcoholic beverages a day and women no more than one. Any smoker should be counseled to quit.

A high-potassium and high-calcium diet, the **Dietary Approaches to Stop Hypertension (DASH) diet plan, reduces blood pressure in an amount**

comparable to single-agent drug therapy. An informational brochure detailing the DASH diet is available from the National Heart, Lung and Blood Institute at www.nhlbi.nih.gov/health/public/heart/hbp/dash/new_dash.pdf. Combining the various lifestyle modifications provides additive benefits, and these efforts should continue even when the decision is made to start medications.

Pharmacologic Management

Lowering blood pressure reduces the risk of adverse outcomes such as strokes and heart attacks. In the primary treatment of hypertension, thiazide diuretics are the recommended first-line therapy in most settings, because they are well-tolerated, inexpensive, and no other medication has superior outcomes in head-to-head studies. Patients with stage 1 hypertension who are inadequately controlled with nonpharmacologic interventions alone should be started on a thiazide diuretic, unless there is a compelling reason to start another class of medication (Table 30–2). Patients with stage 2 hypertension or anyone whose

Table 30–2

INDICATIONS FOR STARTING SPECIFIC CLASSES
OF ANTIHYPERTENSIVE MEDICATION

INDICATION	CLASS OF MEDICATION
Diabetes mellitus	Angiotensin-converting enzyme inhibitor Angiotensin receptor blocker Diuretic Calcium channel blocker β-Blocker
High risk of coronary artery disease	Angiotensin-converting enzyme inhibitor β-Blocker Diuretic Calcium channel blocker
Congestive heart failure	Angiotensin-converting enzyme inhibitor Angiotensin receptor blocker β-Blocker Diuretic Aldosterone antagonist
Postmyocardial infarction	Angiotensin-converting enzyme inhibitor β-Blocker Aldosterone antagonist
Chronic kidney disease	Angiotensin-converting enzyme inhibitor Angiotensin receptor blocker
Prevention of recurrent cerebrovascular accident	Angiotensin-converting enzyme inhibitor Diuretic

blood pressure is above the recommended goal by ≥20/10 mm Hg should be started on combination therapy with two medications given either as separate prescriptions or as a fixed-dose combination of medications.

Comprehension Questions

[30.1] A 62-year-old woman presents for a routine physical examination. She is asymptomatic and is not taking any medications. Her blood pressure is found to be 135/85 mm Hg on two readings. Review of her chart reveals that her blood pressure was 133/84 mm Hg on a visit 4 months ago for a urinary tract infection. Which of the following is the most accurate statement regarding her blood pressure?

A. Her blood pressure is normal and she is at average risk for developing hypertension.

B. She has prehypertension and is at high risk for developing hypertension.

C. She has stage 1 hypertension and should be started on a thiazide diuretic.

D. She has stage 2 hypertension and should be started on multidrug therapy.

[30.2] A patient with stage 1 hypertension does not wish to start medications at this time. What can you tell him about the benefits of lifestyle modifications in the control of his hypertension?

A. The DASH diet can be as effective as single-drug therapy.

B. Diet and exercise is unlikely to lower his blood pressure but can reduce his other risks of cardiovascular disease.

C. A low-potassium diet is recommended for persons with hypertension.

D. When he starts taking medication he doesn't have to worry as much about modifying his lifestyle.

[30.3] A 48-year-old type 2 diabetic has had persistent blood pressure readings of 150/95 mm Hg. Which of the following is the most appropriate treatment for him?

A. DASH diet and recheck blood pressure in 3 months

B. Thiazide diuretic alone

C. Angiotensin-converting enzyme inhibitor alone

D. Combination of angiotensin-converting enzyme inhibitor and thiazide diuretic

Answers

[30.1] **B.** This patient's blood pressure falls in the prehypertensive range. She is at increased risk for developing hypertension and may benefit from the institution of lifestyle modifications to try to reduce her risk of progression.

[30.2] **A.** The DASH diet, a high-potassium and high-calcium diet, is as effective as single-agent antihypertensive therapy. The combination of diet and exercise can both lower blood pressure and other cardiac risk factors. Lifestyle modification efforts should continue along with medication therapy, as the effects will be additive.

[30.3] **D.** This patient's blood pressure goal is <130/80 mmHg. He is >20/10 mmHg above this goal, so a combination of medications is the most appropriate initial therapy.

CLINICAL PEARLS

❖❖ Check every adult patient's blood pressure at every office visit.

❖❖ Thiazide diuretics should be the first-line drug treatment in almost all cases of hypertension. There should be a compelling reason to use another agent before a thiazide.

❖ All patients with hypertension are at risk for cardiovascular and cerebrovascular disease. Be sure to address their other significant risks for these diseases, including lipids, smoking, diabetic control, and obesity.

REFERENCES

National Heart, Lung and Blood Institute. The 7th report of the Joint National Committee on the Prevention, Detection, Evaluation and Treatment of High Blood Pressure. December 2003. Available at: www.nhlbi.nih.gov/guidelines/hypertension/express.pdf.

United States Preventive Services Task Force (USPSTF). High blood pressure screening. Updated July, 2003. Available at: www.ahrq.gov/clinic/uspstf/uspshype.htm.

The mother of a 12-month old male infant calls you at midnight stating that her son has been crying incessantly for the last 6 hours. His bouts of crying last for about 20 minutes, then completely disappear for 15 minutes at a time. Since early afternoon the child has not been eating much and he has started to vomit the small amounts of juice and milk he had ingested. She decided to call you because the vomitus is now green and the bouts of crying seem to be getting worse.

In the emergency room, you recall that the patient does not have any past medical history, was born term without complications, and is up to date on immunizations. On examination his temperature is is 100°F, his respiration rate is 40 breaths/min, his pulse is 155 beats/min, his blood pressure is 109/60 mm Hg, and his weight is 22 lb. He cries inconsolably for 15 minutes, drawing his legs up to his chest, then becomes quiet. You notice he still produces tears, and his mucosae are moist. Heart and lung examinations are normal; abdominal examination reveals markedly decreased bowel sounds with generalized tenderness to palpation. You feel a sausagelike mass in the right side of the abdomen. His diaper holds some amount of bloody stool mixed with mucus. The rest of the examination is normal.

◆ **What is the most likely diagnosis?**

◆ **What is the next diagnostic step?**

◆ **What are the possible complications?**

ANSWERS TO CASE 31: Abdominal Pain and Vomiting in a Child

Summary: This is a 12-month-old infant who had the sudden onset of inter-mittent crying with vomiting that later became bilious. As the day progressed, his bouts of pain became more severe, each lasting about 20 minutes. On examination, the infant does not yet reveal signs of hypovolemia, sepsis, or shock. On palpation of the abdomen, there is generalized tenderness and a sausagelike mass on the right side. Even though not mentioned by the parent, there is a small amount of bloody-mucous stool that is best described as "currant jelly." This patient has an intussusception that has progressed to an obstruction, and is at risk for perforation with ensuing shock and sepsis.

◆ **Most likely diagnosis:** Intestinal obstruction caused by intussusception

◆ **Next diagnostic step:** Abdominal plain x-rays to rule out perforation

◆ **Possible complications:** If perforation occurs, rapid deterioration as a consequence of shock/sepsis.

Analysis

Objectives

1. Become familiar with the most likely causes of intestinal obstruction in the pediatric population.
2. Learn to differentiate between life-threatening abdominal emergencies and urgent conditions.
3. Have a diagnostic approach to the pediatric patient presenting with abdominal pain and vomiting.

Considerations

This 12-month-old infant initially presented with vomiting and intermittent abdom-inal pain. His vomitus was initially the gastric contents of what he had ingested, but later became bilious, which is suggestive of intestinal obstruction. The descrip-tion of his abdominal pain tends to reveal the pathophysiologic nature of intus-susception. The intermittency and "pain-free" intervals correlate with the gradual and slow telescoping of the intussusceptum (proximal or leading part of the intestine) into the intussuscipiens (distal or receiving end of the intestine). As the "telescoping" progresses, the portions of bowel that are trapped within the lumen of the intestine become edematous, which will ultimately lead to obstruc-tion, ischemia, and perforation of the bowel wall. Malrotation with volvulus will also present with a clinical picture of obstruction, and it may be difficult to dif-ferentiate among the two solely on clinical findings.

The sausage-shaped mass felt on examination will not be present in all cases. It represents the portions of bowel that are involved and have become edematous. Another common condition that may reveal a palpable mass is that of pyloric stenosis, with an olive-shaped mass sometimes palpable in the right upper quadrant of epigastrium. However, pyloric stenosis presents in younger patients and does not involve bouts of severe pain. "Currant jelly" stools are basically a mixture of blood and mucus that has sloughed from the affected bowel wall. This is not present in all cases.

Before proceeding to diagnostics, the patient should be stabilized with IV fluid hydration and surgery consultation shouldn't be delayed. A nasogastric tube may need to be placed if obstruction is suspected. A plain film of the abdomen is done to rule out perforation. If perforation has occurred, surgical intervention is required. If no perforation is evidenced, an ultrasound of the abdomen may reveal a "coiled spring" lesion, which reflects layers of intestine within the lumen of a different portion of intestine. However, a **barium enema will be both diagnostic and therapeutic in the case of intussusception.** Although barium is widely used, a water-soluble contrast is preferred if perforation is suspected, because it won't be as irritating to the peritoneum. The therapeutic value of the enema is a result of the constant application of hydrostatic pressure on the intussusceptum, mechanically forcing it to telescope back. Air reduction may also be achieved. This method requires fluoroscopic visualization of bowel-gas patterns until reduction of the intussusceptum is seen. Barium or air reduction is effective in 75–90% of cases, after which a 12–24-hour observation period is needed until bowel function is adequate and a bowel movement has been produced. The risk of recurrence in this patient with idiopathic intussusception is approximately 10%.

APPROACH TO PEDIATRIC ABDOMINAL PAIN WITH VOMITING

The most important aspect of a diagnostic approach in these cases is to be able to rapidly determine whether or not the condition is an emergency. Although the case presented is that of the most common abdominal emergency among the pediatric population, it is by no means the most common cause of intestinal obstruction. **Among the diagnoses that have to be entertained are hypertrophic pyloric stenosis, malrotation with volvulus/obstruction, foreign-body ingestion, and poisoning.**

Clinical Presentation

As described, **intussusception will present with intermittent, severe abdominal pain, associated with vomiting that becomes bilious as obstruction sets in.** The finding of an elongated mass along the right abdomen is very suggestive of this diagnosis. The location of the mass is because most idiopathic intussusceptions occur at the ileocecal junction. They may be entirely in the jejunum, between the jejunum and ileum, or entirely colonic. Currant jelly stool is most often used to describe the finding in this condition and it correlates with the ongoing bowel ischemia as the intussusception and edema progress.

Hypertrophic pyloric stenosis is the most common cause of GI obstruction. It occurs in approximately 3 in 1000 live births, with a male-to-female ratio of 4:1. The usual presenting age is 3–6 weeks old, and is often described as a "hungry baby" with projectile vomiting. Vomiting is nonbilious and occurs immediately after meals. The infant will demand to be refed immediately. On examination, there may be an **olive-shaped mass felt in the right upper quadrant, and peristaltic waves may be seen across the upper abdomen moments before emesis occurs.** Ultrasonography shows the thickened pyloric muscles that are causing to gastric outlet obstruction. An upper GI contrast study usually reveals an elongated pyloric canal and a "double-track sign," which is explained by two thin tracts of barium that are created by compressed pyloric mucosa. Once the diagnosis is made, surgical referral is indicated as it is the definitive management. Because of the early age and dramatic nature of the symptoms, parents will usually seek help before the infant becomes severely ill from not eating.

Malrotation occurs in about 1 in 500 live births, but becomes symptomatic in only 1 in 6000 live births. Approximately **60% of patients will be younger than 1 month of age,** with approximately 10% presenting after 1 year of age, even into adulthood. Because it is primarily a defect that occurs during embryogenesis, the mesentery that is formed will have an abnormally narrow base, which allows the small bowel to move more freely than normal. This creates a problem when the intestinal attachment to the mesentery twists around itself, creating a volvulus. Once obstruction occurs, the **child will present with bilious vomiting and abdominal pain.** If diagnosis is delayed, the involved segments of bowel will eventually become necrotic, leading to fluid losses and sepsis. The diagnostic approach in such cases will depend on the stability of the patient. If the patient is hypovolemic, hypotensive, has GI blood loss, or has signs of peritonitis, quick stabilization with surgical intervention is necessary. However, if the patient is hemodynamically stable, imaging can be performed to confirm a diagnosis. **If malrotation is suspected, an upper GI series is the test of choice.** In 75% of patients, the diagnosis will be clearly seen. Diagnostic findings on an upper GI are an obviously misplaced duodenum, or a duodenal obstruction with the classic "beaklike" appearance of the contrast medium caused by a volvulus. Surgery is the only treatment. Although different surgical techniques are applied to prevent a recurrence, a volvulus can repeat itself in as many as 8% of patients. Malrotation can go undiagnosed if a patient never experiences symptoms from it, and older children may present with intermittent vomiting, episodes of abdominal pain, failure to thrive, or syndromes of malabsorption.

Foreign bodies also need to be considered with abdominal pain and vomiting in a pediatric patient. **Only 10% of patients that ingest a foreign body will need an intervention** either to relieve an obstruction or to prevent GI complications. Approximately 90% of patients will pass a foreign body spontaneously, and parents need only check the stool within 24 hours to confirm passage. Sometimes, if an object can be seen on plain radiographs, a repeat x-ray within 24 hours can be done. **Among objects that require immediate intervention are flat disk batteries in the esophagus.** These batteries will conduct electricity when both poles are in contact with the esophageal wall, which will lead to perforation. Sharp objects also need to be removed. As a general rule, any foreign body in the esophagus needs to be removed in less than 24 hours by upper endoscopy. If a sharp or elongated object (>6 cm) has already passed through the stomach and duodenum, daily x-rays should be done to follow the progress of the object. Those that do not advance within 3 days will require surgical intervention for removal.

Poisoning cannot be overlooked in the evaluation of a child with vomiting and abdominal pain. Among the multiple agents most commonly associated with hospital visits are over-the-counter (OTC) analgesic drugs, cold remedies, insecticides, pesticides, personal care products, and fumes. In a child who presents with vomiting and abdominal pain, a cholinergic syndrome is likely. It is characterized by salivation, lacrimation, diarrhea, vomiting, diaphoresis, intestinal cramps, and seizures. Insecticides and nicotine are among the agents that may induce these symptoms. Antihistamines or tricyclic antidepressants produce dry skin, dry mucosae, urinary retention, and decreased bowel sounds (anticholinergic syndrome). Some medications and substances are radiopaque, such as iron tablets, mercury, lithium, tricyclic antidepressants, Play-Doh, and enteric-coated aspirin. Finding the likely agent of poisoning will mostly depend on the history given.

Treatment

Surgical intervention will almost always be necessary if an anatomical/mechanical defect of the GI tract is present. Intestinal obstruction puts a patient at risk for perforation, which further deteriorates a patient's condition. A nasogastric tube is recommended in cases where obstruction has set in and the patient is ill. Careful monitoring of the patient's fluid status is required because of the likelihood of third spacing into ischemic bowel and decreased oral intake.

Comprehension Questions

[31.1–31.6] Match the following etiologies to the clinical vignette:

    A. Malrotation with intermittent volvulus
    B. Intussusception
    C. Insecticide ingestion
    D. Esophageal foreign body
    E. Pyloric stenosis
    F. Volvulus

[31.1] A 6-year-old boy left alone for 10 hours, now with hematemesis and pneumomediastinum on chest x-ray.

[31.2] A 3-week-old male infant with 2 days of projectile, nonbilious vomiting and constant feeding.

[31.3] A 7-year-old male with three episodes of severe abdominal pain and vomiting in the last month, previously diagnosed with failure to thrive.

[31.4] An 8-month-old female infant with bilious vomiting, constant abdominal pain for 12 hours, and upper GI study showing beaklike appearance of contrast.

[31.5] An 11-month-old male with intermittent bouts of crying and nonbilious vomiting, has a history of Meckel diverticulum. A small, elongated mass is felt on right side of his abdomen.

[31.6] A 4-year-old female with profuse vomiting, sweating, lacrimation, and diarrhea, who seizes in the emergency room.

Answers

[31.1] **D.** The presence of blood in the vomitus and a pneumomediastinum point to an esophageal perforation, most likely from a foreign body in the esophagus.

[31.2] **E.** The young age and presence of projectile, nonbilious vomiting after feeding are the keys to this diagnosis. The diagnosis of pyloric stenosis is much more common in males than females.

[31.3] **A.** This is the presentation of a malrotation that did not cause enough symptoms at a younger age to lead to a diagnosis.

[31.4] **F.** An infant with bilious vomiting and abdominal pain has a volvulus until proven otherwise. The upper GI study is diagnostic of this condition.

[31.5] **B.** The intermittent nature of the symptoms and the palpable mass are highly suggestive of intussusception.

[31.6] **C.** These symptoms are characteristic of a cholinergic syndrome, possibly caused by insecticide or nicotine poisoning.

CLINICAL PEARLS

❖ Most foreign-body ingestions by children will pass spontaneously, but button batteries and sharp objects in the esophagus should be removed endoscopically.

❖ The risk of accidental poisoning with common household products and over-the-counter medications should be a routine part of the anticipatory guidance that occurs in well child visits.

❖ When a child appears critically ill, don't delay your resuscitative efforts or surgical consultation while you wait for lab tests and x-ray results.

REFERENCES

Fonkalsrud E. Rotational anomalies and volvulus. In: O'Neill J, Grosfeld J, Fonkalsrud E, et al. (eds). Principles of pediatric surgery. St. Louis: Mosby, 2003:477.

Hay WW, Levin MJ, Sondheimer JM, et al. Current pediatric diagnosis and treatment. 15th ed. New York: McGraw-Hill, 2004:538, 540, 544, 549–550.

Kitagawa S, Miqdady M. Intussusception in children. Up to Date, version 13.3, updated April 30, 2005. Available at: www.uptodate.com

Mandell GA, Wolfson PJ, Adkins ES, et al. Cost-effective imaging approach to the nonbilious vomiting infant. Pediatrics 1999;103:1198.

An 83-year-old woman is brought to the clinic by her husband who was concerned with his wife's memory problems. He noticed some memory decline a few years ago, but the onset was subtle and didn't interfere with her day-to-day activities. Mainly she has some difficulty remembering details, is repeating things, and is being forgetful. The patient's family noticed her gradually increasing memory problems, particularly over the past year. She is unable to remember her appointments and relies heavily on written notes and appointments books. Recently she got lost while driving and was found by her family 10 hours later. She was unable to use her cell phone and was unsure about her home address and phone number. She has also become more reclusive. She doesn't enjoy her church activities anymore and prefers to stay at home most of the time. She doesn't want to cook, and she is less attentive to her housework. The patient says that she has always been forgetful. Her medical history is significant for well-controlled hypertension and a history of mastectomy secondary to breast cancer diagnosed 20 years ago. She has no significant history of tobacco or alcohol use. She is independent with all activities of daily living but needs assistance with medication administration, banking, and transportation. She is up to date with her health maintenance and immunization. Her vital signs and general physical examination are normal.

◆ **What is the most likely diagnosis?**

◆ **What office testing can help to determine a diagnosis?**

◆ **What laboratory testing and imaging studies are indicated at this time?**

ANSWERS TO CASE 32: Dementia

Summary: An 83-year-old woman is noted by her family to have increasing memory difficulties at home. She is forgetful, repeats questions, and does not remember conversations. She had the very significant episode of getting lost in her home town. She is seemingly unaware that there is a problem that is slowly and progressively worsening.

◆ **Most likely diagnosis:** Dementia of Alzheimer type

◆ **Office-based testing that may be beneficial:** Folstein Mini-Mental Status Examination is the most widely used instrument. Others available include the Clock Test, the Short Portable Mental Status Questionnaire and the Mini-cog test. In addition, a screening test for depression should be performed.

◆ **Laboratory testing and imaging studies:** Screening for vitamin B_{12} and hypothyroidism. Syphilis screening if there is a risk factor or evidence of prior infection, or if patient lives in an area of high incidence. Noncontrast head computed tomography (CT) scan or magnetic resonance imaging (MRI).

Analysis

Objectives

1. Develop a differential diagnosis for dementia.
2. Learn how to appropriately evaluate a complaint of memory loss.
3. Learn about treatment of Alzheimer dementia, the most common specific diagnosis of dementia.

Definition

Executive functions: High-level cognitive abilities that control other, more basic, abilities. Executive functions include the ability to start and stop behaviors, alter behaviors to fit circumstances, and adapt behaviors to new situations.

Considerations

The **essential features of the diagnosis of dementia are a memory loss and impairment of executive function.** Dementia is a clinical diagnosis that can go unrecognized until it is in an advanced stage. **Patients rarely report memory loss;** the informants are usually their family members. However, relatives may fail to recognize signs and symptoms of dementia because many have a tendency to think that memory loss can be a part of normal aging. Studies of aging have showed that nonverbal creative thinking and new problem-solving strategies may decline with age, but information, skills learned with experience and memory retention remain intact.

Clinicians should assess cognitive function whenever cognitive impairment or deterioration is suspected. These concerns may be based upon direct observation, patient report, or concerns raised by family members, friends or caretakers. Patients with dementia may have difficulty with one or more of the following:

- Learning and retaining new information (rely on lists, calendars)
- Handling complex tasks (banking, bills, payments)
- Reasoning (adapting to unexpected situations, unfamiliar environment)
- Spatial ability and orientation (getting loss driving, walking)
- Language (word finding, repetition, confabulation)
- Behavior (agitation, confusion, paranoia)

The evaluation of a patient with suspected dementia should include a mental status exam. The **Folstein Mini-Mental Status Examination** (MMSE) is the most widely used tool in the screening for dementia. The sensitivity of the MMSE for dementia is as high as 92% and the specificity is as high as 96%. The interpretation of the score depends on the patient's education level. It is most accurate in those with at least a high school education.

Another valuable test that can be used in a busy primary care setting is the **Clock Test.** The patient is asked to draw a clock with a specific time. The patient must then accurately draw the clock face with the "big hand" and "small hand" in the correct positions. It is quick, easy to administer, and evaluates executive function in multiple cognitive domains. Other cognitive screening tests, such as the Short Portable Mental Status Questionnaire, Modified MMSE, and Mini-Cog (3-item recall combined with clock drawing) are less popular in primary care setting.

In the evaluation of dementia, it is necessary to get information from people who know the patient well. Useful information can be obtained from informant-based functional tests, such as the Functional Activities Questionnaire (FAQ) and the Instrumental Activities of Daily Living (IADL) and Caregiver Burden assessments. This information can be important for physicians and families in making plans for long-term care.

APPROACH TO DEMENTIA

Alzheimer Disease

Alzheimer's disease is the most common cause of dementia. Although a definitive diagnosis can only be made by the presence of neuritic plaques and neurofibrillary tangles detected on autopsy, clinical diagnostic criteria have been developed (Tables 32–1 and 32–2). **Common diagnostic criteria include the gradual onset and progression of cognitive dysfunction in more than one area of mental functioning that is not caused by another disorder.**

Table 32–1

DSM-IV CRITERIA FOR ALZHEIMER DISEASE

A. Development of multiple cognitive deficits manifested by both memory impairment and one of the following:

1. Aphasia: loss of word comprehension ability.
2. Apraxia: Loss of ability to perform complex tasks involving muscle coordination.
3. Agnosia: Loss of ability to recognize and use familiar objects.

B. The deficits in "A" are a decline from previous functioning and cause significant impairment in social or occupational functioning.
C. The course is of gradual onset and continuing decline.
D. The deficits are not due to other central nervous system, systemic or substance-induced conditions that cause deficits in cognition.
E. The disturbance is not accounted for by another psychiatric diagnosis.

Source: American Psychiatric Association. Diagnosticard Statistical Manual of Mental Disorders, Fourth Edition. Washington, DC: American Psychiatric Association, 1994.

The initial evaluation includes a detailed history, from both the patient and another informant (usually a spouse, child, or other close contact) and complete physical and neurologic examinations to evaluate for any focal neurologic deficit that may be suggestive of a focal neurologic lesion. **A validated test, such as the MMSE, should be used to confirm the presence of dementia.** The results of this test can also be used to follow the clinical course, as a reduction in score over time is consistent with worsening dementia.

A focused evaluation to rule out other causes of dementia must be performed as well. **Depression in the elderly can present with symptoms of memory disturbance.** This is known as "pseudodementia." As depression is common and

Table 32–2

THE NATIONAL INSTITUTE OF NEUROLOGICAL AND COMMUNICATIVE DISORDERS AND STROKE-ALZHEIMER DISEASE AND RELATED DISORDER ASSOCIATION CRITERIA FOR ALZHEIMER DISEASE

A. Probable Alzheimer disease

1. Dementia confirmed by clinical and neuropsychological examination.
2. Problems in at least two areas of mental functioning.
3. Progressive worsening of memory and mental functioning.
4. No disturbances of consciousness.
5. Symptoms beginning between ages 40 and 90 years, usually after age 65 years.
6. No other disorder that could cause the dementia.

Source: www.ninds.nih.gov

treatable, a screening test for depression should be performed when dementia is evaluated. Similarly, hypothyroidism and vitamin B_{12} deficiency are common and treatable conditions that can cause cognitive problems. Thyroid-stimulating hormone (TSH) and vitamin B_{12} levels should be performed as a routine part of the work-up. Neurosyphilis could present in this fashion, but is such an uncommon diagnosis that routine screening would not be recommended. Evaluation for neurosyphilis would be warranted if there were identified high-risk factors, history of the disease, or if the patient lived in an area with a high prevalence of syphilis. Neuroimaging with either a noncontrast CT scan or an MRI of the brain is recommended to rule out other confounding diagnoses. Other testing, such as positron emission tomography (PET), genetic testing, and spinal fluid analysis are not routinely recommended.

When the diagnosis of Alzheimer disease is made, a comprehensive care plan should be initiated. **The management of Alzheimer disease must be directed both at the patient and at the patient's family or caregivers**. The goals of therapy are to maximize the cognition, delay functional decline and prevent or improve the behavioral disturbances.

Table 32–3 lists the medications that are primarily used in the treatment of Alzheimer disease. Family members should understand that the **medications**

Table 32–3
MEDICATIONS USED IN THE TREATMENT OF ALZHEIMER DEMENTIA

CHOLINESTERASE INHIBITORS	INDICATIONS	SIDE EFFECTS/ COMMENTS
Donepezil (Aricept)	Mild-moderate Alzheimer dementia	Common: nausea, vomiting, diarrhea, dizziness, headaches
Galantamine (Razadyne)	Mild-moderate Alzheimer dementia	Severe: arrhythmias, bradycardia, urinary obstruction
Rivastigmine (Exelon)	Alzheimer dementia	
Tacrine (Cognex)	Alzheimer dementia	All of above side effects; risk of hepatotoxicity— must frequently monitor liver enzymes
N-methyl-D-aspartate (NMDA) Antagonist Memantine (Namenda)	Moderate-severe Alzheimer dementia	Side-effect profile comparable to placebo; can be used in combination with cholinesterase inhibitors

may delay the progression of the disease and may not reverse any decline that has already occurred. For that reason, the medications may be more beneficial if started earlier in the course of the disease. Antipsychotic medications have also been used to control hallucinations and agitation in patients with Alzheimer disease. This is an "off-label" use of medication and recent data show a higher death rate associated with the use of the newer antipsychotics.

Behavioral interventions also may be beneficial. These can include scheduled toileting in an effort to reduce episodes of incontinence, writing reminder notes, keeping familiar objects around, providing adequate lighting, and making duplicates of important objects (e.g., keys) in case they get lost. Caregivers also need support and may benefit from appropriate training, support groups, and periodic respite care.

Unfortunately, even with the best of care, Alzheimer disease is relentless and progressive. Families may have significant difficulties and conflicts regarding issues surrounding end-of-life care and placement in assisted living or nursing homes. Resources, such as local chapters of the Alzheimer's Association (www.alz.org), may provide valuable services, information, and support.

Vascular Dementia

Vascular dementia, or multiinfarct dementia, is the second most common cause of dementia. In vascular dementia, there is neuronal loss as a consequence of one or more strokes. The **symptoms are related to the amount and location of the neuronal loss**. Vascular dementia can exist along with Alzheimer disease or other causes of dementia, resulting in a mixed-dementia syndrome. Unlike Alzheimer disease, which is a gradually progressive process, **vascular dementia often has a sudden onset and progresses in a stepwise fashion.** Patients tend to function at a certain level and then show an acute deterioration when the initial, or subsequent, infarcts occur. The risk factors include those for cerebrovascular disease (hypertension, tobacco use, diabetes, etc.). There are no controlled trials showing medication effectiveness in vascular dementia, so the treatment is aimed at reducing the risk of further neurologic damage.

Other Illnesses Associated with Dementia

Numerous other conditions may present with dementia or have dementia as a prominent symptom. **Parkinson disease** commonly has an associated dementia, especially as the overall disease advances. **Normal pressure hydrocephalus** causes the triad of dementia, gait disturbance, and urinary incontinence. **Lewy body** dementia has symptoms similar to Alzheimer disease, but the dementia has a fluctuating course and is often accompanied by hallucinations early in the course of the disease. Dementia can be a complication of **chronic alcohol abuse,** reinforcing the need for a complete history of substance use. Many

prescription and over-the-counter medications can cause memory disturbances. Chief among these are anticholinergic medications, sedatives (benzodiazepines), sleeping pills, and narcotic pain medications. As noted previously,
hypothyroidism, vitamin B_{12} deficiency, and neurosyphilis may present as
dementing illnesses. **Metabolic abnormalities,** such as hyponatremia or
abnormal calcium levels, and other infections, such as **AIDS,** can also cause
dementia.

Delirium

Delirium is an **acute change in mental status that is characterized by fluc-
tuations in levels of consciousness.** It is usually caused by an acute medical
illness, the use of a medication, or the withdrawal from a drug or alcohol.
Delirium affects 10–30% of hospitalized patients, with a higher incidence in
the elderly, in those with an underlying dementia, and in those with multiple
underlying medical conditions. **The treatment of delirium is treatment of
the condition that precipitated it.** Delirium is often reversible if the underlying cause can be found and aggressively managed. Patients with delirium
have significantly longer hospital stays and increased mortality rates.

Comprehension Questions

[32.1] A 63-year-old man is brought in by his family because of memory loss.
They have noted a worsening of his symptoms over several months.
They also report that he has had multiple falls and has had frequent uri-
nary incontinence. Which of the following is the most likely diagnosis?

A. Alzheimer disease
B. Normal pressure hydrocephalus
C. Lewy body dementia
D. Delirium

[32.2] An 82-year-old woman is admitted to the hospital for a urinary tract
infection (UTI). On the second hospital day, her family says that she
has been confused and falling asleep frequently while in the hospital.
She has been hallucinating—talking to people who aren't in the room.
They report that prior to this illness, she was independent and "sharp
as a tack." Which of the following is the most likely diagnosis?

A. Worsening of Alzheimer disease
B. Adverse reaction to the antibiotic she has been given for her UTI
C. Delirium secondary to infection
D. Schizophrenia

[32.3] You decide to prescribe donepezil (Aricept) to a patient for the treatment of Alzheimer disease. Which of the following is true about the medication?

    A. The patient should show a marked improvement in his mental functioning.

    B. This medication would be beneficial even if the dementia is vascular in origin.

    C. This medicine can prevent Alzheimer disease from worsening.

    D. This medication may delay the progression of Alzheimer disease.

[32.4] Which of the following tests should be routinely ordered in the evaluation of dementia?

    A. Head CT or MRI
    B. Lumbar puncture
    C. Rapid plasma reagin (RPR)
    D. Electroencephalogram (EEG)

Answers

[32.1] **B.** Normal pressure hydrocephalus classically causes dementia, incontinence, and gait disturbance. All of the other listed conditions may cause memory disturbance, but the constellation of the three symptoms is most consistent with normal pressure hydrocephalus.

[32.2] **C.** This scenario is one that is commonly seen in hospitals and is consistent with delirium. The patient is elderly and has an infection, causing both an acute change in her mental status and a fluctuating level of consciousness. The treatment is to treat the underlying infection.

[32.3] **D.** The currently available medications for Alzheimer disease may slow the progression of the disease, but cannot prevent its progression or reverse the damage that has already occurred. No medication available improves vascular dementia.

[32.4] **A.** A noncontrast head CT or MRI is recommended by the American Academy of Neurology for the routine evaluation of dementia. All of the other tests may be appropriate if there is a finding on the history or examination that calls for further testing (an exposure to syphilis, episodes suggestive of seizures, or symptoms of normal pressure hydrocephalus for which a spinal tap may be performed)

CLINICAL PEARLS

❖ The presentation of acutely altered mental status (delirium) should prompt an aggressive work-up for an underlying cause, as treatment may result in correction of the mental status.

❖ Alzheimer disease is a disease of the family, not just the individual. It is critical to treat the patient and support the caregivers.

REFERENCES

Alva G, Potkin SG. Alzheimer disease and other dementias. Clin Geriatr Med 2003;19:763–776.

Alzheimer's Association website: www.alz.org.

American Geriatric Society website: www.americangeriatrics.org.

Doody RS, Stevens JC, Beck C, et al. Practice parameters: management of dementia (an evidence-based review). Neurology 2001;56(9):1154–1166.

Galasko D. An integrated approach to the management of Alzheimer's disease: assessing cognition, function and behavior. Eur J Neurol 1998;5(suppl 4):S9–17.

Knopman DS, DeKosky ST, Cummings JL, et al. Practice parameter: diagnosis of dementia (an evidence-based review). Neurology 2001;56(9):1143–1153.

A 20-year-old female comes to clinic for an annual physical examination. She has no complaints. She has no significant medical or surgical history. She is currently taking oral contraceptive pills because of her irregular menstrual cycles. She attained menarche at age 13 years and has had irregular cycles since. She has never been sexually active. Her family history is positive for hypertension and obesity in both her parents. On examination, her blood pressure is 120/85 mm Hg, her pulse is 78 beats/min, and her respiratory rate is 14 breaths/min. Her weight is 188 lb and she is 63 inches tall. Her physical examination is unremarkable except for a brownish/black, velvety thickening of the skin on the back of her neck, hirsutism, and abdominal obesity.

◆ **What are the clinical issues that need to be addressed during this preventive visit?**

◆ **What is your next step in the evaluation of this patient?**

◆ **What are the therapeutic options available for this patient?**

ANSWERS TO CASE 33: Obesity

Summary: A 20-year-old obese female presents for a routine examination. Along with her abdominal obesity, she has irregular menstrual cycles, acanthosis nigricans, and hirsutism.

◆ **Clinical issues to address:** Obesity and possible polycystic ovarian disease.

◆ **Next steps in evaluation:** Calculate a body mass index (BMI), measure waist circumference, repeat blood pressure. Order laboratory tests to measure fasting glucose, lipids, thyroid-stimulating hormone (TSH), and liver enzymes.

◆ **Therapeutic options:** Assess her interest in losing weight. If she is interested, devise weight-loss goals and advise on diet and physical activity to achieve these goals. If she is not interested, advise on the health benefits of weight loss and address other risk factors. In either case, arrange follow-up. At subsequent visits, can consider adding pharmacotherapy therapy as an adjunct to diet and exercise.

Analysis

Objectives

1. Understand the etiology and pathogenesis of obesity
2. Know other comorbid conditions associated with obesity.
3. Learn the diagnostic criteria for obesity and the metabolic syndrome.
4. Understand the therapeutic options available for the management of obesity.

Considerations

Obesity is a chronic and stigmatizing disease that begins early in life. Routine physical examination visits serve as a good platform to address issues related to obesity and its associated comorbid conditions. In this case, this visit should be taken as an opportunity to address obesity and its management.

Increased body weight is a major risk factor for the development of disease and for premature death. In National Health and Nutritional Examination Surveys (NHANES) III, the metabolic syndrome was present in 5% of those at normal weight, 22% of those who were overweight, and 60% of those who were obese. The metabolic syndrome is an important risk factor for subsequent development of type 2 diabetes and cardiovascular disease.

In this case, this patient's BMI is 33.5. Further measurements included a waist circumference of 36 inches and a repeat blood pressure of 125/85 mm Hg. Her laboratory test results included a total cholesterol of 202 mg/dL, high-density lipoprotein (HDL) cholesterol of 35 mg/dL, low-density lipoprotein (LDL) cholesterol of 120 mg/dL, and triglycerides of 172 mg/dL. Her fasting glucose was 104 mg/dL, and she had normal renal and liver function tests. She has metabolic syndrome based on her abdominal circumference, increased triglycerides, low HDL, and mildly elevated LDL cholesterol levels. She may also need further investigation for the presence of polycystic ovarian syndrome (PCOS) because of her obesity and history of irregular cycles.

Both the metabolic syndrome and PCOS are very closely associated with obesity and insulin resistance. In this situation, the key clinical implication of these diagnoses is identification of a patient needing aggressive lifestyle modification focused on weight reduction and increased physical activity.

APPROACH TO OBESITY

Definitions

Body mass index (BMI): A measurement of the relative composition of lean body mass and body fat; calculated as weight in kilograms/(height in meters)^2.

Metabolic syndrome: A state of insulin resistance characterized by abdominal obesity, dyslipidemia, elevated blood pressure, and impaired fasting glucose.

Obesity: An excessive amount of body fat, which increases the risk of medical illness and premature death.

Satiation: Level of fullness during a meal.

Satiety: Level of hunger after a meal.

Clinical Approach

Obesity is a chronic and easily diagnosed disease that is associated with life-threatening morbidity and mortality. Overall, **among adults at least 20 years of age in 1999–2002, 65.1% were overweight or obese, 30.4% were obese and 4.9% were extremely obese.** Approximately 300,000 deaths are attributed to obesity each year with the direct and indirect costs exceeding $100 billion per year.

Diagnostic Tools

BMI is used as a quick and easy measure of overweight and obesity. However, **BMI is not an accurate measure of overweight/obesity in patients with heart failure, pregnant women, body builders, and certain ethnic groups.** Therefore, in addition to BMI, additional measurements, like waist circumference, hip circumference, and waist-to-hip ratio, need to be used to accurately identify the population at risk. Direct measurement of percentage of body fat may also provide additional information. Table 33–1 lists the classification of overweight/obesity based on BMI.

Table 33–1

DEFINITION OF OBESITY BASED ON BMI

	BMI (kg/m^2)	OBESITY CLASS
Underweight	<18.5	
Normal	18.5–24.9	
Overweight	25.0–29.9	
Obesity	30.0–34.9	I
	35.0–39.9	II
Extreme obesity	>40	III

Along with the measurements mentioned above, a physical examination and **focused laboratory work-up** should be performed to look for complications and comorbid conditions. A **fasting glucose** level should be measured to evaluate for diabetes mellitus and impaired glucose tolerance. The presence of acanthosis nigricans—a velvety, hyperpigmented, thickening of the skin commonly found on the neck and axillary regions—may also be a sign of insulin resistance. **Fasting lipids** should also be measured, both to evaluate for the presence of metabolic syndrome and for the assessment of the patient's risk for cardiovascular disease. **TSH** should be measured to screen for hypothyroidism. **Liver enzymes** should be requested, as abnormal results may indicate the development of a fatty liver.

Pathogenesis

Energy balance is the relationship of energy intake to energy expenditure. When more energy is expended than taken in, weight loss ensues. When the intake of energy exceeds the amount expended, weight gain occurs. In all persons, **obesity is caused by ingesting more energy than is expended over a period of time.** Energy balance is affected by both genetic and environmental factors.

It has been **estimated that genetic background can explain 40% or more of the variance in body mass in humans.** The genetic component is complex and involves the interaction of multiple genes. However, the marked increase in obesity cannot be completely attributed to genetics. An **increase in energy consumption with a decrease in physical activity is thought to be the main contributor to the current obesity epidemic.** Among numerous issues, the availability of convenience foods and the increase in palatability and serving size, compounded with industrialization leading to decreased physical activity, has led to an altered energy balance.

Health Hazards Associated with Obesity

Obesity is a risk factor for the development of numerous medical conditions (Table 33–2). The more complications that develop, the greater the mortality risk for the individual. Also, the more complications that develop, the more

Table 33–2
COMMON MEDICAL COMPLICATIONS OF OBESITY

Cardiovascular disease
Cerebrovascular disease
Cholelithiasis
Degenerative joint disease
Eating disorders
Hyperlipidemia
Hypertension
Infertility/reduced fertility
Malignancies
Menstrual cycle irregularities
Mood disorders
Polycystic ovary syndrome
Sleep apnea
Type 2 diabetes mellitus

difficult it becomes to manage the underlying obesity. For example, a person with degenerative arthritis and heart disease may have significant symptoms during exercise, impairing his or her ability to expend more energy in an effort to lose weight.

Treatment

Treatment of obesity should begin in patients with a BMI >25 or who have visceral obesity, documented by increased waist circumference or a waist-to-hip ratio >0.9 in men and >0.85 in women. Weight loss of as little as 5 lb reduces the risk of developing comorbid conditions. Developing a **treatment plan** for obesity is complex and should use a **combination of dietary restrictions, increased physical activity, and behavior therapy** as a gold standard.

Dietary intervention is the cornerstone of weight-loss therapy. Most diets work in two principal dimensions: energy content and nutrient composition. **A calorie deficit of 500–1000 calories per day produces a weight loss of 1–2 lb per week.** There are different kinds of specific dietary modifications recommended, but they all work based on calorie restriction. Calorie restriction should not compromise the nutrient content of the diet; patients should still aim for a balanced meal.

The addition of exercise training to a diet program can add to the weight loss. However, **physical activity alone is not an effective method for achieving weight loss.** Although increasing physical activity is not effective for initial weight loss, physical activity is very important for long-term weight management. Patients should engage in moderate to vigorous physical activity for at least 30 minutes per day, 5 days per week, both to maintain weight loss and for the independent health benefits of exercising.

The **purpose of behavior modification therapy is to help patients identify and modify eating and physical activity habits that contribute to obesity.** The targets of behavior modification are avoiding triggers, maintaining dietary diaries, avoidance of high-risk situations and breaking repetitive behaviors, such as watching TV while eating.

Pharmacotherapy

Table 33–3 lists the medications commonly used in the treatment of obesity. Only sibutramine and orlistat are approved for long-term use. With the exception of orlistat, which inhibits the absorption of dietary fat, all medications approved for obesity act as anorexiants. Anorexiant medications increase satiation, satiety, or both, by affecting the monoamine system in the hypothalamus. Increasing satiation results in a reduction in the amount of food eaten, whereas increasing satiety reduces the frequency of eating.

Table 33–3
MEDICATIONS USED IN THE TREATMENT OF OBESITY

DRUG NAME (TRADE NAME)	MECHANISM OF ACTION	NOTES
Dextroamphetamine (Dexedrine)	Sympathomimetic (increased norepinephrine release)	All: Numerous drug interactions; stimulant side effects include insomnia, agitation, tachycardia; additive effects with other stimulants (caffeine, cold medications, etc.); can be addicting; avoid with monoamine oxidase-inhibitors
Phendimetrazine (Bontril)	Sympathomimetic (increased norepinephrine release)	
Diethylpropion (Tenuate)	Sympathomimetic (increased norepinephrine release)	
Phentermine (Fastin, Ionamin, Adipex-P)	Norepinephrine reuptake inhibitors	
Sibutramine (Meridia)	Serotonin-norepinephrine reuptake inhibitor	Can result in severe blood pressure elevation; should not be used in combination with selective strotonin reoptake inhibitors or triptans (increased risk of serotonin syndrome)
Orlistat (Xenical)	Selective inhibitor of pancreatic lipase, results in reduced intestinal digestion of fat	GI side effects common: diarrhea, bloating, gas, oily stools; must follow low-fat diet to reduce side effects

Bariatric Surgery

Patients with a **BMI >40, or >35 with comorbid conditions, are potential candidates for surgical treatment of obesity.** The two most common surgeries done are Roux-en-Y gastric bypass and "lap banding." The Roux-en-Y gastric bypass involves the construction of a small (10–30-mL) gastric pouch that empties into a segment of jejunum. This is mostly a restrictive procedure, but there is some degree of associated malabsorption. In lap banding, an adjustable silicone gastric band is laparoscopically placed around the upper stomach just distal to the gastroesophageal junction. The band has a balloon connected to a subcutaneously implanted port, which can be inflated or deflated to reduce the circumference of the band. Complications of the banding procedure are less common and less severe than in gastric bypass, but the weight loss may also be less.

Metabolic Syndrome

Guidelines from the 2001 National Cholesterol Education Program (Adult Treatment Panel [ATP] III) suggest that the clinical identification of the metabolic syndrome should be based upon the presence of any three of the following traits:

- Abdominal obesity, defined as a waist circumference in men >102 cm (40 in) and in women >88 cm (35 in). ATP III recognized that some men develop multiple metabolic risk factors when waist circumference is only marginally increased (94–102 cm [37–39 in]); such patients may have a genetic predisposition to insulin resistance.
- Serum triglycerides ≥150 mg/dL (1.7 mmol/L).
- Serum high-density lipoprotein (HDL) cholesterol <40 mg/dL (1 mmol/L) in men and <50 mg/dL (1.3 mmol/L) in women.
- Blood pressure ≥130/85 mm Hg.
- Fasting plasma glucose ≥110 mg/dL (6.1 mmol/L).

Current minimum estimates are that the prevalence of metabolic syndrome in the United States is at least 22%. The metabolic syndrome is an important risk factor for subsequent development of type 2 diabetes and cardiovascular disease. Thus, the key clinical implication of a diagnosis of metabolic syndrome is identification of a patient needing aggressive lifestyle modification focused on weight reduction and increased physical activity.

Comprehension Questions

[33.1] Which of the following patients would be a candidate for bariatric surgery as initial treatment for obesity?

A. A man with a BMI of 32 and arthritis of the knees.
B. A woman with a BMI of 30 and type 2 diabetes.
C. A woman with a BMI of 42 but no identifiable complications.
D. Any obese patient who desires bariatric surgery should have it offered.

[33.2] For which of the following patients is a BMI measurement most likely to be an accurate assessment of obesity?

A. A bodybuilder with a BMI of 38.
B. A pregnant woman with a BMI of 31 in her 37th week of gestation.
C. A man with congestive heart failure, pitting edema, and a BMI of 30.
D. A hypertensive woman with a BMI of 32.

[33.3] Which of the following medications may be used for the long-term management of obesity?

A. Orlistat
B. Phendimetrazine
C. Dextroamphetamine
D. Phentermine

Answers

[33.1] **C.** Bariatric surgery can be effective but carries significant risks. It is indicated for people with a BMI of 40 or greater or with a BMI of 35 or greater and obesity-related complications.

[33.2] **D.** A BMI reading will not accurately assess the ratio of lean body mass to body fat in highly muscled persons (weightlifters, athletes), in pregnant women, and in symptomatic congestive heart failure.

[33.3] **A.** Only orlistat and sibutramine are indicated for the long-term treatment of obesity. All of the other medications should be for short-term use only.

CLINICAL PEARLS

❖ Obesity is a chronic disease that is reaching epidemic status in the United States and worldwide.

❖ BMI is a common tool used to grade obesity but in certain cases, it may be inadequate.

❖ Obesity treatment should include dietary restriction, increased activity, and behavioral modifications.

REFERENCES

Allison DB, Fontaine KR, Manson JE, et al. Annual deaths attributable to obesity in the United States. JAMA 1999;282:1530.

Bray GA. Contemporary diagnosis and management of obesity and the metabolic syndrome. 2nd ed. Newton, PA: Handbooks in Healthcare, 2003.

Centers for Disease Control and Prevention. Available at: www.cdc.gov/obesity.

National Heart, Lung and Blood Institute. The third report of the National Cholesterol Education Program Expert Panel on the Detection, Evaluation and Treatment of High Blood Cholesterol in Adults. NIH Publication No. 01-3760. May 2001.

World Health Organization. Preventing and managing the global epidemic of obesity. Report of the World Health Organization Consultation of Obesity. Geneva: WHO, 1997.

A 33-year-old female presents with a complaint of headaches. She has had headaches since she was a teenager but they have become more debilitating recently. The episodes occur once or twice each month and last for up to 2 days. The pain begins in the right temple or at the back of the right eye and spreads to the entire scalp over a few hours. She describes the pain as a sharp, throbbing sensation that gradually worsens and is associated with severe nausea. Several factors aggravate the pain, including loud noises and movement. She has taken several over-the-counter medications for the pain, but the only thing that works is going to sleep in a quiet, darkened room. A thorough history reveals that her mother suffers from migraine headaches. Her vital signs, general physical examination, and a thorough neurologic examination are all within normal limits.

◆ **What is the most likely diagnosis?**

◆ **What imaging study is most appropriate at this time?**

◆ **What are the most appropriate therapeutic options?**

ANSWERS TO CASE 34: Migraine Headache

Summary: A 33-year-old female presents with classic migraine headaches, without aura. Her headaches have occurred since she was a teenager and have progressively worsened. She has not found relief from over-the-counter preparations.

◆ **Most likely diagnosis:** Migraine without aura.

◆ **Most appropriate imaging study:** No imaging is indicated at this time as there are no "red flag" symptoms or signs.

◆ **Most appropriate therapy:** A "triptan" medication given in a means that does not have to be swallowed (e.g., subcutaneous, intranasal, or orally dissolving tablet).

Analysis

Objectives

1. Know the differential diagnosis of chronic headache.
2. Learn the "red flag" symptoms and signs that should prompt rapid, specific diagnostic and treatment interventions.
3. Know how to manage common headache syndromes.

Considerations

Migraine headaches are the most common headaches of vascular origin. They **typically cause recurrent episodes of headache, nausea, and vomiting.** They can also be associated with other neurologic symptoms such as photophobia, light-headedness, paresthesia, vertigo, and visual disturbances. In the patient described in this case, the history and lack of physical findings can reasonably lead to the diagnosis of migraine headaches without aura ("common migraine"), the most frequently occurring form. Other classifications of migraines include migraine with aura ("classic migraine"), ophthalmoplegic migraine, retinal migraine, and childhood periodic syndromes that may be precursors to or associated with migraines.

According to the International Headache Society, symptoms diagnostic of migraine headache include **moderate to severe headache with a pulsating quality; unilateral location; nausea and/or vomiting; photophobia; phonophobia; worsening with activity; multiple attacks lasting for 4 hours to 3 days; and absence of history or physical examination findings that would make it likely that the headache is the result of another cause.** Common triggers of migraine headaches include menses, fatigue, hunger, and stress.

APPROACH TO MIGRAINE HEADACHES

Headaches are an extremely common complaint in primary care, urgent care, and emergency settings. The vast majority of adults have at least one headache each year, although most do not present for medical care. **The role of the practitioner is to attempt to accurately diagnose the cause of the headache, rule out secondary causes of headaches ("red flags") that may signify a serious underlying pathology, provide appropriate acute management, and assist with headache prevention when needed.**

The medical history in a patient with headaches should focus on several important areas. The quality and characteristics of the headache and its specific location and radiation should be identified. The presence of associated symptoms, especially neurologic symptoms that may suggest the presence of a focal neurologic lesion or increased intracranial pressure, must be documented. The age at which the patient first developed the headaches, the frequency and duration of the headaches, and the amount of disability and distress that is caused to the patient should be explored. It is also important to note what the patient has done to try to treat the headaches in the past, including as much detail as possible regarding medication usage (both prescription and over-the-counter [OTC]).

The examination should include both a general examination and a detailed neurologic examination. A funduscopic examination revealing papilledema may be supportive of the presence of increased intracranial pressure. **Identifying a focal neurologic deficit increases the likelihood of finding a significant CNS pathology as the cause of the headache.**

A patient with symptoms and signs consistent with migraine and who does not have any "red flag" findings (Table 34–1) does not require any further testing prior to instituting treatment. Neuroimaging should be performed if there is an unexplained neurologic abnormality on examination or if the headache syndrome is not typical of either migraines or some other primary headache disorder. The **presence of rapidly increasing headache frequency or a history of either lack of coordination, focal neurologic symptom, or headache awakening the patient from sleep, raises the likelihood of finding an abnormality on an imaging test.** Magnetic resonance imaging (MRI) may be more sensitive than computed tomography (CT) scanning for the identification of abnormalities, but it may not be more sensitive at identifying *significant* abnormalities. Other testing (e.g., blood tests, electroencephalogram [EEG]) should only be performed for diagnostic purposes if there is a suspicion based on the history or physical examination.

The treatment of headache is best individualized based on a thorough history, physical examination, and the interpretation of any additional study results. Nonpharmacologic measures and cognitive-behavioral therapy are worth considering in most patients with primary headache disorders. The U.S. Headache Consortium lists the following general management guidelines for the treatment of migraine headaches:

Table 34–1

"RED FLAG" SYMPTOMS AND SIGNS IN THE EVALUATION
OF HEADACHES

RED FLAG	DIFFERENTIAL DIAGNOSIS	WORK-UP STUDIES
Sudden-onset headache	Subarachnoid hemorrhage, pituitary apoplexy, hemorrhage into a mass lesion or vascular malformation, mass lesion	Neuroimaging first; lumbar puncture if neuroimaging negative
Headaches increasing in severity and frequency	Mass lesion, subdural hematoma, medication overuse	Neuroimaging, drug screen
Headache beginning after age 50 years	Temporal arteritis, mass lesion	Neuroimaging, Erythrocyte sedimentation rate level
New-onset headache in patient with risk factors for HIV infection or cancer	Meningitis, brain abscess (including toxoplasmosis), metastasis	Neuroimaging first; lumbar puncture if neuroimaging negative
Headache with signs of systemic illness (fever, stiff neck, rash)	Meningitis, encephalitis, Lyme disease, systemic infection, collagen vascular disease	Neuroimaging, lumbar puncture, serology
Focal neurologic signs or symptoms of disease (other than typical aura)	Mass lesion, vascular malformation, stroke, collagen vascular disease	Neuroimaging, collagen vascular evaluation (including antiphospholipid antibodies)
Papilledema	Mass lesion, pseudotumor cerebri, meningitis	Neuroimaging, lumbar puncture
Headache subsequent to head trauma	Intracranial hemorrhage, subdural hematoma, epidural hematoma, posttraumatic headache	Neuroimaging of brain, skull, and cervical spine

Adapted from South-Paul JE, Matheny SC, Lewis EL, et al. Current diagnosis and treatment in family medicine. New York: McGraw-Hill, 2004:330.

- Educate migraine patients about their condition and its treatment, and educate them to participate in their own management.
- Use migraine-specific agents (e.g., triptans, dihydroergotamine, ergotamine) in patients with more severe migraines, and in those whose headaches respond poorly to treatment with nonsteroidal antiinflammatory drugs (NSAIDs) or combination analgesics, such as aspirin plus acetaminophen plus caffeine.
- Select a nonoral route of administration for patients whose migraines present early with nausea or vomiting as a significant component of the symptom complex.
- Consider using a self-administered rescue medication for patients with severe migraine who do not respond well to other treatments.
- Guard against medication-overuse or rebound headaches. Patients who require acute treatment on two or more occasions per week should probably be on prophylactic treatment.

The goal of therapy in migraine prophylaxis is a reduction in the severity and frequency of headache by 50% or more. The strongest evidence supports the use of amitriptyline, propranolol, timolol, and divalproex sodium for migraine headache prevention.

Other Headache Syndromes

Tension-type Headache

Tension headache is the most prevalent form of primary headache disorder, typically presenting with pericranial muscle tenderness and a description of a bilateral bandlike distribution of the pain. Headaches can last from 30 minutes to 7 days and there is no aggravation by walking stairs or similar routine physical activity. There is no associated nausea or vomiting. Photophobia and phonophobia are both absent, or one, but not the other, is present. They can be either episodic (less than 180 days per year) or chronic (greater than 180 days per year).

Initial medical therapy of episodic tension-type headache includes aspirin, acetaminophen, and NSAIDs. Because of the significant risk of developing drug dependency or medication-overuse headache, avoiding caffeine-containing over-the-counter or prescription drugs and codeine- or ergotamine-containing preparations (including combination products) is recommended. The general management principles for the treatment of migraine headaches can also be applied to the treatment of chronic tension-type headaches. In frequent headache sufferers, the combination of antidepressant medications and stress management therapy reduces headache activity significantly. Other prophylactic treatments of chronic tension-type headaches include calcium channel blockers and β-blockers.

Cluster Headache

Cluster headache is strictly unilateral in location and can be located in the orbital, supraorbital, or temporal region. It is generally described as a deep, excruciating pain lasting from 15 minutes to 3 hours. The frequency can vary from one every other day to eight attacks per day. Cluster headaches are associated with ipsilateral autonomic signs and symptoms, and have a much greater prevalence in men. Compared to migraine sufferers who often desire sleep and a quiet, dark environment during their headache, individuals with cluster headache pace around, unable to find a comfortable position. The acute treatment of cluster headache involves 100% oxygen at 6 L/min, dihydroergotamine and the triptans. Verapamil, lithium, divalproex sodium, methysergide, and prednisone may be used for prophylactic treatment. Because of side effects related to chronic use, methysergide and prednisone need to be used with caution.

Chronic Medical Conditions

Patients with certain underlying medical conditions have a greater incidence of having an organic cause of their headache. Patients with cancer may develop headaches as a consequence of metastases. Someone with uncontrolled hypertension (with diastolic pressures >110 mm Hg) may present with the chief complaint of headache. Patients with HIV infection or AIDS may present with central nervous system metastases, lymphoma, toxoplasmosis, or meningitis as the cause of their headache.

Medication-Related Headache

Numerous medications have headache as a reported adverse effect. Medication-overuse headache (formerly drug-induced or "rebound" headache) may occur following frequent use of any analgesic or headache medication. This includes both nonprescription (e.g., acetaminophen, NSAIDs) and prescription medications. Caffeine use, whether as a component of an analgesic or a beverage, is another culprit in this category. The duration and severity of the withdrawal headache following discontinuation of the medication vary depending on the medication(s) involved.

Comprehension Questions

[34.1] A 28-year-old male presents for evaluation of headaches. He has had several episodes of unilateral throbbing headaches that last 8–12 hours. When they occur, he gets nauseated and just wants to go to bed. Usually they are relieved after he lies down in a dark, quiet room for the remainder of the day. He is missing significant amounts of work because of the headaches. He has a normal examination today. Which of the following statements is true regarding this situation?

   A. He needs a CT scan of his head to evaluate for the cause of his headache.
   B. When he gets his next headache, he should breathe in 100% oxygen and use a triptan medication.
   C. If he has not already done so, he should use aspirin 650 mg orally every 4 hours as needed and take a stress-management class.
   D. An injectable or nasal spray triptan is most appropriate.

[34.2] A 52-year-old woman presents to the office for an acute visit complaining of 2 hours of headache. She says that it came on suddenly and is the worst headache she has ever had. Her blood pressure is elevated at 145/95 mm Hg, but otherwise she has no focal neurologic abnormalities on examination. Which of the following is the most appropriate management at this time?

   A. Prescribe a triptan medication.
   B. Schedule a noncontrast head CT scan for tomorrow morning.
   C. Call 911 and transfer the patient to the nearest emergency room.
   D. Prescribe an antihypertensive medication and follow-up in 2 weeks.

[34.3] A 43-year-old male presents with headaches that he has had daily for several months. Every morning at work, usually between 9 and 10 A.M., he has to take 650 mg of acetaminophen to relieve the headache. This has been going on for the past 3 months and he is at the point of looking for a new job, as he thinks that job stress is the cause of his symptoms. His examination is normal. Which of the following is the most appropriate advice for him?

   A. Continue with the as-needed acetaminophen and find a less stressful career.
   B. He should start an antidepressant for headache prophylaxis.
   C. His headaches are most likely to improve if he stops taking the acetaminophen.
   D. A triptan is a more appropriate treatment for him.

Answers

[34.1] **D.** This patient gives a history very consistent with common migraine headaches. There are no red flags found on history or examination, so no further testing is necessary at this point. As he has significant nausea, he may benefit from nonoral medication. A triptan delivered by injection or nasal spray is a reasonable starting point for him.

[34.2] **C.** The acute onset of the most severe headache in a patient's life is concerning for the presence of a subarachnoid hemorrhage. This is a medical emergency. This patient should be transported by emergency medical services to the nearest emergency facility for stabilization and management.

[34.3] **C.** This situation is typical of a medication-related headache. While finding a new, less-stressful job may be beneficial, the problem will not resolve until he discontinues the daily use of his over-the-counter analgesic.

CLINICAL PEARLS

❖ Migraine headaches can occur in children and adolescents, as well as adults.

❖ Most patients presenting for the evaluation of headaches don't need diagnostic testing beyond the history and physical. However, the presence of focal neurologic deficits or other red-flag symptoms/signs should prompt an immediate work-up or referral.

REFERENCES

Rakel RE. Essentials of family practice. Philadelphia: WB Saunders, 1993.
Silberstein SD for the U.S. Headache Consortium. Evidence-based guidelines for migraine headache (an evidence-based review). Neurology 2000;55:754–762.
South-Paul JE, et al. Current diagnosis and treatment in family medicine. New York: McGraw-Hill, 2004.

A 56-year-old male comes in for a routine health maintenance visit. He is new to your practice and has no specific complaints today. He has hypertension for which he takes hydrochlorothiazide and he occasionally takes an aspirin because someone told him that it was good for him. He has no other significant medical history. He does not smoke cigarettes, occasionally drinks alcohol, and does not exercise. His father died of a heart attack at age 60 years and his mother died at age 72 years of cancer. He has two younger sisters who are in good health. On examination, his blood pressure is 130/80 mm Hg and his pulse is 75 beats/min. He is 6 feet tall and weighs 200 lb. His complete physical examination is normal. You order a fasting lipid panel, which subsequently returns with the following results: total cholesterol 242 mg/dL; triglycerides 138 mg/dL; high-density lipoprotein (HDL) cholesterol 48 mg/dL; and low-density lipoprotein (LDL) cholesterol 155 mg/dL.

◆ **What is this patient's LDL-cholesterol goal?**

◆ **What other laboratory testing is indicated at this time?**

◆ **What is the recommended management at this point?**

ANSWERS TO CASE 35: Hyperlipidemia

Summary: A 56-year-old male with well-controlled hypertension is found to have elevated cholesterol on a screening blood test as part of a physical examination. He has no known history of coronary artery disease or of any coronary artery disease risk equivalent.

◆ **Goal for LDL-cholesterol:** <130 mg/dL

◆ **Further testing at this time:** blood glucose, creatinine, liver function tests, thyroid-stimulating hormone

◆ **Initial management of his elevated cholesterol:** therapeutic lifestyle changes

Analysis

Objectives

1. Know the risk factors for cardiovascular disease.
2. Know the Adult Treatment Panel (ATP) III guidelines for the diagnosis, evaluation, and management of hyperlipidemia.
3. Be able to counsel patients on therapeutic lifestyle changes to lower their cholesterol levels.

Considerations

It is important to remember that cholesterol is not a disease; however, high cholesterol is a risk factor for coronary heart disease (CHD). As such, **an individual's cholesterol levels must be interpreted in the context of their overall risks for CHD.** The recommended intensity with which we want to lower someone's cholesterol level should be proportionate to their risk of CHD: the higher one's risk, the lower the cholesterol goal. To do this, one must first learn what these major risks are.

Someone with known CHD has a greater than 20% risk of having another CHD event in 10 years. Persons with other forms of atherosclerotic disease (peripheral arterial disease, cerebrovascular disease, or abdominal aortic aneurysm), type 2 diabetes, or multiple risk factors that together raise the risk of CHD to ≥20% in 10 years, are said to have a CHD risk equivalent. **People with known CHD or CHD risk equivalents have the highest risk of future CHD events and, therefore, their cholesterol targets are the lowest.** Similarly, someone with one or fewer risk factors for CHD is at low risk of having a CHD event. These people usually have a less than 10% risk of a CHD event in 10 years. In this population, the recommended lipid levels are not as low.

A third population is one with intermediate risk when compared to the previous two groups. They have two or more risks factors but a CHD risk between 10%

and 20%. In this population, an individual risk should be calculated. Numerous risk calculators are available online or for download into a PDA (personal digital assistant). One is available from the National Heart, Lung and Blood institute at www.nhlbi.nih.gov/guidelines/cholesterol/index.htm. By determining the individual risk of CHD, one can then determine an appropriate lipid goal for that patient.

APPROACH TO HIGH CHOLESTEROL

Definitions

ATP III: The third report of the National Cholesterol Education Program Expert Panel on the Detection, Evaluation and Treatment of High Blood Cholesterol in Adults.

HDL cholesterol: High-density lipoprotein cholesterol.

LDL cholesterol: Low-density lipoprotein cholesterol.

Statin: Medication in the beta-hydroxy-beta-methylglutaryl-coenzyme A (HMG-CoA)-reductase inhibitor class. These are the most widely used medications for lowering LDL cholesterol.

Clinical Approach

Determination of Lipid Goal

Numerous studies show that **LDL cholesterol is a major risk for developing CHD and that lowering LDL cholesterol can reduce this risk.** For these reasons, the ATP III guidelines focus on the identification of those with high LDL cholesterol, the determination of that individual's risk of CHD, and development of an appropriate management plan to reach LDL cholesterol goals.

These guidelines recommend measuring lipid levels in all adults older than age 20 years every 5 years. The test performed can be either a fasting lipid panel (total, LDL and HDL cholesterol; triglycerides) or a nonfasting total and HDL cholesterol, with subsequent fasting lipid panel if either total cholesterol is over 200 mg/dL or if HDL cholesterol is less than 40 mg/dL. Table 35–1 lists the ATP III classification of lipid levels.

LDL cholesterol is the primary goal of management. Along with the presence of CHD or a CHD risk equivalent, the following **five factors are considered to determine the LDL goal** of a given individual:

- **Cigarette smoking**
- **Hypertension** (blood pressure ≥140/90 mm Hg or on antihypertensive medication)
- **Low HDL**
- **Age** (≥45 years for men; ≥55 years for women)
- **Family history of premature CHD** (male first-degree relative ≤55 years of age; female first-degree relative ≤65 years of age)

Table 35–1
ATP III CLASSIFICATION OF LIPID LEVELS

LDL Cholesterol (mg/dL)
<100	Optimal
100–129	Near optimal/above optimal
130–159	Borderline high
160–189	High
190 or greater	Very high

Total cholesterol (mg/dL)
<200	Desirable
200–239	Borderline high
240 or greater	High

HDL cholesterol (mg/dL)
<40	Low
60 or greater	High

Information from ATP III report.

A high HDL level is considered a negative risk, which removes one other risk factor from the total.

The LDL cholesterol goal is based upon the evaluation of these risks. A person with **CHD or a CHD risk equivalent has an LDL goal of 100 mg/dL or less.** Someone with **0–1 identified risks has an LDL goal of 160 mg/dL or less.** An individual with 2 or more risks should have an individual risk assessment performed, using a risk calculator. If someone has **2 or more risk factors and an individual risk of between 10% and 20%, that person's LDL goal is 130 mg/dL or less.** However, if the individual risk is ≥20%, that person should be treated as having a CHD equivalent, with a goal LDL of <100 mg/dL (Table 35–2).

An update to the ATP III was issued in 2004 with an interpretation of some more recent clinical trials. This update suggests a **"therapeutic option" of a very low LDL goal of <70 mg/dL for those patients at very high risk of CHD.** This very-high-risk category includes people with CHD and either multiple major risk factors (especially diabetes), poorly controlled risk factors (especially smoking), multiple risk factors of metabolic syndrome (see Case 33), or an acute coronary syndrome.

Evaluation

When high blood cholesterol is identified, an investigation should be performed to evaluate for **secondary causes of dyslipidemia.** Included among these causes are **diabetes, hypothyroidism, obstructive liver disease, and chronic renal failure.** Consequently, a reasonable laboratory work-up includes a fasting

Table 35–2

MANAGEMENT GUIDELINES TO REACH LDL GOALS

RISK CATEGORY	LDL GOAL	LDL LEVEL TO START THERAPEUTIC LIFESTYLE CHANGE	LDL LEVEL TO CONSIDER MEDICATION
CHD or CHD equivalent	<100	≥100	≥130 (optional for 101–129)
2 or more risks factors	<130	≥130	10-yr risk 10–20% ≥160 10-yr risk <10% ≥190
0–1 risk factors	<160	≥160	≥190

All LDL levels in mg/dL. Information from ATP III report.

blood glucose, thyroid-stimulating hormone (TSH), liver enzymes, and a creatinine level. Certain medications, including progestins, anabolic steroids, and corticosteroids, also can result in elevated cholesterol. Consideration should be given to changing or discontinuing these when possible.

Management

Therapeutic lifestyle changes (TLCs) are the cornerstone of all treatments for hyperlipidemia. All patients should be educated on healthier living, including dietary modifications, increased physical activity, and smoking cessation. Weight reduction should be encouraged.

Specific dietary recommendations should include a **reduction of saturated fats to less than 7% of total calories and an intake of less than 200 mg/d of cholesterol.** Total dietary fat should be kept to no more than 35% of total calories, with less than 10% polyunsaturated fat. Trans fats should be kept as low as possible.

When dietary restriction alone does not lead to adequate LDL reduction, the addition of dietary soluble fiber and plant stanols/sterols can be beneficial. Soluble fiber 10–25 g and of plant stanols/sterols 2 g can be added to aid in cholesterol reduction. Referral to a dietician may be helpful as well.

When TLC is instituted, regular follow-up must be arranged. Fasting lipids should be rechecked in approximately 6 weeks. If adequate reduction has occurred, reinforcement of the lifestyle changes should be given and the patient followed every 4–6 months.

Pharmacotherapy may be considered in patients who do not reach their LDL goals with TLC alone. **TLC should continue to be reinforced and encouraged even when starting medications.** In someone who does not have CHD or a risk equivalent (primary prevention), medications should be considered after the third visit of TLC management. In someone with CHD or an equivalent (secondary prevention), the more stringent LDL goals often require earlier institution of drug treatment.

The first-line pharmacotherapy for LDL cholesterol reduction is a statin. **Statins not only reduce LDL cholesterol but also reduce the rates of coronary events, strokes, cardiac death, and all-cause mortality.** When statin therapy is started, fasting lipids should be rechecked in 6 weeks. If LDL goals are not met, the dose of the statin can be increased or a second agent added. These other medications include fibric acids, nicotinic acids, bile acid sequestrants, and cholesterol absorption blockers (Table 35–3). When taking statins, liver enzymes must be monitored as well (6–12 weeks after initiation or dosage change, then every 6–12 months). When goal levels are met, regular follow-up should be arranged to reinforce lifestyle changes, medication compliance, and overall risk factor reduction.

Table 35–3
MEDICATIONS USED TO LOWER CHOLESTEROL

DRUG CLASS/ MEDICATION	EFFECTS	SIDE EFFECTS	CONTRAINDICATIONS
Statin Lovastatin Pravastatin Fluvastatin Atorvastatin Cerivastatin Simvastatin	LDL ↓ 18–55%; HDL ↑ 5–15%; triglytrides (TG) ↓ 7–30%	Myopathy, myalgia, increased liver enzymes	Active or chronic liver disease; relative contraindication with cytochrome P450 inhibitors, cyclosporine, macrolides, antifungals
Bile acid sequestrants Cholestyramine Colestipol Colesevelam	LDL ↓ 15–30%; HDL ↑ 3–5%; TG no change; or increase	GI distress, constipation, decreased absorption of other mes	Dysbetalipoproteinemia; TG >400
Nicotinic acids Immediate-release, sustained-release, or extended- release nicotinic acid	LDL ↓ 5–25%; HDL ↑ 15–35%; TG ↓ 20–50%	Flushing, hyperglycemia, hyperuricemia, upper GI distress, hepatotoxicity	Absolute: chronic liver disease, severe gout; relative: diabetes, hyperuricemia, peptic ulcer disease
Fibric acids Gemfibrozil Fenofibrate Clofibrate	LDL ↓ 5–20%; HDL ↑ 10–20%; TG ↓ 20–50%	Dyspepsia, gallstones, myopathy, unexplained non-CHD deaths in WHO study	Severe renal disease, severe hepatic disease
Cholesterol absorption blocker Ezetimibe	LDL ↓ 13–25%; HDL ↑ 3–5%; TG ↓ 5–14%	Abdominal pain, diarrhea	Hepatic insufficiency/active liver disease

Information from ATP III report and ezetimibe product information.

Comprehension Questions

[35.1] A 62-year-old male smoker with no known history of CHD presents for follow-up of intermittent claudication. He has normal blood pressure and no family history of premature CHD. His HDL cholesterol is 48 mg/dL. According to the ATP III guidelines, what is his goal LDL?

    A. 70 mg/dL
    B. 100 mg/dL
    C. 130 mg/dL
    D. 160 mg/dL

[35.2] A 55-year-old woman presents to your office for follow-up. She was discharged from the hospital 1 week ago following a heart attack. She has quit smoking since then and vows to stay off cigarettes forever. Her lipid levels are total cholesterol 240; HDL 50 mg/dL; LDL 150 mg/dL; triglycerides 50 mg/dL. What is the most appropriate management at this time?

    A. Institute therapeutic lifestyle changes alone
    B. Institute TLC and a statin
    C. Institute a statin alone
    D. Institute TLC, a statin, and nicotinic acid

[35.3] A 48-year-old man with no significant medical history and no symptoms is found to have elevated cholesterol at a health screening. Which of the following tests is part of the routine evaluation of this problem?

    A. EKG
    B. Stress test
    C. Complete blood count (CBC)
    D. Thyroid-stimulating hormone (TSH)

Answers

[35.1] **B.** This patient has symptomatic peripheral arterial disease, which is considered a CHD risk equivalent. His LDL goal is 100 mg/dL or less.

[35.2] **B.** This patient has known CHD, documented by her recent myocardial infarction. Her goal LDL is 100 mg/dL or less. As her starting level is above 130 mg/dL, it would be reasonable to start both TLC and a statin to help her to reach her goal. Nicotinic acid may be a reasonable addition if the TLC and statin do not lead to adequate LDL reduction.

[35.3] **D.** Hypothyroidism is a potential cause of secondary dyslipidemia. A TSH is a reasonable test to perform in this setting. There is no indication to screen for CHD with an EKG or stress test in this asymptomatic person. Other tests to perform could include a fasting sugar, liver enzymes, and a measurement of renal function.

CLINICAL PEARLS

❖ Lipid levels must always be interpreted in the context of the individual's overall risk factors for CHD.

❖ Statins have the best data to support improvement in outcomes that are clinically significant, such as heart attacks, strokes, and death. Except when there is a contraindication, a statin should be the first medication used for cholesterol reduction.

❖ Remind patients who are taking lipid-lowering medications that lifestyle modifications are still necessary. Medications are not a substitute for a healthy lifestyle.

REFERENCES

Grundy SM, Cleeman JI, Merz CN et al. NCEP report: implications of recent clinical trials for the National Cholesterol Education Program Adult Treatment Panel III guidelines. Circulation 2004;110:227–239.

National Cholesterol Education Program. The third report of the NCEP Expert Panel on the detection, evaluation and treatment of high blood cholesterol in adults. NIH Publication No. 01–3670. 2001.

A 20-month-old girl, new to your practice, is brought in by her mother because she's been crying and not walking for the past day. Her mother reports that the child is "very clumsy and falls a lot." She says that the little girl may have injured her leg by falling off the sofa because, she repeats, "she really is clumsy and falls a lot." Upon review with the mother, she states that the child has no significant medical history and takes no medications regularly. There are two older children in the family, ages 4 and 6 years, who are in good health but also are "clumsy and forever hurting themselves." The husband lives in the home. Without any questioning or prompting, the mother states that her husband is "a good man but he's under a lot of stress." You ask the mother to undress the child for an examination and she quickly replies, "Do you really have to undress her? She's very shy." You politely, but firmly, say that you need to examine her and she removes the child's pants. You see that her right knee is visibly swollen and tender to palpation on the medial bony prominences. You also note numerous bruises of the buttocks and posterior thighs, which appear to be of different ages. There are also several small, circular scars on the legs, each about a centimeter in size. "See how clumsy she is?" the mother says, pointing to her bruises. An x-ray of the child's knee shows a corner fracture of the distal femoral metaphysis.

◆ **What is the likely mechanism of this child's injuries?**

◆ **What further evaluation is necessary at this time?**

◆ **What legal obligation must a physician fulfill in this circumstance?**

ANSWERS TO CASE 36: Family Violence

Summary: A 20-month-old girl is brought to the office for evaluation of crying and not walking. On examination, she is found to have multiple bruises and circular wounds that are suspicious for cigarette burns. Her knee x-ray shows a metaphyseal corner fracture, an injury that is inconsistent with the stated history of "falling off the sofa."

◆ **Most likely mechanism of injuries:** Inflicted injuries, including leg injury from forceful pulling, bruising from hitting the child's legs, and cigarette burns.

◆ **Further evaluation at this time:** Complete, unclothed physical examination of child (including ophthalmoscopic and neurologic exams); radiographic skeletal survey.

◆ **Legal obligation of physician:** Report of suspected child abuse to the appropriate child protective services organization.

Analysis

Objectives

1. Learn the symptoms and signs suggestive of abuse.
2. Know the situations in which the risk of family violence increases.
3. Learn some of the medicolegal requirements involved in situations of family violence.

Considerations

Family violence can occur in families of any socioeconomic class and in households of any composition. The term *family violence* **includes child abuse, partner abuse, and elder abuse.** The abuse that occurs can be physical, sexual, emotional, psychological, or economic. It can take the forms of battering, raping, threatening, intimidating, isolating from others, stealing, and preventing the earning of money, among many others.

In the case presented here, there are several signs of intentionally inflicted injuries to the child. The presence of numerous bruises of varying ages, especially on relatively protected areas such as the buttocks and upper posterior thighs, should raise suspicions. Finding injuries inconsistent with the reported history also can be a clue. Certain types of fractures, such as metaphyseal corner fractures (caused by forceful jerking or twisting of the leg) are usually a result of abuse. The identification of wounds consistent with cigarette burns is highly specific for abuse.

Physicians often find these situations extremely difficult and uncomfortable to deal with. They may feel caught between two partners—both of whom are patients—but who give conflicting stories. They may have concerns about the legal implications of their findings and fear legal actions if they make reports to authorities. They may have frustrations in dealing with a person who won't leave an abusive spouse and may feel ill-trained to deal with many of these situations. By knowing situations in which family violence is more likely to occur, knowing the laws regarding disclosure and reporting, and learning to recognize the signs of family violence, physicians can be better prepared to address these situations when they occur.

APPROACH TO FAMILY VIOLENCE

Definitions

Neglect: Failure to provide the needs required for functioning or for the avoidance of harm.
Physical abuse (battery): Intentional physical actions (e.g., biting, kicking, punching) that can cause injury or pain to another person.

Clinical Approach

Partner Abuse

Family violence is an abuse of power, in which a more-powerful person exerts control over a less-powerful person or persons. This abuse can take the form of **physical violence (battery), sexual violence, intimidation, emotional and psychological abuse, economic control, and isolation from others.** Although it is most common to think of this as a man abusing a woman, abuse can occur both in homosexual relationships and in heterosexual relationships with a male victim. It is estimated that **more than 1 million women are abused annually in the United States and that approximately 1 in 3 women are abused at some time in their lives.**

Abuse can occur in any relationship or in any socioeconomic class. Certain situations increase the likelihood, or escalate the occurrences, of abuse. These situations include changes in family life (such as pregnancy, illnesses, deaths), economic stresses, and substance abuse. Personal and family histories of abuse also increase the likelihood of family violence.

Numerous professional organizations, such as the American Medical Association and the American College of Obstetricians and Gynecologists, advocate for the routine screening of women for abuse by direct questioning. Numerous tools exist for screening, from simple questioning ("Do you feel safe in your home?") to more formal inventory tools. The United States Preventive Services Task Force (USPSTF) has found insufficient evidence to make a recommendation for or against screening for domestic violence because they did not find studies that directly looked at the impact of screening on reducing adverse outcomes. The USPSTF does recommend that **all clinicians should be alert to physical and behavioral signs and symptoms associated with abuse and neglect.**

Victims of abuse can present with varied symptoms and signs suggestive of the problem. Direct physical findings can include obvious traumatic injuries, such as contusions, fractures, "black eyes," concussions and internal bleeding. Genital, anal, or pharyngeal trauma, sexually transmitted diseases (STDs), and unintended pregnancy may be signs of sexual assault. Depression, anxiety, post-traumatic stress disorder, and suicide attempts can also result from abusive relationships.

Some signs and symptoms may be less obvious and may require numerous encounters until the finding of family violence is made. **Victims of abuse may present to doctors frequently for health complaints or have physical symptoms that cannot otherwise be explained.** Chronic pain, frequently abdominal or pelvic pain, is commonly a sign of a history of abuse. The development of substance abuse or eating disorders may prompt inquiry into family violence as well.

When abuse is identified, an initial priority is to assess the safety of the home situation. Direct questioning regarding the presence of weapons in the home, as well as the need for a plan for safety for the victim and others at home (children, elders), is critical. Resources, such as shelters, should be provided. It may be helpful to allow the patient to contact a shelter, law enforcement, family members or friends, while still in the doctor's office. Multidisciplinary interventions, including family, medical, legal, mental health, and law enforcement, are often necessary.

The **laws regarding clinician reporting partner violence varies from state to state.** It is important to know the statutes in your locality. Many states do not require contacting legal authorities if the victim of the abuse is a competent adult.

Child Abuse

Approximately 1 million cases of child abuse, with more than 1000 deaths, are reported each year in the United States; the number of unreported cases makes the overall prevalence much higher. The situations that increase the risk of child abuse are similar to those that increase the likelihood of other family violence. Children who are chronically ill or who have physical or developmental disorders may be at even higher risk.

Certain history and physical examination findings raise the suspicion for child abuse. **Injuries that are inconsistent with the stated history or a history that repeatedly changes with questioning should raise the suspicion of abuse.** Children who are taken to numerous different physicians or emergency rooms, or who are brought in repeatedly with traumatic injuries, may be victims. Delay in seeking medical care for an injury may also be a clue to abuse.

Neglect is also a form of child abuse. An injury or illness that occurred because of lack of appropriate supervision may be a sign of neglect. Failure to provide for basic nutritional, healthcare, or safety needs may be other forms of neglect.

Children frequently have bruises, fractures, and other injuries that occur accidentally and it can be difficult to distinguish with certainty whether an injury is accidental or intentional. However, **certain types of injuries are uncommon as accidents** (Table 36–1). The presence of these injuries is highly suggestive of child abuse.

When an injury suspicious for child abuse is identified, attention should initially focus on treatment and protection from further injury. A complete examination should be performed and all injuries documented with drawings or photographs. An x-ray skeletal survey can be performed to look for evidence of current or previous bony injuries. Ophthalmologic examination should be performed to look for retinal hemorrhages. The progress note should be documented carefully and legibly.

All 50 states require reporting of suspected child abuse to the appropriate authorities (refer to local laws to determine the appropriate authority). Parents should be informed that a report is going to be made and the process that is likely to occur after the report is made. Consideration must also be given to the possibility that there are other victims of abuse in the home (spouse, other children, elders). **Any healthcare provider who makes a good-faith report of suspected abuse or neglect is immune from any legal action, even if the investigation reveals that no abuse occurred.** Providers may be held liable for failure to report child abuse.

Table 36–1
INJURIES SUGGESTIVE OF CHILD ABUSE

- Stocking-and-glove burns of the extremities (immersion in scalding water)
- Burns of the buttock and groin that spare the intertriginous areas (immersion in scalding water)
- Centimeter-sized circular burns (cigarettes)
- Multiple bruises of differing ages
- Unexplained injury to buttocks, thighs, ears, neck
- Bruises in the shape of a hand, belt buckle, or loops of a cord
- Retinal hemorrhages ("shaken baby syndrome")
- Corner or "bucket-handle" fractures of metaphysis of long bones
- Spiral fracture of femur or humerus
- Posterior rib fractures
- Scapular fractures
- Spinous process fractures
- Sternal fractures
- Complex, bilateral, or wide skull fractures
- Injury to external genitalia
- Sexually transmitted diseases, genital warts
- Circumferential hematoma of anus (forced penetration)

Elder Abuse

Many types of elder abuse may occur, including physical, sexual, and psychological abuse, neglect, and financial exploitation. An estimated 2 million elders are abused in some form annually in the United States. Along with the other risks for domestic violence, several factors unique to the care of elders may play a role. Caregiver frustrations and burnout are commonly heard excuses for abuse. **Persons who are older, more cognitively and physically debilitated, and have less access to resources are more likely to be abused or exploited.**

A history of abuse may be difficult to obtain, as the patient may fear worsening of the abuse or may not have the cognitive ability to make an accurate report. If feasible, it is **helpful to interview the patient without the presence of the caregiver.** The physical examination, like in child abuse, should carefully document any injuries that are found. Suspicions of dehydration or malnutrition should be confirmed with appropriate laboratory testing and radiographs should be performed as necessary.

By law, elder abuse should be reported to the appropriate adult protective services, but the reporting requirements vary by state. A multidisciplinary approach, involving medical providers, social workers, legal authorities, and families is usually necessary to address the issues involved.

Comprehension Questions

[36.1] A 42-year-old woman presents to your office for evaluation of chronic abdominal pain. She has been to see you multiple times for this complaint, but the work-up has always been negative. On examination today, she also is found to have a black eye, which she says that she got by bumping into a door. Which of the following statements is true?

A. You should ask your patient about physical abuse and report your suspicions to the local police.

B. You should ask your patient about physical abuse, make an assessment of her immediate danger, and provide her with information about local support services.

C. You should only discuss abuse if she brings up the topic.

D. You should refer the patient to a psychiatrist for further evaluation and treatment.

[36.2] A 7-month-old male is found to have a spiral fracture of the femur that his father says he got by climbing onto a chair and then jumping off. Which of the following statements is true regarding this situation?

    A. You cannot report this to child protective services because the history provides a legitimate possible mechanism of injury other than abuse.

    B. The father can sue you if you report this to the authorities and they determine that no abuse occurred.

    C. You should anonymously report the abuse to the authorities.

    D. You can be held legally liable for failing to report child abuse.

[36.3] Which of the following injuries is most likely to be caused by abuse of a toddler?

    A. Three or four bruises on the shins and knees

    B. Spiral fracture of the tibia

    C. A displaced posterior rib fracture

    D. A forehead laceration

Answers

[36.1] **B.** It is appropriate to discuss your concerns in a nonaccusatory, non-judgmental fashion with your patient. Waiting for her to bring up the subject may result in her suffering further abuse. The reporting of the abuse of competent adults (not elders) is not mandated by law in most states. You should offer assistance, evaluate her safety, and provide her with information regarding available services in the area.

[36.2] **D.** This injury is highly suspicious for abuse. It is the type of injury often associated with abuse and the history given is inconsistent with the developmental abilities of a 7-month-old child. The law in every state requires that child abuse be reported and a physician who fails to report abuse could be held legally liable.

[36.3] **C.** A posterior rib fracture is often the result of grabbing and squeezing the chest violently. It is very suspicious for abuse. A spiral fracture of the tibia is known as a "toddler's fracture" and is a common injury that is often confused with abuse, but not often caused by abuse. Bruises on the shins and knees and forehead injuries are common from falls while learning to walk.

CLINICAL PEARLS

❖ Suspected child and elder abuse must be reported. Good-faith reports of suspected abuse are a shield to lawsuits; failure to report can result in legal action against the physician.

❖ When seeing a suspected abuse victim, always consider the possibility that there could be other abuse victims in the household.

REFERENCES

Eyler AE, Cohen M. Case studies in partner violence. Am Fam Physician 1999;60: 2569–2576.

Johns Hopkins: the Harriet Lane handbook: A manual for pediatric house officers. In: Robertson J, Shilkofski N, et al. (eds). 17th ed. St. Louis: Mosby, 2005:120–123.

Pressel DM. Evaluation of physical abuse in children. Am Fam Physician 2000;61: 3057–3064.

Swagerty DL, Takahashi PY, Evans JM. Elder mistreatment. Am Fam Physician 1999;59(10):2804–2808.

United States Preventive Services Task Force. Screening for family and intimate partner violence. March, 2004. Available at: www.ahrq.gov.

A 12-year-old boy is brought to the office with right thigh pain and a limp. His mother has noticed him limping for the past week or so. He denies any injury to his leg but says that it hurts some when he plays basketball with his friends. He denies back pain, hip pain, or ankle pain. He occasionally gets some pain in the right knee but doesn't have any swelling or bruising. He has no significant medical history, doesn't take any medications regularly, and otherwise feels fine. On examination, he is an overweight adolescent. His vital signs and a general physical examination are normal. When you have him walk, he has a prominent limp. You note that he seems to keep his weight on his left leg for a greater proportion of his gait cycle than he does on the right leg. Examination of his back reveals a full range of motion, no tenderness, and no muscle spasm. He gets pain in the right hip when it is passively internally rotated. When the hip is passively flexed there is a noticeable external rotation. There is no thigh muscle atrophy. His right knee and the remainder of his orthopedic examination are normal.

◆ **What is the most appropriate test to order first for this patient?**

◆ **What is the most likely diagnosis?**

◆ **What complication could occur if this problem is not diagnosed and treated?**

ANSWERS TO CASE 37: Limping and Pain in Children

Summary: An overweight 12-year-old boy presents for evaluation of a limp and thigh pain. There is no history of injury or trauma. He is found to have pain on internal rotation of the hip and his hip externally rotates when passively flexed. He bears weight more on his left leg than his right while walking.

◆ **Most appropriate test to order:** X-ray of the right hip

◆ **Most likely diagnosis:** Slipped capital femoral epiphysis

◆ **Complication for which he is at risk:** Avascular necrosis of the hip

Analysis

Objectives

1. Develop a differential diagnosis of the most likely causes of leg pain and limping in children.
2. Know common causes of leg pain and limping in children of different ages.

Considerations

Leg pain is a common complaint in childhood. The most common causes of leg pain in children are acute injuries—sprains, strains, contusions, etc. However, leg pain and limping can be a sign of a more serious, even life-threatening, pathology. Learning an approach to the evaluation and the common diagnoses involved may help in the identification of these problems earlier, when a better outcome is more likely.

To understand a limp, it is first important to understand the normal gait. Gait is composed of two phases: the "swing" and the "stance" phases. The stance phase is the weight-bearing phase and accounts for approximately 60% of the gait cycle. The swing phase is the non–weight-bearing phase, when the foot lifts off the ground and is propelled forward. The **antalgic gait occurs when the stance phase of gait is shortened, usually because of pain during weight bearing.** Antalgic gait is the most common type of limp and is the type of gait described in this case.

There are many causes of limb pain in children; some of the more common causes may be broadly categorized as being primarily orthopedic, reactive, infectious, rheumatologic, neoplastic and congenital (Table 37–1). The prevalence of the specific diagnoses also varies by age.

In the specific case presented, there are several symptoms and signs that make the diagnosis of slipped capital femoral epiphysis (SCFE) likely. The absence of a specific injury is significant, as SCFE is the most common nontraumatic

Table 37–1
COMMON CAUSES OF LIMB PAIN IN CHILDREN

Orthopedic
  Fracture
  Stress fracture
  Sprain/strain/contusion
  Chondromalacia patellae
  Slipped capital femoral epiphysis
  Legg-Calvé-Perthes disease
Reactive
  Toxic synovitis
  Transient synovitis following viral infection
  Rheumatic fever
Infectious
  Septic arthritis
  Osteomyelitis
  Cellulitis
  Discitis
  Gonococcal arthritis
Rheumatologic
  Juvenile rheumatoid arthritis
  Systemic lupus erythematosus
Neoplastic
  Leukemia
  Lymphoma
  Bone tumors (benign and malignant)
Congenital
  Hip dysplasia
  Sickle cell disease
Other
  "Growing pains"
  Neuropathies

Information from Hollister JR. Rheumatic diseases. In: Hay WW, Levin MJ, Sondheimer JM, et al. (eds). Current pediatric diagnosis and treatment. 15th ed. New York: McGraw-Hill 2001:734; and Leet AI, Skaggs DL. Evalution of the acutely limping child. Am Fam Physician 2000;61: 1011–1018.

hip pathology in adolescents. The initial complaint of thigh pain may lead to other considerations, but **hip pathology will frequently present with pain in the groin, thigh, or even the knee.** The patient's age and body habitus are typical for SCFE, which is classically described as occurring most often in overweight adolescent males. Pain with internal rotation of the hip and the finding of external rotation on passive flexion of the affected hip are also suggestive of SCFE.

APPROACH TO LIMPING AND LOWER-EXTREMITY PAIN IN CHILDREN

Definitions

Avascular necrosis: Death of living bone tissue caused by disruption of blood flow.
Dysplasia: Abnormal growth or development.

Infants and Toddlers

Common causes of limping in children in this age group are septic arthritis, fractures, and complications of congenital hip dysplasia. **Septic arthritis** is usually monoarticular and associated with systemic signs such as fever. In young infants, the symptoms may be less obvious, such as crying, irritability, and poor feeding. Children who are ambulatory (crawlers or walkers) will often refuse to do anything that puts weight on the affected joint because of pain. Infection of a joint causes a septic effusion, which raises the pressure inside of the joint capsule. **Children with a septic hip joint will often lay with their hip flexed, abducted, and externally rotated,** which helps to reduce the pain, and they will have significant pain with any internal rotation or extension of the joint. Children with a septic joint will usually have an elevated white blood cell count, erythrocyte sedimentation rate (ESR) and C-reactive protein (CRP). Definitive diagnosis comes from joint aspiration. **Any suspected septic joint must be aspirated.** In younger infants (4 months or younger), group B streptococcus and *Staphylococcus aureus* are the most common pathogens involved. In older infants and children under the age of 5 years, *S. aureus* and *Streptococcus pyogenes* are the usual causes. Treatment is urgent surgical irrigation and debridement, along with antibiotics.

Unsuspected **fractures**—either stress fractures or traumatic fractures—can present with pain and limping. Abuse must be suspected if the injury is inconsistent with the history presented, if the history changes with repeated questioning, if the child is said to have performed an act outside of his developmental ability, or if a fracture usually associated with abuse is found (see Case 36). However, the **history may not reveal the source of the injury,** as a child may fall outside of the view of the parent. **A traumatic injury may not result in limping or in complete immobility, but may cause a change in how the child ambulates.** For example, a child who previously walked and now refuses to walk but will crawl, may have an injury of the lower leg or foot.

A **toddler's fracture** is one example of an unsuspected fracture that may present primarily as a limp or a refusal to walk. This fracture is a **spiral fracture of the tibia that results from twisting while the foot is planted.** The diagnosis may be suspected in the setting of an acute limp or change in ambulation, a normal examination of the knee and upper leg and tenderness of the tibia. It can be confirmed with a plain film x-ray. Undiagnosed **congenital dysplasia of**

the hip may present as a painless limp that is present from the time that the child learns to walk. All newborns and infants should have their hips examined for instability or dislocation. If undiagnosed, contractures may form that limit movement of the hip. When the child learns to walk, the child will have a painless limp. The diagnosis may be confirmed by x-rays showing abnormal hip alignment. If the problem is found in the first few weeks of life, the child can be treated with splinting of the hip and normal development usually follows. If diagnosed late, the treatment is often surgical.

Young Children

Transient synovitis is a self-limited inflammatory response that is a common cause of hip pain in children. It occurs typically in children ages 3–10 years, is more common in boys than in girls, and **often follows a viral infection.** It is frequently seen as gradually increasing hip pain that results in a limp or refusal to walk. These children have a low-grade or no fever, a normal white blood cell (WBC) count, and a normal ESR. On examination, there is pain with internal rotation of the hip and the overall range of motion is limited by pain. X-rays are either normal or show some nonspecific swelling. In a situation where the patient is afebrile, has a normal WBC count, normal ESR, and short-term follow-up can be assured, the patient can be followed clinically and should improve in a few days. If these conditions are not met and the diagnosis of a septic joint is considered, or if a patient followed expectantly continues to worsen, an aspiration should be done. **A septic joint will have a purulent aspirate with a WBC count >50,000/μL; transient synovitis will have a yellow/clear aspirate with a lower WBC count (<10,000/μL).**

Legg-Calvé-Perthes (LCP) disease is an **avascular necrosis of the femoral head** that typically occurs in children ages 4–8 years. It is much more common in boys than in girls. Any disruption of blood flow to the femoral capital epiphysis, such as trauma or infection, may cause avascular necrosis. In LCP disease, the etiology of the disruption of blood flow is unknown. Children typically have a gradual onset of hip, thigh, or knee pain, and limping over a few months. Early in the course, x-rays of the hip may appear normal. Later radiographic findings include collapse, flattening, and widening of the femoral head. Bone scans or magnetic resonance imaging (MRI) may be necessary to confirm the diagnosis. The **treatment is usually conservative,** with protection of the joint and efforts to maintain range of motion. Children who develop more severe necrosis or who develop the disease at older ages may have a worse outcome and a higher risk of developing degenerative arthritis.

Adolescents

The capital femoral epiphysis is the growth plate that connects the metaphysis (femoral head) to the diaphysis (shaft of the femur). A **slipped capital femoral epiphysis** is a separation of this growth plate, which results in the femoral head being medially and posteriorly displaced. This may be caused by an acute injury, but more often is not. It is most often seen in overweight adolescent boys and presents as pain in the hip, thigh, or knee along with a limp. Examination reveals **limited internal rotation** and obligate **external rotation when the hip is passively flexed.** Early x-rays may show only widening of the epiphysis; later x-rays can show the slippage of the femoral head in relation to the femoral neck. The treatment is surgical pinning of the femoral head. These patients must be closely followed, as approximately 33% will develop avascular necrosis and 33% will develop SCFE in the contralateral hip.

Other causes of limb pain are common in adolescents. Sprains, strains, and overuse injuries are the most common cause of limb pain in this population, and are usually readily diagnosed on history and examination (see Case 12). Sexually active adolescents or teens are at risk for sexually transmitted diseases (STDs) and their complications, including gonococcal arthritis. In this population, an appropriate history, sexual history, and review of systems are necessary.

Comprehension Questions

[37.1] A 6-year-old male is brought in for evaluation of a painful hip. He has been limping and not wanting to walk for the past 2 days. He has had no obvious injury. He feels a little better if he is given some ibuprofen. He has not had a fever and does not have any other current symptoms, although he had "the flu" last week. On examination, his vital signs are normal. His right hip has some pain with internal rotation. He walks with a pronounced limp. Which of the following statements is most appropriate?

A. He can be sent home with a prescription for ibuprofen.
B. He should have a complete blood count (CBC) and ESR.
C. He should have an aspiration of his hip in the office.
D. If he has a normal x-ray, no further work-up is needed.

[37.2] An 18-month-old African-American girl is brought into your office because she has been crying and stopped walking today. She will crawl, however. Her mom denies any injury to the child. On examination, she is crying but consolable in her mother's arms. She has bruising and swelling just proximal to the left ankle. An x-ray reveals a spiral fracture of the tibia. At this time you advise the mother that:

A. You are going to report this to child protective services as suspected abuse.
B. You are going to refer the child for a bone biopsy because this is a pathologic fracture that may represent a neoplasm.
C. This is a common fracture resulting from twisting on a planted foot.
D. You should draw blood to evaluate for sickle cell disease, which may cause infarction of the bone.

[37.3] A 2-year-old boy is brought in with fever and poor feeding. He started getting sick yesterday and has worsened significantly today. He has had no recent illnesses or injuries, and no known ill contacts. On examination, his temperature is 101°F, he is tachycardic, and he appears ill. He is laying on his back with his left leg flexed and abducted at the hip. An head, ears, eyes, nose, and throat (HEENT) examination is normal, the heart is tachycardic but regular, and the lungs are clear. The abdomen is nontender and has normal bowel sounds. He screams in pain when you move his left leg from its resting position. Blood work reveals an elevated WBC count of 15,000 mm³ and an ESR of 45 mm/h (normal: 0–10). An x-ray of his left hip shows a widened joint space but no fractures. What is your next step at this point?

A. Oral antibiotic and follow-up in 1 day
B. MRI of the hip and referral to an orthopedist
C. Antiinflammatory medication and close follow-up
D. Hip joint aspiration

Answers

[37.1] **B.** The case presented is suspicious for transient synovitis following a viral illness. A CBC and ESR should be drawn. With a normal CBC and ESR, and if follow-up can be assured, this child could be treated expectantly, given an oral nonsteroidal antiinflammatory drug (NSAID) with the expectation of a recovery in a few days.

[37.2] **C.** The case presented is classic for a toddler's fracture. Spiral fractures of other long bones (femur, humerus) are more suspicious for abuse. Orthopedic referral is appropriate for management, but a bone biopsy or further work-up is not necessary at this time.

[37.3] **D.** The child in this case has all of the symptoms and signs of a septic hip joint. This situation demands a joint aspiration to confirm the diagnosis. If it is confirmed, he should be promptly referred for urgent surgical management.

CLINICAL PEARLS

❖ Hip pathology may not cause hip pain; it may cause groin, thigh, or knee pain instead.

❖ Because of the high risk of bilateral disease, follow-up in SCFE cases should include examination and x-rays of the unaffected hip until the growth plate closes.

REFERENCES

Adkins SB, Figler RA. Hip pain in athletes. Am Fam Physician 2000;61:2109–2118.

Hollister JR. Rheumatic diseases. In: Hay WW, Levin MJ, Sondheimer JM, et al. (eds). Current pediatric diagnosis and treatment. 15th ed. New York: McGraw-Hill, 2001.

Leet AI, Skaggs DL. Evaluation of the acutely limping child. Am Fam Physician 2000;61:1011–1018.

Smith SM. Physical examination of the patient in pain. In: Raj PP (ed). Practical management of pain. 3rd ed. Philadelphia: WB Saunders, 2002.

On the third postoperative day following an uneventful open appendectomy under spinal anesthesia, a 70-year-old male with history of hypertension and benign prostatic hyperplasia (BPH) suddenly developed a temperature of 102.5°F accompanied by chills and vomiting. Just before surgery, a urethral catheter was placed, which was removed 24 hours later, only to be replaced when he was unable to urinate on his own on the second postoperative day. Physical examination is unremarkable except for costovertebral angle tenderness and suprapubic tenderness. He has no abdominal guarding or rebound tenderness.

◆ **What is the most likely cause of postoperative fever?**

◆ **What is the next diagnostic step?**

◆ **What is the most appropriate treatment at this time?**

ANSWERS TO CASE 38: Postoperative Fever

Summary: A 70-year-old male with history of hypertension and BPH who underwent open appendectomy under spinal anesthesia develops fever, chills, and vomiting on the third postoperative day. Physical examination shows costovertebral tenderness and suprapubic tenderness. He has a urethral catheter in place because of a problem in voiding.

◆ **Most likely cause of postoperative fever:** Urinary tract infection (UTI)

◆ **The next diagnostic step:** Urinalysis and urine culture

◆ **Treatment:** IV antibiotic

Analysis

Objectives

1. Identify the different causes of postoperative fever based on the timing of onset, nature of surgery, and patient's risk factors.
2. Understand the different clinical presentations that point to the etiology of postoperative fever.

Considerations

This 70-year-old male with history of hypertension and BPH is at high risk for UTI because he recently underwent a pelvic procedure under spinal anesthesia and because he has urinary retention secondary to BPH. In addition, the use of a urethral catheter poses an additional risk for bacterial seeding of the urinary bladder. Suprapubic pain and costovertebral tenderness are physical findings suggestive of UTI, most likely acute pyelonephritis. For those without a urethral catheter, symptoms such as dysuria, urgency, and frequency are common.

UTI is high on the list of causes of fever in the third postoperative day, although it could also occur anytime during the postoperative period. Urinalysis may detect presence of bacteriuria, pyuria, nitrites, and leukocyte esterase. Urine culture would determine the type of offending organism, the most common of which are *Escherichia coli, Proteus, Klebsiella, Staphylococcus epidermidis, Pseudomonas,* and *Candida.*

In this patient, the urethral catheter needs to be changed now and discontinued as soon as he is able to void on his own. Symptomatic patients and those who are at high risk for infection are usually treated with appropriate IV antibiotics according to the most likely pathogens. The antibiotics subsequently can be adjusted based on culture results. Blood culture should be ordered if urosepsis is suspected. Most importantly, it is crucial to address and treat the cause of urinary retention (e.g., BPH, kidney stone) to prevent recurrence and avoid complications.

APPROACH TO POSTOPERATIVE FEVER

Definitions

Drug fever: Fever that coincides with the administration of a particular drug and cannot otherwise be explained by clinical and laboratory findings. Resolution of the fever occurs with discontinuation of the suspected drug. Drugs that are usually implicated are β-lactams, sulfa derivatives, heparin, and amphotericin B.

Malignant hyperthermia: A rare autosomal dominant disorder characterized by fever of greater than 104°F, tachycardia, metabolic acidosis, and calcium accumulation in skeletal muscle leading to rigidity. This may occur up to 24 hours after exposure to certain anesthetic agents such as halothane and succinylcholine. Treatment includes supportive therapy, such as antipyretics, oxygen, cooling blankets, and dantrolene IV.

Surgical site infection (SSI): A concept introduced by the Centers for Disease Control and Prevention (CDC) and various consensus panels to replace the term surgical wound infection. This refers to any infection that occurs in the site of surgery and classified as superficial, deep, or organ/space SSI.

Clinical Approach

Fever is the most common postoperative complication, occurring in 40% of major surgery in the immediate postoperative period. **As an integral part of informed consent prior to surgery, patients need to be made aware by the physician of the possibility of experiencing postoperative febrile episodes.** In addition, adequate preoperative evaluation, which includes performing a history and physical examination to identify risk factors, medications, nutritional status, and comorbid conditions, is imperative to avoid possible life-threatening situations during the perioperative period. Fortunately, postoperative fever typically resolves spontaneously and most of the time does not necessarily indicate the presence of infection.

The etiology of postoperative fever could be infectious or noninfectious (Tables 38–1 and 38–2). The mnemonic **"5 Ws"** helps in remembering the most common causes of postoperative fever in roughly the order of frequency: **Water** (UTI), **Wind** (pneumonia), **Wound** (SSI), **Walk** (deep venous thrombosis [DVT]), and **Wonder drugs** (drug fever). When a surgical patient develops fever, the differential diagnosis and investigative methods are directed by the timing of the fever, the type of surgery performed, the preexisting clinical conditions, and the presenting symptoms. A thorough physical examination should be initiated, followed by inspection of the surgical site, review of all medications, and request for necessary laboratory tests. If three or more of the

Table 38–1
COMMON CAUSES OF POSTOPERATIVE FEVER

APPROXIMATE ONSET OF FEVER	INFECTIOUS	NONINFECTIOUS
Intraoperative up to 24 h after surgery	Preexisting infection Bacteremia from urologic instrumentation Intraperitoneal leak (up to 36 h) Invasive soft-tissue infection Toxic shock syndrome	Surgical trauma Medications Blood products Malignant hyperthermia
1 day to 1 week from surgery	UTI Pneumonia SSI Catheter-related infection Preexisting infection	Acute myocardial infarction Alcohol withdrawal Gout Pancreatitis Pulmonary embolism DVT
1–4 weeks after surgery	SSI Thrombophlebitis Pseudomembranous colitis Catheter-related infection Device-related infections Abscess	Medications DVT Pulmonary embolism
More than 1 month after surgery	Blood-transfusion Organ transplant-related infection Infective endocarditis SSI Device-related infections Vascular graft infection	Postpericardiotomy syndrome

following risk factors are present, the likelihood of infection as the source of fever approaches 100%:

- Preoperative trauma
- American Society of Anesthesiologists (ASA) score >2 (patient with mild systemic disease or worse)
- Onset on the second postoperative day
- White blood cell (WBC) count >10,000 cells/mm^3
- Blood urea nitrogen (BUN) >15 mg/dL
- Systemic manifestations such as chills and rigors

Table 38–2
OTHER CAUSES OF POSTOPERATIVE FEVER WITH VARIABLE TIMING OF ONSET

INFECTIOUS	NONINFECTIOUS
Abscess	Withdrawal reaction from drugs/alcohol
Sinusitis	Subarachnoid hemorrhage
Otitis media	Bowel infarction
Parotitis	Pancreatitis
Meningitis	Hyperthyroidism/hypothyroidism
Acalculous cholecystitis	Dehydration
Osteomyelitis	Acute hepatic necrosis
Bacteremia	Hypoadrenalism
Empyema	Neoplastic fever
Fungal sepsis	Suture reaction
Hepatitis	Systemic inflammatory response syndrome (SIRS)
Decubitus ulcers	Pheochromocytoma
Perineal infections	Lymphoma
Peritonitis	Hematoma
Pharyngitis	Seroma
Tracheobronchitis	

Tissue trauma during surgery stimulates an inflammatory response that leads to release of pyrogenic cytokines (e.g., interleukins, tumor necrosis factor, interferon) from the tissues. Elevated levels of bacterial endotoxins and exotoxins that are released from the colon as a result of surgical complications also elicit the same inflammatory response. This reaction leads to elevation of the thermoregulatory set point and production of fever (temperature >100.5°F). This explains why suppression of cytokine release by nonsteroidal antiinflammatory drugs (NSAIDs) and steroids reduces the fever and could lead to earlier recovery. The surgical patient goes through a considerable degree of stress, both physically and emotionally, making it appropriate to administer antipyretics to alleviate further distress on the patient's body and to minimize unwarranted expenditure of energy caused by fever.

There are very **few causes of fever in the immediate postoperative period.** One of them is **malignant hyperthermia,** which is characterized by markedly elevated temperature, up to 104°F, shortly after induction of anesthesia with agents such as halothane and succinylcholine. Another cause of immediate postoperative fever is **bacteremia,** which occurs more commonly in urologic procedures that involve instrumentation, for example, transurethral resection of the prostate. Gram-negative bacteria are the most common pathogen. Within 30–45 minutes, the patient develops chills and temperature that could exceed 104°F. Accompanying symptoms such as tachycardia, tachypnea, oliguria, and hypotension are common.

If fever occurs within 36 hours postlaparotomy, there are two important infectious etiologies to be kept in mind—**bowel injury with leakage of gastrointestinal contents into the peritoneum** and **invasive soft-tissue wound infection** caused by *β-hemolytic streptococci* or *Clostridium* species. The former is accompanied by hemodynamic instability. Least common in this setting is **toxic shock syndrome** caused by *Staphylococcus aureus*.

Within the first 48–72 postoperative hours, **atelectasis** (partial collapse of peripheral alveoli) causes 90% of pulmonary complications of surgery. Contrary to popular beliefs, recent literature disputes its association with fever and found their coexistence to be merely coincidental. The alveolar collapse is compounded by the loss of functional residual capacity in almost all patients, and 50% reduction of vital capacity intraoperatively. Chest x-ray may reveal discoid infiltrate and an elevated hemidiaphragm. Certain conditions make atelectasis more likely, including heavy cigarette smoking, prior lung resection, old age, malnutrition, asthma, chronic obstructive pulmonary disease (COPD), prolonged procedure, abdominal distension, and thoracic or abdominal incision.

The use of narcotics and anesthesia could also affect the patient's breathing pattern. Instructing the patient on deep inspiration and coughing, the use of incentive spirometry and the provision of adequate pain control can facilitate the opening of the alveoli.

Without resolution of atelectasis, **pneumonia** may ensue, on the third postoperative day, when the build up of secretions facilitates growth of bacteria. Patients who are on mechanical ventilators are at highest risk for pneumonia (ventilator-associated pneumonia). Fever associated with productive cough, pulmonary crackles, elevation of WBCs, positive sputum culture, and infiltrates in chest x-ray are the usual indicators of pulmonary infection. Appropriate use of broad-spectrum IV antibiotic therapy is the treatment. **Aspiration** as the possible cause of pneumonia should be suspected in the elderly, those who reside in a nursing home, and those with neurologic dysphagia, altered mentation, and gastroesophageal reflux disease (GERD). **Gram-negative coverage is required for aspiration pneumonia,** such as third-generation cephalosporins, fluoroquinolones, and piperacillin. It is also around this time that **UTI** should be entertained as part of differential diagnosis.

The patient with persistent fever 5–7 days after surgery needs to have a thorough examination of the operative site to check for signs of infection, which include erythema, pain, local edema, and purulent discharge. **Surgical site infection** has markedly decreased through wide practice of aseptic technique. Patients at high risk of wound infection are those who underwent lengthy surgical procedure, who received blood transfusion, those who are malnourished, and those who have diabetes mellitus.

Purulent drainage and fluctuance indicate the presence of abscess, which requires incision and drainage. When cellulitis is confirmed, treatment with antibiotic is warranted. Gram-positive bacteria, such as *S. aureus, S. epidermidis* (especially with implants or devices), *Streptococcus pyogenes,* and *Enterococcus,* are important pathogens. Fungal etiology should not be ruled out in patients with severe comorbid conditions. On rare occasions, deep abscesses produce fever 10–15 days after surgery. A high level of suspicion leads to diagnostic imaging such as computed tomography (CT) scan of the body region most likely to be infected, which depends on the location of the surgery. Interventional radiology specialists could be called upon for radiologically guided drainage of the abscess, which is the definitive treatment. Antibiotics should include coverage for Gram-negative enteric bacilli and anaerobes.

Intravascular catheter or line-associated infection needs to be entertained when the patient has had IV devices for 3 days or more, even when the site appears clean. Any unnecessary lines should be discontinued, as they are potential sites of infection. The catheter tip is cultured to reveal the offending organism that would direct treatment.

Fever caused by **deep venous thrombosis** usually occurs on the fifth postoperative day. Half of the time patients with DVT are asymptomatic. Common complaints are leg edema, tenderness, pain, and warmth. **Homan sign** (pain in the calf on foot dorsiflexion) is demonstrated in some cases. When possible, surgical patients are encouraged to ambulate early; otherwise, compression devices and low-molecular-weight heparin are useful prophylactic measures. Diagnosis is made by duplex ultrasound, but most accurately confirmed with venography. Patients who develop **pulmonary embolism** usually have concomitant DVT. The treatment of DVT and pulmonary embolism is initiated with low-molecular-weight heparin or unfractionated heparin, followed by warfarin.

The type of surgery also provides a clue as to the associated risks of fever-associated surgical morbidity. In general, laparoscopic surgery comparatively causes fewer cases of fever than open surgery. Pleural effusion develops in all patients undergoing cardiothoracic surgery and 5% of those patients acquire pneumonia. Particularly unique to abdominal surgery is deep abdominal abscess and pancreatitis. Obstetric and gynecologic surgery could be complicated by postpartum endometritis, deep pelvic abscess, and pelvic thrombophlebitis. SSI is the most common infectious cause of fever in orthopedic surgery. Prostatic and perinephric abscess are more commonly seen in urologic procedures. Patients undergoing genitourinary procedure are at greater risk of having UTI. Meningitis is a common cause of fever following a neurosurgical procedure. Neurosurgery patients, who are usually immobilized and less aggressively anticoagulated to avoid brain hemorrhage, have the highest incidence of DVT.

Comprehension Questions

[38.1] A 60-year-old male with adenocarcinoma of the colon underwent left hemicolectomy with primary anastomosis. Thirty hours after surgery, he was found to have a fever of 102°F, blood pressure of 90/60 mm Hg, heart rate of 140 beats/min, respirations of 24 breaths/min, and low urine output. Physical examination showed diffuse abdominal tenderness. The surgical site is clean and Gram stain did not show any organism. Urinalysis (UA) was negative and the complete blood count (CBC) showed leukocytosis. What is the most likely cause of this patient's fever?

A. Pneumonia
B. Intraperitoneal leak from bowel injury
C. Surgical site infection
D. Deep tissue abscess

[38.2] An 84-year-old female nursing home resident with advanced Alzheimer disease, hypertension, and diabetes, and who was receiving nutrition via nasogastric tube (NGT), underwent emergency open cholecystectomy under general anesthesia. On the second postoperative day, she was noted to be coughing and vomiting. The following day, she had a temperature of 102°F, heart rate of 90 beats/min, respiratory rate of 25 breaths/min, blood pressure of 120/70 mm Hg, and oxygen saturation of 87% on room air. Lung auscultation showed crackles bilaterally and chest radiograph revealed bilateral lower lobe infiltrates. D-dimer was negative. Sputum Gram stain showed Gram-positive cocci. Regarding this patient's clinical condition, which statement is most accurate?

A. Tube feeding prevents aspiration pneumonia.
B. In patients with dementia who are fed via NGT, prolonged periods in supine position is a risk factor for aspiration of gastric content.
C. Mortality from the patient's condition is minimal.
D. The greater the degree of unconsciousness, the less likely the possibility of aspiration.

[38.3] A 42-year-old male underwent open reduction and internal fixation of a comminuted fracture of the right femur. He was doing well until the fifth postoperative day, when he complained of pleuritic chest pain and he developed fever of 101°F, hear rate of 118 beats/min, respiration of 30 breaths/min, blood pressure of 130/85 mm Hg, and oxygen saturation of 85% on room air. His left ankle became edematous, warm, and tender. Which of the following is a risk factor for his condition?

A. Having an IV in his arm for more than 3 days
B. Failure to adequately use his incentive spirometer
C. Urinary bladder catheterization
D. Prolonged immobility

[38.4] A 50-year-old female with diabetes was recuperating from left inguinal hernia repair. Her glycosylated hemoglobin (HbA1c) prior to surgery was 10%. During postoperative follow-up a week after surgery, the surgical site was markedly erythematous, warm, and tender with pus. What is the next step in treatment?

    A. Apply topical antibiotic to the surgical site.
    B. Warm compresses alone will relieve the inflammation.
    C. Open the surgical site and drain the infected material.
    D. Send the patient home with prescription for oral antibiotics for 7 days.

Answers

[38.1] **B.** In the presence of severe hemodynamic changes and diffuse abdominal tenderness, intraperitoneal leak is the most common cause of fever in the first 36 hours after laparotomy.

[38.2] **B.** This patient presumably had silent aspiration pneumonitis that eventually led to secondary bacterial pneumonia, most commonly by *Haemophilus influenzae* or *Streptococcus pneumoniae*. Studies show that feeding tubes offer no protection from aspiration pneumonia. Aspiration pneumonia is the most common cause of death in patients on gastrostomy tube feedings.

[38.3] **D.** This patient has DVT and concomitant pulmonary embolism (PE). Risk factors include prolonged immobility, vascular damage, and hypercoagulability.

[38.4] **C.** Incision and drainage is the most important therapy for SSI. Antibiotics are used solely in cases of significant systemic involvement.

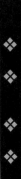

CLINICAL PEARLS

❖ Pulmonary complications, especially atelectasis, are the largest single cause of postoperative morbidity.

❖ Pneumonia is currently the leading cause of mortality from nonsurgical postoperative nosocomial infection. Mortality rate is 20–50%. Mechanical ventilation is the most important risk factor.

❖ UTI is the most common cause of nonsurgical postoperative nosocomial infection.

❖ The most common noninfectious cause of postoperative fever is drug fever.

REFERENCES

Dayton M. Surgical complications. In: Townsend C, Beauchamp RD, Evers BM, Mallox K (eds). Sabiston textbook of surgery. 17th ed. Philadelphia: WB Saunders, 2004:297–330.

Dellinger EP. Surgical infections. In: Mulholland M, Lillemoe K, Doherty G, Maier R, Upchurch G (eds). Greenfield's surgery: scientific principles and practice. Philadelphia: Lippincott Williams and Wilkins, 2006:163–176.

Engoren M. Lack of association between atelectasis and fever. Chest 1995;107: 81–84.

Harrison GW, Baddour L. Postoperative fever. In: Rose DR (ed). UpToDate, version 14.1. Available at: www.UpToDate.com. Last accessed March 17, 2006.

Mangram AJ, Horan TC, Pearson ML, et al. Guideline for the prevention of surgical site infection, 1999. Available at: http://www.cdc.gov/ncidod/hip/SSI/SSI.pdf. Last accessed March 17, 2006.

Marik P. Aspiration pneumonitis and aspiration pneumonia. N Engl J Med 2001; 344:665–671.

Paulman A, Paulman P. Perioperative care. AAFP Home Study Self-Assessment Monograph Series, No. 263. American Academy of Family Physicians, Leawood, KS, 2001.

CASE 39

You were busy seeing patients in your outpatient clinic when you heard a commotion coming from the waiting room. You went to check and found a very frantic mother and her 2-year-old son who is clutching his throat, coughing, drooling, and visibly struggling to breathe. The mother endorses that just a few minutes ago, the child was running around while eating grapes when she suddenly heard him gagging and wheezing. Her son has an appointment for well child examination and he is apparently doing well. He has no significant history of respiratory illness. The toddler is still conscious but unable to talk, and his cough is becoming weaker. Breath sounds are decreased bilaterally, with wheezing and stridor heard on auscultation. You tried to ventilate the patient with the chin-lift maneuver but the chest fails to rise. You opened the mouth but you are unable to see any foreign object.

◆ **What is the most likely diagnosis?**

◆ **What is the next step in the management of this patient?**

ANSWERS TO CASE 39: Acute Causes of Wheezing Other Than Asthma in Children

Summary: A 2-year-old boy had acute onset of coughing, choking, drooling, and wheezing while eating grapes. He is unable to speak and his cough is weak. He was in a good state of health prior to the incident and has no history of respiratory illness. Physical examination reveals decreased breath sounds, wheezing, and stridor. There is no chest rise on ventilation attempt. No foreign object could be seen on his mouth.

◆ **Most likely diagnosis:** Foreign-body airway obstruction

◆ **Next step in the management for this patient:** Heimlich maneuver (subdiaphragmatic abdominal thrusts)

Analysis

Objectives

1. Identify the illnesses, other than asthma, that cause acute wheezing in children.
2. Understand the steps in the diagnosis and management of a wheezing child.

Considerations

Acute onset of wheezing in an otherwise healthy child similar to the above case should raise the suspicion for **foreign-body airway obstruction (FBAO).** Witnessed swallowing followed by choking is not necessary for diagnosis, but as much information should be gathered surrounding the onset of symptoms. FBAO is common among children age 6 months to 3 years old, accounting for approximately 70% of cases. Small toys and objects, balloons, and food (e.g., nuts, grapes, candies) are high-risk objects for aspiration. Older children may be able to identify the object they swallowed and assume the posture of clutching their neck with their hand **(universal choking sign).** Symptoms such as weak cough, inability to speak or cry, high-pitched sounds or no sounds during inhalation, cyanosis, choking, vomiting, drooling, wheezing, blood-streaked saliva, and respiratory distress are clues to the diagnosis of FBAO. Physical findings of unilateral wheezing, unequal or decreased breath sounds, and stridor are common. In children, the foreign body could lodge on either side of the airway. If the foreign body lodges in the esophagus, acute wheezing is still possible when the obstruction compresses on the airways.

One should not attempt to remove the foreign object in a child who is actively coughing. Blind finger sweep is not recommended because of the danger of further obstruction or injury. Although the patient mentioned above is still conscious, he seems to have ineffective coughing and is beginning to get tired. Ventilation should be attempted while opening the airway with the head-tilt maneuver, which could also relieve the obstruction. In the above case, an attempt to remove the foreign object was initiated when ventilation was unsuccessful.

Since no foreign object is visualized, a series of **abdominal thrusts (Heimlich maneuver)** should be the next step to try to expel the foreign body. In infants, back blows and chest thrusts are performed instead of abdominal thrusts, which could cause iatrogenic trauma to the liver and stomach that are not protected by the rib cage at that age. If the child continues to deteriorate even after 1 minute of resuscitative efforts and the above maneuvers fail to expel the foreign object, the emergency medical services (EMS) system should be activated while continuing cardiopulmonary resuscitation (CPR).

In the hospital setting, a bronchoscopic procedure is the treatment of choice. Chest x-ray is often normal, but in some cases shows a radiopaque foreign object or identifies localized hyperinflation and/or atelectasis. Most deaths from FBAO occur in children younger than 5 years of age; 65% are infants.

APPROACH TO WHEEZING

Definitions

Heimlich maneuver: Performed by standing or sitting behind the person who is choking and placing the thumb side of one fist between the navel and the xiphoid process. The other hand grasps the fisted hand and a series of upward abdominal thrusts are delivered to create an "artificial cough" in a choking victim in an effort to dislodge the object blocking the airway.

Stridor: Wheezing coming from obstruction of the large airway that has a constant pitch and intensity throughout the entire inspiratory effort.

Wheezing: A musical sound heard on pulmonary auscultation produced by the oscillating walls of airways that had been narrowed by mucus, inflammation, etc.

Clinical Approach

Among the many causes of wheezing in children, asthma and viral infections are most common. Worldwide studies show that approximately 10–15% of infants wheeze in the first 12 months of life. The diagnosis of wheezing hinges on accurate history, physical examination, laboratory tests, and even response to treatments. It is also important to gather information regarding the age of onset, exposure to cigarette smoke, presence of allergic signs and symptoms, frequency of wheezing, association with vomiting or feeding, and other accompanying symptoms.

The etiology of **acute wheezing** in children could be infectious (e.g., bronchiolitis) or mechanical obstruction (e.g., FBAO). **Recurrent wheezing,** on the other hand, encompasses anomalies of the tracheobronchial tree (e.g., bronchomalacia), cardiovascular disease (e.g., vascular rings and slings), gastroesophageal reflux, and immunologic disorders (e.g., bronchopulmonary dysplasia, cystic fibrosis). This case concentrates on acute onset of wheezing other than asthma in children (Case 6 provides a more detailed discussion of asthma).

Bronchiolitis is the most common acute cause of wheezing in children younger than 2 years of age, especially in infants who are 1–3 months old. It is a viral infection causing nonspecific inflammation of the small airways and peaks during the winter months. **Respiratory syncytial virus (RSV) accounts for 70% of cases;** the rest are caused by parainfluenza, adenovirus, *Mycoplasma*, and metapneumovirus. These viruses elicit inflammatory and immune responses that produce mucus, edema, and cellular debris that block the small airways. The introduction of the influenza vaccine reduced the incidence of bronchiolitis caused by the flu virus.

Initially, the child develops rhinorrhea and wheezing followed by low-grade fever. On succeeding days, rhinorrhea will be more copious and the child may also experience cough, irritability, and varying degrees of dyspnea. As a result, the infant may have poor oral intake and possibly dehydration. Physical examination may reveal wheezing, fine crackles, prolonged expiratory phase, and increased work of breathing as evidenced by nasal flaring, intercostals retraction, and even apnea.

Diagnosis of bronchiolitis is clinical and current literature does not support the routine use of laboratory tests as they do not alter clinical outcomes. If the diagnosis is doubtful or the clinical presentation is unusual, one may request a chest x-ray that might reveal hyperinflation and/or atelectasis brought about by air trapping caused by severe obstruction. A complete blood count (CBC) is usually normal. There are available assays for RSV and influenza that often are unnecessary, unless the patient is to be admitted and placed in a room with other RSV-positive infants. Sputum culture is requested if bacterial superinfection or pneumonia is suspected. Patients who are in respiratory distress, younger than 3 months old, or premature, those with comorbid conditions, lethargy, hypoxemia, or hypercarbia, and those with atelectasis or consolidation in chest radiograph need to be hospitalized.

The Agency for Healthcare Research and Quality (AHRQ), in collaboration with the American Academy of Family Physicians (AAFP) and the American Academy of Pediatrics (AAP), recommends supplemental oxygen and supportive care as the modes of treatment with clear evidence of effectiveness. They also found nebulized epinephrine, nebulized ipratropium bromide with or without salbutamol, oral or parenteral corticosteroids (preferably dexamethasone), and inhaled corticosteroids (preferably budesonide) to be potentially efficacious. They recommend inhaled helium-oxygen for severely ill children and surfactant for those on ventilators. The AAP, however, does not agree with the use of corticosteroids. Furthermore, a recent randomized controlled trial demonstrated that nebulized epinephrine does not decrease the length of hospital stay and should be discontinued if an initial therapeutic trial fails to show significant clinical improvement.

Symptomatic treatment includes head elevation, suctioning of secretions after spraying the nasal passages with saline; antipyretics for fever; cool, humidified oxygen for hypoxemia; and adequate hydration. If the infant is at high risk for aspiration, IV fluids may be the safest way to deliver nutrients. A therapeutic trial with albuterol, especially in infants with personal or family history of allergies, could identify a few responders. Parents of infants with bronchiolitis should be instructed not to expose the infant to cigarette smoke and educated on frequent handwashing to prevent transmission of the disease.

For infants with congenital heart disease or chronic lung disease, the antiviral agent ribavirin via aerosol has been used but has not been proven to alter mortality and length of illness. Administration of RSV immunoglobulin (RespiGam) and palivizumab (Synagis) just before the beginning of RSV season are proven effective preventive therapy for children younger than 2 years old who were born prematurely or who suffer from chronic lung disease. The cost-effectiveness of prophylaxis, however, is still debatable. In most cases, the illness is self-limited with median duration of about 12 days. Mortality is approximately 1% and could be attributed to apnea, respiratory acidosis, and severe dehydration. Children who had experienced bronchiolitis are at higher risk of developing asthma.

Croup is the most common cause of airway obstruction in children ages 6 months to 6 years old, and is the leading cause of hospitalization for children younger than 4 years old. It is **a viral infection that causes inflammation of the subglottic region** of the larynx that produces the characteristic barking cough, hoarseness, stridor, and different degrees of respiratory distress that are more severe at night. The croup syndrome encompasses **laryngotracheitis, laryngotracheobronchitis, laryngotracheobronchopneumonitis, and spasmodic croup.**

Croup usually occurs during fall and winter. Common organisms involved are parainfluenza, adenovirus, RSV, rhinovirus, Enterovirus, influenza viruses, and rarely, *Mycoplasma pneumoniae*. The prodrome is characterized by 12–72 hours of runny nose and low-grade fever. Hypoxia only occurs in severe cases. These symptoms peak from 1–2 days, and in most cases, resolve in 1 week. Diagnosis is made through clinical presentation. Radiographic picture of the neck occasionally features the classic **steeple sign** (narrowing column of air in the subglottic region). When diagnosis is doubtful, computed tomography (CT) scan of the neck offers a more sensitive evaluation. Children who are hospitalized with croup should be monitored closely and frequent physical examination needs to be performed. Mainstays of treatment are cool-mist therapy, corticosteroids (nebulized, IM, or oral), and nebulized racemic epinephrine in moderate to severe cases. Mortality is rare.

Epiglottitis is a **bacterial infection of the supraglottic tissue** and surrounding areas that causes rapidly progressive airway obstruction. It usually affects children younger than 5 years old and is most commonly caused by bacteria such as *Haemophilus influenzae, H. parainfluenzae, Streptococcus pneumoniae, Staphylococcus aureus,* and *β-hemolytic streptococcus* A, B, and

C. With the introduction of the *H. influenzae* type b (Hib) vaccine, there has been a steady decline in cases of epiglottitis. Within 24 hours, the patient with epiglottitis would appear "toxic" and develop fever, severe sore throat, muffled speech ("hot potato voice"), drooling, and dysphagia. The child usually is noticeably anxious and assumes the sitting position, leaning forward on out-stretched arms with chin thrust forward and neck hyperextended (tripod posi-tion) so as to increase the airway diameter.

With progression of airway obstruction, the patient may begin to have wheezing and stridor. **Epiglottitis is a medical emergency and visualization to confirm the presence of severely erythematous epiglottis is preferably done in the operating room** with experienced surgeon or anesthesiologist. The patient should be kept in a calm environment to prevent sudden airway obstruc-tion. CBC usually shows leukocytosis, neutrophilia, and bandemia. The radi-ographic finding that is characteristic of epiglottitis is the **"thumb sign"** or protrusion of the enlarged epiglottis from the anterior wall of the hypophar-ynx seen on a lateral neck x-ray. Cultures of the blood and epiglottis yield the pathogenic bacteria. Treatment consists of appropriate antibiotics (oxacillin or nafcillin; cefazolin; clindamycin and ceftriaxone or cefotaxime) and airway management, usually in an ICU setting with a team ready to respond for intu-bation or tracheostomy. Death results from hypoxia, hypercapnia, and acidosis that lead to cardiorespiratory failure.

Deep abscesses of the neck are less-common causes of acute wheezing, but they have the potential to be very serious. They are located in the peritonsillar, retropharyngeal, and pharyngomaxillary spaces. **Retropharyngeal abscess** affects children 2–4 years old and manifest as severe odynophagia, dysphagia, stiff neck, drooling, and airway obstruction. The posterior pharyngeal wall may show swelling or fluctuant mass. **Peritonsillar abscess** is an infection of the superior pole of the tonsils and is more common in young teenagers. Fever, severe sore throat, muffled voice, drooling, trismus, and neck pain are typical symptoms. Enlarged tonsils with abscess, cervical adenopathy, and deviation of the uvula may be obvious on physical examination. CT scan of the neck is the most help-ful diagnostic modality for identifying deep neck abscesses. The predominant pathogens are *Streptococcus pyogenes, S. aureus,* and anaerobes. Ampicillin-sulbactam or clindamycin for 14 days is appropriate treatment. Drainage of the abscess is indicated either as first-line treatment or when antimicrobial agents fail to produce adequate result. Serious complications from deep abscesses result from airway obstruction, septicemia, aspiration, jugular vein thrombosis/throm-bophlebitis, carotid artery rupture, and mediastinitis.

Comprehension Questions

[39.1] A 7-month-old female was brought by her mother to an outpatient clinic because of a 2-day history of fever, copious nasal secretions, and wheezing. The mother volunteered that the baby has been healthy and has not had these symptoms in the past. The infant's temperature is noted to be 100.7°F, her respiratory rate is 50 breaths/min, and her pulse oximetry is 95% on room air. Physical examination reveals no signs of dehydration, but wheezing is heard on lung auscultation. The infant shows no improvement after three treatments with nebulized albuterol. Which of the following is the recommended treatment?

A. Continued nebulized albuterol every 4 hours
B. Antihistamines and decongestants
C. Antibiotics for 7 days
D. Initiate synagis
E. Supportive care with hydration and humidified oxygen

[39.2] Which of the following is true regarding the diagnosis of epiglottitis?

A. Child usually prefers to be in prone position
B. Radiographic finding of "steeple sign"
C. Every effort should be made to visualize the epiglottis in the office to confirm the diagnosis
D. Diagnosis is decreasing in incidence

[39.3] Antibiotic therapy is one of the mainstays of treatment for which of the following causes of wheezing?

A. Asthma
B. Epiglottitis
C. Croup
D. Bronchiolitis
E. Foreign-body aspiration

[39.4] A 12-year-old girl was brought to the emergency department because of severe sore throat, muffled voice, drooling, and fatigue. She had been sick for the past 3 days and is unable to eat because of painful swallowing. The parents deny any history of recurrent pharyngitis. The patient still managed to open her mouth and you were able to see an abscess at the upper pole of the right tonsil with deviation of the uvula toward the midline. Examination of the neck reveals enlarged and tender lymph nodes. Which of the following is the most appropriate management?

A. Analgesics for pain and follow up in 24 hours
B. A prescription for oral antibiotics and follow-up in 1 week
C. Nebulized racemic epinephrine
D. Incision and drainage of the abscess
E. Tonsillectomy and adenoidectomy

Answers

[39.1] **E.** Bronchiolitis is the most likely diagnosis in this case. There is no established treatment for bronchiolitis except for supportive management of the patient's symptoms. Because the infant did not respond to an albuterol trial, there is no justification for continuing its use. Antihistamines, decongestants, and antibiotics are not effective. Synagis is not helpful in the acute setting.

[39.2] **D.** The incidence of epiglottitis has markedly reduced since the introduction of the Hib vaccine. Children with epiglottitis are more likely to be in the tripod position than prone. The "steeple sign" is seen in croup; the "thumb" sign is seen in epiglottitis. Visualization of the epiglottis should preferentially occur in an operating room, where immediate intubation or tracheostomy can occur.

[39.3] **B.** Epiglottitis is usually a bacterial infection treated with antibiotics.

[39.4] **D.** This patient is suffering from peritonsillar abscess. Of the choices listed, incision and drainage is the most appropriate. Tonsillectomy is only indicated if there are confirmed cases of **recurrent** pharyngitis and peritonsillar abscess.

CLINICAL PEARLS

❖ Sufficient airflow is required for the airway to produce a wheezing sound. Disappearance of wheezing in a patient who initially presents with wheezing is an ominous sign that suggests complete blockage of the airway or imminent respiratory failure.

❖ Bronchiolitis is the most common lower respiratory disease of infants and the most common reason for hospitalization for infants younger than 1 year old.

❖ Never perform a blind finger sweep of a foreign object aspirated by an infant or child.

❖ Epiglottitis is a medical emergency.

REFERENCES

Agency for Healthcare Research and Quality. Management of bronchiolitis in infants and children. Evidence report/technology assessment no. 69. AHRQ publication no. 03-E009. Rockville, MD: Agency for Healthcare Research and Quality, 2003. Available at: http://www.ahrq.gov/downloads/pub/evidence/pdf/bronchio/bronchio.pdf. Last accessed March 19, 2006.

Cincinnati Children's Hospital Medical Center. Evidence based clinical practice guideline for medical management of bronchiolitis in infants less than 1 year of age presenting with a first time episode. 2001. Available at: http://www.guideline.gov/summary/summary.aspx?doc_id=7665&nbr=004464&string=bronchiolitis. Last accessed March 19, 2006.

Eisen GM, Baron TH, Dominitz JA, et al. Guideline for the management of ingested foreign bodies. Gastrointest Endoscopy 2002;55(7):802–806.

Kuntson D, Aring A. Viral croup. Am Fam Physician 2004;69:3.

Mathers LH, Frankel L. Stabilization of the critically ill child. In: Behrman RE, Kliegman RM, Jenson HB (eds). Nelson textbook of pediatrics. 17th ed. Philadelphia: WB Saunders, 2004:286–288.

Roosevelt GE. Acute inflammatory upper airway obstruction. In: Behrman RE, Kliegman RM, Jenson HB (eds). Nelson textbook of pediatrics. 17th ed. Philadelphia: WB Saunders, 2004:1405–1409.

Ward ER. Peritonsillar and retropharyngeal abscess in children. In: Rose DR (ed). UpToDate version 14.1. Available at: www.uptodate.com.

A 28-year-old White female presents to your office with a chief complaint of constipation and abdominal pain. On further questioning, she reports she has had this problem since beginning college at the age of 18 years. Her symptoms have waxed and waned since this time, but never have worsened. She describes her abdominal pain as dull, crampy, and nonfocal but more prominent in the left lower quadrant, and sometimes relieved with defecation. She denies radiation of pain, nausea, vomiting, fever, chills, weight loss, heartburn, or bloody or dark stool. She reports having a bowel movement every 1–2 days that is hard and feels incomplete. She has tried over-the-counter remedies, including stool softeners and antacids, but only experienced minimal improvement in her symptoms. She only takes birth control pills and denies any use of herbs or laxatives. Her family history is negative, including for colorectal cancer and inflammatory bowel disease, and she reports that her parents and siblings are healthy. She is currently engaged and reports significant stress in preparing for the wedding. On physical examination, you note her to be somewhat anxious but otherwise in no apparent distress. Her vital signs and a general physical examination are normal. Her abdomen has normal bowel sounds, no tenderness on superficial and deep palpation, and no rebound, rigidity, or guarding. Liver and spleen size are within normal limits and no masses are palpable. Pelvic examination is normal. Rectal examination shows normal sphincter tone, no masses, and brown stool that is occult blood negative.

◆ **What is your most likely diagnosis?**

◆ **What is your next diagnostic step?**

◆ **What is the next step in therapy?**

ANSWERS TO CASE 40: Irritable Bowel Syndrome

Summary: A 28-year-old female presents with a several-year history of abdominal pain and constipation. She denies any fever, weight loss, heartburn, or bloody stools. Her past medical history and family history are otherwise unremarkable. The physical examination, including abdominal and pelvic examination, are grossly within normal limits.

◆ **Most likely diagnosis:** Irritable bowel syndrome

◆ **Most appropriate next step:** In the absence of any GI alarm features, a complete blood count and stool Hemoccult test for initial screening

◆ **What is the next step in therapy?** Trial of fiber supplementation

Analysis

Objectives

1. Describe the epidemiology, clinical manifestations, and pathophysiology of irritable bowel syndrome
2. Learn the diagnostic approach to irritable bowel syndrome and rationale for ordering diagnostic studies based on symptom subtype and/or presence of "alarm features."
3. Review current therapeutic strategies in the patient with irritable bowel syndrome.
4. Recognize the role of psychosocial factors in irritable bowel syndrome.

Considerations

This is a young female patient with long-standing abdominal pain and constipation. She denies any "alarm features" like weight loss, bloody stools, fever, and refractory diarrhea, and her family history is negative for colon cancer or inflammatory bowel disease. The chronicity and lack of worsening of her symptoms coupled with her young age points to a functional GI disorder, such as irritable bowel syndrome.

APPROACH TO SUSPECTED IRRITABLE BOWEL SYNDROME

Irritable bowel syndrome (IBS) is a functional GI disorder characterized by chronic abdominal pain and altered bowel habits. The prevalence of IBS is approximately 10–15% of the U.S. population and accounts for a large proportion of GI complaints seen both by primary care physicians and gastroenterologists. **IBS affects women 2–3 more times often than men** and patients typically present in the second or third decades of life, although virtually any age group can be affected. Despite studies to elucidate the underlying physiologic abnormalities seen in IBS, the pathophysiology of IBS remains unclear. Several studies show abnormal gut hypersensitivity to visceral perception and pain, altered gastrointestinal motility, and dysregulation of the brain–gut axis through increased reactivity to stress. A high prevalence of psychopathology is seen in patients who are eventually diagnosed with IBS. Although the association between psychological disturbances and IBS are complicated and not clearly defined, psychiatric symptoms appear to predict illness behavior rather than directly cause IBS.

Patients with IBS complain of constipation, diarrhea, alternating constipation with diarrhea, and periods of normal bowel habits that alternate with either constipation and/or diarrhea. The abdominal pain associated with IBS is frequently in the lower part of the abdomen, with the left lower quadrant being the most common location. However, both the location and the nature of the pain in IBS is subject to great variability. The pain is described as a cramping sensation of intermittent frequency and variable intensity, often improved or relieved with defecation. Other gastrointestinal symptoms seen in IBS include the passage of mucus with stool, bowel urgency, bloating, dyspepsia, gastroesophageal reflux, and the sensation of incomplete stool evacuation.

Diagnosis

In an effort to objectively diagnose a patient with IBS, the Rome Criteria (Table 40–1) were developed and subsequently revised. Based on the presence of positive symptoms and the absence of structural or biochemical explanation of the symptoms, a patient may be diagnosed with IBS. Physicians are encouraged

Table 40–1

ROME II DIAGNOSTIC CRITERIA FOR IRRITABLE
BOWEL SYNDROME

At least 12 weeks or more, which need not be consecutive, in the preceding 12 months of abdominal discomfort or pain that is accompanied by at least two of the following features:

1. It is relieved with defecation, and/or
2. Onset is associated with a change in frequency of stool, and/or
3. Onset is associated with a change in form (appearance) of stool.

Other symptoms that are not essential but support the diagnosis of IBS:

- Abnormal stool frequency (greater than 3 bowel movements per day or less than 3 bowel movements per week);
- Abnormal stool form (lumpy/hard or loose/watery stool);
- Abnormal stool passage (straining, urgency, or feeling of incomplete evacuation);
- Passage of mucus;
- Bloating or feeling of abdominal distension.

Source: Olden KW. Diagnosis of irritable bowel syndrome, *Gastroenterology.* 2002;122(6):1701–14.

to avoid unnecessary and expensive studies and instead to use judicious cost-effective diagnostic testing.

A thorough history should be obtained using open-ended, nonjudgmental questions. The physical examination should focus on ruling out organic patho-logic processes that are inconsistent with IBS. Importance should be paid to all medications and dietary habits that may worsen or mimic the symptoms of IBS.

Patients should be asked for the presence of "alarm features," which include fever, anemia, involuntary weight loss greater than 10 lb, hematochezia, melena, refractory or bloody diarrhea, and a family history of colon cancer or inflammatory bowel disease. The **presence of alarm features usually points to an underlying organic etiology** and may warrant further work-up, includ-ing laboratory, endoscopic, and/or radiographic testing.

In the patient with typical features of IBS and the absence of alarm features, a complete blood count and stool Hemoccult are appropriate initial screening tests. Because of the high pretest probability of neoplasm in patients age 50 years or older, a colonoscopy is recommended in addition to any other diagnostic work-up. A sigmoidoscopy or colonoscopy can be performed on the younger patient if inflammatory bowel disease is suspected, or if the patient has additional alarm features, such as refractory diarrhea or unintentional weight loss.

Treatment

Based on the predominant symptom subtype, empiric therapy can be initiated to control a patient's symptoms. For abdominal pain, the use of antispasmod-ics, such as dicyclomine and hyoscyamine, on an as-needed basis have shown benefit, especially when pain is mild and infrequent. Low-dose tricyclic anti-depressants (TCAs) should be considered when pain is more frequent and severe. Selective serotonin reuptake inhibitors (SSRIs) may be beneficial when depression or anxiety disorders are comorbid with IBS.

For constipation-predominant IBS, increasing fiber intake, either via dietary fiber, synthetic fiber, or natural fiber, is recommended. For diarrhea-predominant IBS, loperamide may reduce the frequency of loose stools, as well as decrease bowel urgency.

Two novel agents acting at the serotonin (5-HT) receptor show benefit in treat-ing pain associated with IBS. If the stool habit is primarily constipation, tegaserod is indicated. In IBS with predominant diarrhea, alosetron is recommended.

Pharmacologic agents should be used as adjuncts in the overall treatment plan. A multifactorial approach, including modification of diet and lifestyle, providing patient education and reassurance, and medication therapy is often required. For patients with significant psychosocial issues, psychotherapy, stress management, and treatment of underlying psychiatric disorders appear to be helpful in overall symptom management. As always, a therapeutic physi-cian–patient relationship is critical to maximizing the best clinical outcome.

Comprehension Questions

[40.1] A 65-year-old male patient reports a lifelong history of IBS with alternating bouts of constipation and diarrhea. He denies any so-called alarm symptoms, but does report that his symptoms have worsened over the last several months. What is the most important next step?

A. Esophagogastroduodenoscopy (EGD)
B. Begin trial of the 5-HT agonist tegaserod
C. Explore possible underlying psychiatric symptoms
D. Colonoscopy

[40.2] Which of the following agents is clinically indicated as a first-line treatment for mild to moderate abdominal pain associated with IBS?

A. Amitriptyline
B. Alosetron
C. Dicyclomine
D. Fluoxetine

[40.3] As regards to comorbid psychiatric disorders and IBS, which of the following statements is most accurate?
A. IBS is usually caused by the underlying psychiatric disorder.
B. Psychiatric conditions may worsen coexisting IBS but do not cause IBS.
C. Successfully treating the comorbid psychiatric disorder resolves all IBS symptoms.
D. There is no relationship between psychiatric disorders and IBS.

[40.4] For the patient with constipation-predominant IBS, what is the best first-line therapy?

A. Hyoscyamine
B. Sertraline
C. Psyllium fiber supplementation
D. Loperamide

Answers

[40.1] **D.** Age-appropriate cancer screening (colonoscopy) is indicated, even in the setting of an established diagnosis of IBS, because of the high pretest probability of detecting an underlying neoplasm.

[40.2] **C.** Dicyclomine, an antispasmodic anticholinergic medication, can be used on an as-needed basis for mild to moderate abdominal pain associated with IBS. For more persistent and severe pain, low-dose TCAs, like amitriptyline, are beneficial.

[40.3] **B.** Comorbid psychiatric disorders typically worsen IBS symptomatology but have not been shown to cause IBS directly. Successfully treating an underlying psychiatric disorder may improve symptoms of IBS, but will not likely resolve all symptoms of IBS.

[40.4] **C.** Fiber supplementation is considered first-line therapy in constipation-predominant IBS. It is effective and safe, and available without prescription.

CLINICAL PEARLS

❖ The pathophysiology of IBS is not clearly elucidated. However, altered gut motility, visceral hypersensitivity, and dysregulation of the brain gut axis, coupled with psychosocial factors, appear to influence IBS symptoms in varying degrees.

❖ The symptom complex of altered bowel habits and chronic abdominal pain is the hallmark of IBS. Symptoms typically begin early in life, wax and wane, and occur in the absence of any organic cause.

❖ Alarm features may indicate an underlying organic pathology and require additional diagnostic work-up that may include laboratory, radiologic, and/or endoscopic studies.

❖ Treatment should be symptom specific and should include appropriate use of medication, dietary and lifestyle changes, and examination of any psychosocial factors that contribute to IBS symptoms.

REFERENCES

American College of Gastroenterology Functional Gastrointestinal Disorders Task Force. Evidence-based position statement on the management of irritable bowel syndrome in North America. Am J Gastroenterol 2002;97(Suppl):S1–S5.

American Gastroenterological Association. Medical position statement: irritable bowel syndrome. Gastroenterology 2002;123:2105–2107.

Thompson WG, Longstreth GF, Drossman DA, Heaton KW, Irvine EJ, Muller-Lissner SA. Functional bowel disorders and functional abdominal pain. Gut 1999;45(Suppl II): II43–II47.

A 30-year-old woman presents to the clinic complaining of feeling depressed and jittery. She has been feeling this way on and off for the last year, since her husband divorced her. She has 3 children, ages 12, 5, and 2 years. She reports an increase during the past 3 months of headaches, difficulty sleeping, loss of appetite, crying spells, and increased irritability. When asked about substance use, she says she drinks wine at night to help her sleep. Further questioning leads her to disclose that she started drinking more after her husband left, and she currently drinks, on average, 1.5 bottles of wine every evening, and sometimes more on the weekends. She does not use illicit drugs. She has no prior history of psychiatric disorders. The patient's physical examination is unremarkable with the exception of an elevated blood pressure (140/90 mm Hg). Routine lab tests from her last visit 1 month ago indicate an elevated γ-glutamyltransferase (GGT) (220 IU/L).

◆ **What is the most likely diagnosis?**

◆ **What is your next step?**

ANSWERS TO CASE 41: Alcohol Dependence/ Substance-Induced Depressive Disorder

Summary: A 30-year-old, physically healthy woman presents to an outpatient clinic with depressive symptoms that became clinically significant after increased use of alcohol to cope with stress. There is no previous history of psychiatric disorder or physical illness that could account for the symptoms.

 Most likely diagnosis: Alcohol dependence with a secondary substance-induced depressive disorder.

 Next steps: Assess severity of alcohol problem using standardized screening questions; assess for suicidality; assess social support network; deliver a brief intervention consisting of recommendation for reducing or quitting drinking and referral for substance abuse and/or mental health treatment.

Analysis

Objectives

1. Know brief alcohol screening questions (and cut point) for use in clinical practice.
2. Know the diagnostic criteria for alcohol abuse and dependence.
3. Know the definition of "at-risk" drinking.
4. Know what constitutes a standard drink.
5. Understand the distinction between substance-induced and non-substance-induced depression.
6. Know the signs and dangers of alcohol withdrawal.
7. Know components of a brief, office-based intervention for alcohol abuse and dependence.

Considerations

In patients reporting depressive symptoms, it is important to assess for current substance abuse, particularly alcohol, cocaine, and methamphetamine. If used in excess, these substances and their associated withdrawal syndromes can result in depression. Whether determined to be substance-induced or not, the depressive symptoms should be taken seriously. An assessment for suicidality (current and past) and current sources of family/social support should be conducted. The potential for significant alcohol withdrawal should also be assessed. If depressive symptoms persist longer than 4 weeks after discontinuation of alcohol, consider other potential causes of depression.

APPROACH TO SUSPECTED ALCOHOL DEPENDENCE

Assessment

Alcohol Screening

Brief screening instruments have been developed in order to identify potential alcohol abuse or dependence. The **most commonly used instrument is the CAGE.** The CAGE was designed for rapid verbal screening for alcohol dependence in clinical practice. CAGE **is a mnemonic representing the following four items**: (a) Have you ever felt you should **C**ut down on your drinking?; (b) Have people **A**nnoyed you about your drinking?; (c) Have you ever felt bad or **G**uilty about your drinking?; (d) Have you ever had a drink first thing in the morning to steady your nerves or get rid of a hangover (**E**ye-opener)? Based on a positive response to two or more items, the CAGE has been found to have a sensitivity ranging from 72–91%, and a specificity from 77–96%.

Substance Abuse Versus Dependence

A diagnosis of *substance abuse* is given if a patient does not meet DSM-IV (*Diagnostic and Statistical Manual of Mental Disorders,* Fourth Edition) criteria for substance dependence and one or more of the following is evident: (a) failure to fulfill major role obligations (work, school, home); (b) recurrent use in physically hazardous situations (e.g., driving intoxicated); (c) legal problems; (d) continued use despite persistent or recurrent social or interpersonal problems caused or made worse by the substance. Table 41–1 describes substance dependence.

At-Risk Drinking

Patients may not meet DSM-IV criteria for alcohol abuse or dependence, but may still be considered "at risk" for problems related to alcohol, particularly health-related problems. The National Institute on Alcoholism and Alcohol Abuse (NIAAA) defines at-risk drinking as follows:

- Men age 65 years or younger
- More than 4 standard drinks in a day and/or
- More than 14 standard drinks in a week
- Men older than age 65 years and *all* women
- More than 3 standard drinks in a day and/or
- More than 7 standard drinks in a week

Standard Drink Measurement

A standard drink represents 14 g of pure alcohol, typically 1 (12 oz) beer, 1 (5 oz) glass of wine, or 1 shot (1.5 oz) of spirits (e.g., whiskey, gin, vodka). When assessing for at-risk drinking, it is important to clarify the number of standard drinks a patient is consuming in a day or week. For example, a patient

Table 41–1
DSM-IV DIAGNOSTIC CRITERIA FOR SUBSTANCE DEPENDENCE

A maladaptive pattern of substance use, leading to clinically significant impairment or distress, as manifested by three or more of the following occurring at any time in the same 12-month period:

1. Tolerance, either:
   a. need for markedly increased amounts of the substance to achieve intoxication or desired effect, or
   b. markedly diminished effect with continued use of the same amount of the substance.
2. Withdrawal, either:
   a. the characteristic withdrawal syndrome for the substance, or
   b. the same (or a closely related) substance is taken to relieve or avoid withdrawal symptoms.
3. Substance is often taken in larger amounts or over a longer period than was intended.
4. Persistent desire or unsuccessful efforts to cut down or control substance use.
5. A great deal of time is spent in activities necessary to obtain the substance or recover from its effects.
6. Important social, occupational, or recreational activities are given up or reduced because of substance use.
7. Substance use is continued despite knowledge of having a persistent or recurrent physical or psychological problem caused or made worse by the substance (e.g., alcohol use despite high liver enzymes).

Source: DSM-IV, Diagnostic and statistical manual of mental disorders, 4th ed. Washington, DC: American Psychiatric Association (APA). 1994.

may report he drinks only 2 beers each day, but the beers to which he is referring may be large, 48 oz cans, equaling 4 standard drinks each.

Substance-Induced Depression Versus Primary Depression

A substance-induced mood disorder is distinguished from a primary Mood Disorder typically by considering the onset and course of the two disorders. **Depression only arising in association with alcohol intoxication or withdrawal states is likely to be substance-induced.** If depressive episodes are reported prior to substance use or occur during times of sustained abstinence or are substantially in excess of what would be expected given the type or amount of the substance used or the duration of use, then the mood disorder is likely to be primary. Withdrawal states can be relatively protracted and substance-induced mood symptoms may be evident up to 4 weeks after the cessation of substance use. The importance of this distinction lies in the chosen treatment plan. **Antidepressant medication is likely to be ineffective, if not harmful, to a patient with a significant alcohol (or other substance) problem.** Referral to substance abuse treatment should be the first choice of treatment in such cases, with follow-up for reassessment of depressive symptoms, about 1 month postabstinence.

Alcohol Withdrawal

Alcohol withdrawal may not be immediately obvious if a patient has ingested alcohol in the past 12 hours. Signs and symptoms to notice or assess for include tremulousness ("shake" or "jitters," which can occur within 6 hours of abstinence), insomnia, anxiety, depressed mood, gastrointestinal upset, heart palpitations, and sweating. More severe symptoms associated with a long history of chronic alcoholism include generalized tonic-clonic seizures (within 6–48 hours), hallucinations (within 12–48 hours; typically visual but can be auditory or tactile), and delirium tremens (DTs; within 48–72 hours), which is characterized by hallucinations, agitation, tremor, sleeplessness, and sympathetic hyperactivity. DTs only occur in approximately 5% of patients with withdrawal symptoms, but this is a serious condition with an in-hospital mortality of 5–10%, usually from arrhythmias or infections. Benzodiazepines are the drugs of choice for managing alcohol withdrawal.

Intervention

Brief, Office-Based Intervention for Alcohol Abuse and Dependence

Research indicates that a brief **5–10 minute discussion between physician and patient can lead to significant reductions in risky and hazardous drinking.** The Brief Negotiation Interview is a brief intervention for substance abuse that can be conducted in fewer than 10 minutes and is ideally suited for use in busy clinical settings. The main point to keep in mind is that this approach is nonconfrontational, nonjudgmental, and proceeds based on how ready the client is to make any changes with regard to alcohol use. Rather than lecturing and reprimanding, a physician can initiate a discussion about the patient's drinking and provide feedback so as to increase a patient's *own* internal motivation and to help resolve ambivalence about changing. There are five components to this intervention:

1. Establish rapport
2. Ask permission to discuss alcohol use
3. Provide feedback
4. Assess readiness
5. Enhance motivation, negotiate, and advise

Establishing rapport and asking permission to discuss alcohol use ("I have some concerns about your alcohol use and I'm wondering if we can discuss this today") will reduce patient resistance. Information or feedback about the patient's current drinking level, associated risks to one's health, and recommended drinking levels should be provided. Many patients are unaware of the healthy drinking limits established by the NIAAA. In the current case, it would also be important to express empathy with the stressors the patient is facing, and to note that some people use alcohol to cope, and this can lead to alcohol-induced depression.

The next step is to ask patients to rate how ready they are to reduce their drinking to below-risk levels, or to quit drinking entirely (which is recommended for people diagnosed with alcohol dependence). Ask patients to rate how ready they are to reduce or quit using alcohol on a scale from 1 to 10, where 1 is "not at all ready" and 10 is "completely ready and wants help making a plan."

For patients who are not currently motivated to change their alcohol use, make sure their viewpoint is acknowledged, using statements such as, "it sounds like you are not quite ready to change right now." Questions like, "what might have to happen for you to decide to work on changing," are also appropriate and will prompt further thinking about the issue. Another effective strategy is to ask clients who rate their readiness in the low range, "Why did you rate yourself a 3 (or 4 or 2) and not a 1?" This question usually elicits "change talk," or causes the patient to talk about why change would be beneficial. After a brief discussion, offer a phone number or brochure for available treatment options, and explain that if they do decide to seek help, services are available.

For patients who are ready to make changes, ask whether they can make a commitment to a goal, what that goal is, and what they can use to help them achieve this goal. Things to consider include social support (e.g., church) or treatment options including free community support groups (e.g., 12-step meetings), psychotherapy, and medication management. Writing down the plan to which they agree and asking them to sign it is a final tool that can help solidify their commitment to making the change. It is important to assess the risk of withdrawal symptoms based on quantity and chronicity of alcohol use and make appropriate arrangements for supervised, medically assisted detoxification, when appropriate.

In summary, it is important to clearly convey, in a nonjudgmental manner, the levels at which drinking is risky, concern about the impact of a patient's alcohol use, and to provide a recommendation to reduce drinking. For patients with a substance-induced mood or anxiety disorder, physicians should suggest that stopping or reducing alcohol use may reduce or eliminate problematic psychological symptoms (e.g., depression). Offering referrals for psychotherapy, 12-step meetings, or alcohol detoxification/treatment programs is a final and critical component of care.

Comprehension Questions

[41.1]   For which of the following does the mnemonic **CAGE** (a brief alcohol screening questionnaire) stand?

    A. **C**ut down? **A**ge? **G**uilt? **E**ver blacked out?

    B. **C**areful? **A**nnoyed? **G**uilt? **E**ye-opener?

    C. **C**ut down? **A**nnoyed? **G**uilt? **E**ye-opener?

    D. **C**rafty? **A**ge? **G**randiose? **E**ver blacked out?

[41.2] Which of the following are signs of alcohol withdrawal?

A. Laziness and apathy
B. Hallucinations and seizures
C. Excessive sleepiness and low heart rate
D. Systemic rash and increased blood pressure

[41.3] A 35-year-old man states that he drinks about 16 ounces of beer each morning. Approximately how many standard drinks does this amount of beer equal?

A. 1
B. 1.3
C. 2
D. 2.5

[41.4] A 45-year-old man presents for his annual physical with high blood pressure and a slight hand tremor. He admits that he drinks more than he probably should, but has no interest in changing his behavior. Which of the following should the physician do?

A. Scream at him as loudly as possible about the risks of heavy drinking.
B. Tell him repeatedly in a nice way that it's obvious he needs to quit drinking.
C. Not discuss the issue until he is ready to change.
D. Acknowledge the patient's choice not to change his drinking, engage him in a brief discussion or negotiation, and offer referrals in case he changes his mind.

Answers

[41.1] **C.** Has the patient ever tried to **cut down** his/her drinking? Has the patient ever been **annoyed** by others asking about his/her drinking? Has the patient felt **guilty** about drinking? Has the patient ever had a drink first thing in the morning (an **eye-opener**)?

[41.2] **B.** Hallucinations, seizures, and DTs are the more severe symptoms of alcohol withdrawal and are typically associated with long-term alcohol dependence.

[41.3] **B.** One 16 oz beer = 1.3 standard drinks (one 12 oz beer = 1 standard drink).

[41.4] **D.** With patients who are not motivated to change, arguing or insisting they change is unlikely to be effective. Their opinions and choices should be acknowledged, followed by a brief discussion of the patient's drinking and potential consequences, a recommendation to cut down or stop, and a referral.

CLINICAL PEARLS

❖ Alcohol and other drug abuse can significantly impact both physical and mental health.

❖ Assess whether the onset of depression or other mental health/behavioral problems preceded or followed significant alcohol or other drug abuse or dependence, to determine the primary problem and associated treatment.

❖ Alcohol dependence is characterized by tolerance; withdrawal; drinking larger amounts or for longer periods over time; desire or unsuccessful efforts to control use; much time spent drinking; reduction in other life activities; and continued use despite drinking-related physical and psychological problems.

❖ Alcohol withdrawal symptoms can be life-threatening. Supervised, medically assisted detoxification may be necessary for long-term, chronic alcoholism.

❖ Brief, physician-delivered alcohol interventions are effective for reducing problematic drinking.

❖ "Finger wagging," scolding, or lecturing patients tends to engender resistance to changing; a physician's advice can have a much more powerful effect if delivered in a nonjudgmental, nonconfrontational manner.

REFERENCES

Bertholet N, Daeppen JB, Wietlisbach V et al. Reduction of alcohol consumption by brief alcohol intervention in primary care: systematic review and meta-analysis. Arch Intern Med 2005;165(9):986–995.

D'Onofrio G, Bernstein E, Rollnick S. Motivating patients for change: a brief strategy for negotiation. In: Bernstein E, Bernstein J (eds). Case studies in emergency medicine and the health of the public. Boston: Jones and Bartlett, 1996: 295–304.

Ewing JA Detecting alcoholism: the CAGE Questionnaire. JAMA 1984;252: 1905–1907.

A 35-year-old woman presents to your office complaining of skipped or "irregular beats" for the past few weeks. She paid little attention to her symptoms because she had been under job-related stress and she thought these symptoms would disappear. Instead, her occasional skipped beats increased in frequency to twice a day, lasting up to 2 minutes. Her father, who suffered from heart disease, urged her to see a doctor. There had been no chest pain, shortness of breath, or dizziness. She consumes about 2 cups of coffee a day. She recently tried some diet pills to lose weight but stopped this medicine when her symptoms became more frequent. On examination, she is average build. Her blood pressure is 130/85 mm Hg, her heart rate is 92 beats/min, and her temperature is 98.6°F. Head, ears, eyes, nose, and throat (HEENT) examination is normal. No conjunctival pallor noted. Neck examination is supple. No jugular venous distension. Thyroid gland is normal size without nodules and is nontender. There are no associated thyroid bruits. Lung examination is normal. Cardiac examination reveals regular rate and rhythm with normal S_1 and S_2. No midsystolic click is heard. Abdominal and extremity examinations are normal. Neurologic examination reveals no resting tremor. Reflexes are normal.

◆ **What is your most likely diagnosis?**

◆ **What is your next diagnostic step?**

◆ **What is the next step in therapy?**

ANSWERS TO CASE 42: Palpitations

Summary: A 35-year-old woman presents to your office with a few weeks worth of palpitations that have increased in frequency. Her symptoms are not associated with chest pain, syncope, dyspnea, or dizziness. She has no pertinent past medical history. She has the potential triggers of caffeine consumption, diet pill use, and stress. Family history of heart disease also noted. Her examination is normal.

◆ **Most likely diagnosis:** Cardiac dysrhythmia, benign

◆ **Next diagnostic step:** Obtain 12-lead EKG

◆ **Next step in therapy:** Restrict caffeine, alcohol, and drugs (especially amphetamine-based stimulants and diuretics) for next 2 weeks; keep a diary of symptoms or possible triggers; follow-up with patient in 2 weeks. If symptoms persist, additional work-up may be required.

Analysis

Objectives

1. Define palpitations.
2. Identify benign rhythm disturbances and those associated with sudden cardiac death.
3. Identify the most common structural heart diseases associated with sudden cardiac death.
4. Develop a rational approach that takes into account cardiac and non-cardiac causes for palpitations.

Considerations

This 35-year-old woman gives a history of frequent palpitations and otherwise appears healthy (normal physical exam) without associated dizziness or syncope. Because she is also younger than the age of 50 years (thus a low risk for coronary artery disease), she is most likely to have a nonthreatening cause for her symptoms and can be worked up on an outpatient basis.

This history is the most important part of the work-up. We are given clues to noncardiac factors that may contribute to palpitations, including caffeine consumption, use of diet pills, job-related stress, and possibly stress surrounding her father's own health problems. Anemia should be considered if there is a history of fatigue, light-headedness, GI blood loss, or menorrhagia.

Family history can be very important because some dysrhythmias, such as familial prolonged QT syndrome, can run in families. A family history of premature cardiac death (or unexplained sudden death) should be sought, as hypertrophic cardiomyopathy is autosomal dominant and may not demonstrate a heart murmur when examined.

If this woman were to have a midsystolic click associated with or without a late systolic murmur, we would need to consider the presence of **mitral valve prolapse** (MVP) syndrome. Usually asymptomatic, it is the **most common valvular heart defect** in the United States, occurring in 3–6% of the population. Because MVP is common, the presence of palpitations may or may not be the result of this condition. Still, people may present with palpitations, fatigue, chest discomfort (not typical of angina), and dyspnea with this valvular finding. This symptom complex is defined as mitral valve prolapse syndrome. These patients may also present with panic attacks or manic-depressive syndromes. Two percent of MVP patients will have complications resulting in progression to mitral regurgitation with subsequent left-sided two-chamber enlargement, atrial fibrillation (if left atrium becomes enlarged), left ventricular dysfunction leading to heart failure, pulmonary hypertension, and infective endocarditis. For these reasons, a two-dimensional echocardiogram is recommended at least once when MVP is identified.

APPROACH TO PALPITATIONS

Definition

Palpitations: A subjective sensation of unduly strong, slow, rapid, or irregular heart beats that may be related to cardiac arrhythmias. The sensation may last seconds, minutes, hours, or days. They are common and usually not dangerous. They usually are the result of a change in the heart's electrical system.

Clinical Approach

Etiologies

Approximately 40% of patients complaining of palpitations have a primary rhythm disturbance. An underlying mental health problem (anxiety or panic disorder) is the cause in 31% of symptomatic patients. Drugs (prescription, recreational, or over-the-counter) cause 6% of palpitations; intrinsic structural problems with the heart are the cause of 3%; 4% have noncardiac causes; and the remaining 16% have no identifiable cause.

The largest group has some type of primary rhythm disorder, including sinus bradycardia, sinus tachycardia, Wolf-Parkinson-White (WPW) syndrome, sick sinus syndrome, premature atrial contractions, supraventricular tachycardias, premature ventricular contractions, advanced atrioventricular block, and ventricular tachycardia. These rhythm disturbances can be seen in childhood and adulthood.

Patients with **long Q-T interval syndrome** are at increased risk for ventricular arrhythmias and sudden cardiac death (SCD). The long QT syndrome follows an **autosomal dominant pattern and is seen more commonly in females.** Patients with this syndrome will present with either palpitations and/or syncope and have a family history of syncope or sudden death. Prolonged QT interval is defined as QT_C* 470 msec in men or >480 msec in women. **Any patient with a QT interval >500 msec is at increased risk for dangerous dysrhythmias.** Prolonged QT intervals may also be the result of the use of certain medications.

Benign rhythm disturbances include premature atrial contractions, sinus tachycardia, and sinus bradycardia appropriate for activity/stress level, sinus pauses less than 3 seconds and isolated unifocal premature ventricular contractions (PVCs). However, PVCs in the presence of known cardiac disease, metabolic disease, or the presence of worrisome symptoms (such as dizziness, syncope or seizures) require aggressive work-up because of the risk of ventricular tachycardia or fibrillation. PVCs occurring at rest and disappearing with exercise are usually benign, commonly seen in athletes, and require no investigation.

Supraventricular tachycardia (SVT) is not life-threatening but can be frightening to the patient and may require medical management or catheter ablation. Typically, a cardiologist or cardiac electrophysiologist becomes involved in managing this type of patient. Symptomatic atrial flutter or fibrillation, in isolation or as part of WPW, are also worrisome rhythm disturbances and may require consultation with a cardiologist.

Psychiatric causes are always considered in the differential diagnosis for palpitations and may be missed if not screened for in the initial history. Panic disorder is seen more often in women of childbearing age. Patients with panic attacks commonly present to emergency departments. They will report brief episodes of overwhelming panic or sense of impending doom associated with tachycardia, dyspnea, or dizziness. Still, these complaints may be identical to primary rhythm disturbances and deserve formal work-up.

Cardiac or structural problems include cardiomyopathy, atrial or ventricular septal defects, congenital heart disease, mitral valve prolapse, pericarditis, valvular heart disease (e.g., aortic stenosis, aortic insufficiency), and congestive heart failure. The presence of restrictive, hypertrophic or dilated cardiomyopathies may lead to sudden cardiac death.

Hypertrophic cardiomyopathy is the most common cause of sudden cardiac death in adolescents in the United States. These patients may present with chest pain, syncope, and palpitations. Hypertrophic cardiomyopathy may be passed down as an autosomal dominant trait. A heart murmur, if present, will usually be systolic and will be accentuated by Valsalva maneuver. Echocardiography demonstrating a thickened intraventricular septum remains the gold standard for diagnosis.

Marfan syndrome should be suspected in patients who are tall and have scoliosis, pectus excavatum, arachnodactyly, high arched palate, and an arm span exceeding their height. Mitral valve prolapse may be seen in patients with Marfan

---

*QT_C is defined as measured QT interval corrected for heart rate:

$$QT_C = \frac{QT \text{ (in msec)}}{\sqrt{RR \text{ interval (in msec)}}}$$

syndrome. These patients often have aortic root dilations and are at risk for aortic arch aneurysm rupture. The diagnosis can be confirmed by echocardiography.

Noncardiac causes of palpitations may be suggested by the history and exam. Noncardiac etiologies include anemia, electrolyte disturbances, hyperthyroidism, hypothyroidism, hypoglycemia, hypovolemia, fever, pheochromocytoma, pulmonary disease, and vasovagal syncope. **Laboratory screening includes a complete blood (CBC), chemistry panel, and thyroid-stimulating hormone (TSH).** If a pheochromocytoma is suspected, a 24-hour urine collection for catecholamines and metanephrines is required.

Numerous medications and substances may contribute to palpitations. Among these are alcohol, caffeine, street drugs (cocaine), tobacco, ephedra (found in weight loss drugs), diuretics (causing electrolyte disturbances), digoxin, β-agonists (e.g., albuterol), theophylline, and phenothiazine. Patients should be questioned about their use of over-the-counter medications, herbs, and supplements, as they often will not provide this information unless specifically asked.

Clinical Presentation

Evaluation of a patient presenting with palpitations should take into account numerous factors. The patient's age at symptom onset is important, as an **age older than 50 years should always lead to the consideration of coronary artery disease.** Possible triggers should be pursued, such as medication use, exercise, and stress. Pay particular attention to palpitations associated with collapse, as these are usually pathologic and hospitalization should be considered.

The clinical examination should focus on vital signs (blood pressure and heart rate), including orthostatic readings if suggested by history. The thyroid gland should be examined for abnormalities such as goiter, nodule, or bruit. The presence of resting tremor or brisk reflexes should also lead one to the consider hyperthyroidism.

The cardiac examination should be thorough. The point of maximum impulse should be palpated, as displacement may suggest cardiomegaly. The rate and rhythm should be noted, particularly if there are any irregularities. For example, an irregularly irregular rhythm is suggestive of atrial fibrillation whereas an occasional extra beat may be PVCs. Extra sounds, such as the midsystolic click of mitral valve prolapse or any murmurs consistent with valvular pathology, should also be documented.

A 12-lead electrocardiogram is appropriate in all patients with palpitations, even if they are symptom-free during physician encounter. The presence of left ventricular hypertrophy, atrial enlargement, atrioventricular block, old myocardial infarction, and delta waves (as seen in Wolf-Parkinson-White syndrome) should trigger additional testing. Prolonged QT intervals increase the risk for dangerous rhythm disturbances and usually require consultation with a cardiologist or cardiac electrophysiologist.

Other cardiac testing may be appropriate based on the history, examination, and results of the initial evaluation. **Ambulatory electrocardiographic**

rhythm monitoring can be accomplished **for periods of 24–72 hours using a Holter monitor**. A cardiac **event monitor can be worn by a patient for up to 30 days** and might be useful when the palpitations do not occur daily. The monitor is worn continuously and activated by the patient when palpitations are felt.

An echocardiogram might be useful in identifying patients with suspected structural abnormalities of their heart chambers or heart valves which could trigger heart rhythm disturbances. These findings could be missed on physical examination. Exercise stress tests in age-appropriate patients may be important for identifying dysrhythmias triggered by exercise. This may be of particular importance in patients with suspected coronary artery disease. Anyone with suspected structural problems should be evaluated by an echocardiogram before undergoing exercise. Patients with suspected hypertrophic cardiomyopathy or severe aortic stenosis should avoid exercise stress testing, as they may develop heart rhythm disturbances which may be nonrecoverable. Finally, electrophysiology studies may be the needed to recreate rhythm disturbances and subsequently treat using ablative techniques. These studies require referral to a cardiac electrophysiologist.

Treatment

The treatment of a given patient's symptoms is dependent on the etiology. If medication related, the offending agent should be stopped. Anxiety may be treated by a combination of pharmacologic and nonpharmacologic interventions. If the problem is structural cardiac disease, referral to a cardiologist is usually indicated.

Primary supraventricular rhythm disturbances may respond nicely to β-blockers or calcium channel blockers. Digoxin can be used to slow down rapid ventricular responses to atrial fibrillation and flutter. If symptoms are short-lived or episodic, short-acting negative chronotropics, such as short-acting β-blockers, can be used on an as-needed basis.

Symptomatic SVT can often be self-treated by patients with recurrent episodes by several vagal stimulation techniques. Carotid sinus massage, Valsalva maneuver, and cold applications to the face ("diver's reflex") can trigger vagus nerve stimulation, which may break an episode of SVT. When these are unsuccessful, IV injection of adenosine is often successful.

Chronic atrial fibrillation should be treated with medication to keep the ventricular rate below 100 beats/min; these agents are often β-blockers or calcium channel blockers. **Most patients with atrial fibrillation will also require anticoagulation with warfarin,** as they are at an increased risk of embolic stroke from blood clots that form in the cardiac atrium.

Ventricular arrhythmias require the services of an electrophysiologist. This is especially true in patients where medications might not work or worse lead to disastrous results. Electrophysiologists can create short circuits to accessory pathways and stop aberrantly conducted myocardial contractions using precise destructive techniques called ablation. An implanted defibrillator may also be placed, which can provide life-saving cardioversion when a ventricular arrhythmia is detected.

Comprehension Questions

[42.1] Which of the following is the most common cause of underlying etiology in patients who complain of palpitations?

A. Medication
B. Structural heart disease
C. Coronary artery disease
D. Primary rhythm disturbance
E. Idiopathic

[42.2] Which of the following is the most appropriate initial treatment for an episode of supraventricular tachycardia?

A. Rubbing over area of carotid artery.
B. Placing a warm pack to the face.
C. IV injection of anxiolytic medication
D. Electrophysiology studies and ablation

[42.3] Which of the following is an indication for referral to a cardiologist or cardiac electrophysiologist?

A. PVCs on a resting EKG that resolve with exercise
B. QT_C interval >500 msec.
C. Isolated unifocal PVCs found on EKG
D. Sinus arrhythmia

[42.4] Which of the following patients should undergo an exercise stress test for evaluation of his condition?

A. A 60-year-old with symptomatic PVCs
B. A 35-year-old with hypertrophic cardiomyopathy seen on an echocardiogram
C. A 32-year-old, tall, slender man with pectus excavatum and mitral valve prolapse on examination
D. A 68-year-old with suspected aortic stenosis

Answers

[42.1] **D.** Primary rhythm disturbances are the most common cause of palpitations, making up approximately 40% of cases. Other common causes include anxiety, medications, and structural heart disease. Many cases of palpitations remain undiagnosed in spite of appropriate evaluation.

[42.2] **A.** Vagal stimulation techniques, such as carotid sinus massage, Valsalva maneuver, and cold applications to the face, are usually the first things to try when SVT is diagnosed. IV adenosine may be useful when these are unsuccessful.

[42.3] **C.** The presence of a QT_C of >500 msec puts a patient at an increased risk for ventricular arrhythmias and should prompt a referral to an electrophysiologist for further evaluation.

[42.4] **A.** A 60-year-old with PVCs, especially if they are of new onset, may be showing the initial presentation of coronary artery disease and should undergo stress testing. All of the other conditions listed are contraindications to stress testing.

CLINICAL PEARLS

❖ Consider Marfan syndrome in a tall patient with long arms, long fingers, who wears glasses.

❖ A 24–72-hour Holter monitor is appropriate in a patient with frequent (i.e., daily) palpitations; a 30-day event monitor is a better test in someone with infrequent episodes.

❖ Hypertrophic cardiomyopathy is the most common cause of sudden cardiac death in adolescents. An adolescent with a systolic heart murmur that increases in intensity with Valsalva maneuver should have his/her activity restricted until a diagnostic echocardiogram can be performed.

REFERENCES

Abbott AV. Diagnostic approach to palpitations. Am Fam Physician 2005;71(4): 743–750.

Batra AS, Hon AR. Consultation with the specialist: palpitations, syncope, and sudden death in children: who's at risk? Pediatric Rev 2003;24(8):269–275.

Bouknight DP, O'Rourke RA. Current management of mitral valve prolapse. Am Fam Physician 2000;61(11):3343–3350, 3353–3354.

Rowland T. Evaluating cardiac symptoms in the athlete: is it safe to play? Clin J Sport Med 2005;15(6):417–420.

Zipes DP, Ackerman MJ, Mark Estes NA, et al. Arrhythmias. J Am Coll Cardiology 2005;45:1354–1363.

The mother of a 16-year-old girl calls you when you are on call on a Saturday afternoon. The mother states that her daughter was stung by a wasp about 2 hours ago on her left arm. The patient has no known history of previous allergic reactions to insect bites or stings. She is having no difficulty breathing or swallowing, nor has she been dizzy or light-headed. The mother's primary concern is that the area of the sting is red and swollen. The daughter says that it hurts and itches. She says that the site of the injury was the midpoint of the forearm and there is now redness and swelling extending in a circular pattern that is about 3 inches across. The red area is hot to the touch, so the mother is concerned that it is infected. She gave her daughter some ibuprofen for the pain and would like you to phone in some antibiotic and something to prevent the reaction from spreading.

◆ **Which antibiotic should you prescribe to treat this condition?**

◆ **What other treatments might be beneficial at this point?**

◆ **What immunization is appropriate for this patient?**

ANSWERS TO CASE 43: Sting and Bite Injuries

Summary: A 16-year-old female has been stung by a wasp and is having a painful, itchy local reaction. She has no history of previous allergic reactions. The patient's mother is calling and asking you to manage the situation over the phone.

◆ **Most appropriate antibiotic to use:** No antibiotic treatment is indicated, as this is a local reaction.

◆ **Other therapy that may be beneficial:** Local applications of ice, nonsteroidal antiinflammatory drug (NSAID) or acetaminophen for pain, and antihistamine for itching.

◆ **Immunization that is appropriate:** Tetanus-diphtheria booster, if not up to date.

Analysis

Objectives

1. Know the insects that commonly cause bite and sting injuries.
2. Be able to differentiate local from systemic reactions to bites and stings.
3. Know the management of common animal-bite injuries.

Considerations

The insect order Hymenoptera includes wasps, yellow jackets, hornets, honeybees, bumblebees, and fire ants. These insects cause the majority of cases of sting- or bite-induced anaphylaxis and cause more mortality than all other types of insect bites and stings. Local reactions occur as a result of the toxic properties of the venom whereas more severe reactions tend to be caused by allergic reaction to venom allergens.

Several types of bee stings result in retention of the stinger in the victim, which can result in continued injection of the bee venom. Stingers should be promptly removed. Grasping the base of the stinger may result in compression of a venom-containing sac, resulting in increased venom release. Thus it is suggested that scraping or brushing the stinger off of the skin is preferable to grasping the stinger. However, **rapidly removing the stinger is preferable to taking the time to locate a scraping implement** if one (such as a credit card or driver's license) is not immediately at hand.

APPROACH TO BITES AND STINGS

Insect Stings

Local Reactions

Almost all hymenoptera stings will result in a **local reaction**, which includes redness, swelling, pain, and itching at the site of the injury. These reactions **tend to occur almost immediately and last for a few hours.** The local tissue response is a consequence of a histaminelike reaction caused by the venom that is released by the sting. Local reactions can be treated with ice and antihistamine for itching. Tetanus prophylaxis should be provided for those who have not been vaccinated.

Delayed Reactions

Large local reactions are immunoglobulin (Ig) E-mediated allergic reactions to the hymenoptera venom. These reactions are often confused with cellulitis, as large areas ($\geq$10 cm in diameter) of redness and warmth develop over 24–48 hours. These reactions are not infectious and will not respond to antibiotics. These reactions are **best treated with oral steroids** initiated early after the sting. Tetanus prophylaxis should be reviewed and updated, if needed. A person with a history of a large local reaction to a bee sting is likely to have similar reactions to subsequent stings. However, the history of this type of reaction does not result in an increased risk of anaphylaxis to subsequent stings.

Anaphylaxis

Up to 4% of the population may have a systemic reaction to a hymenoptera sting. Those who have had a systemic reaction have a 50% or greater risk of having a systemic reaction to future stings. These systemic reactions can vary from milder symptoms of nausea, generalized urticaria, or angioedema to severe and life-threatening hypotension, shock, and airway edema. Severe immediate-hypersensitivity reactions usually occur within minutes of the sting.

Treatment of anaphylaxis should include assessment and management of the ABCs (Airway, Breathing, and Circulation), with intubation, if necessary, IV access, and fluid resuscitation. **Subcutaneous or intramuscular injection of 0.3–0.5 mL of 1:1000 solution of epinephrine should be given as quickly as possible** and repeated in 10–15 minutes if needed. Antihistamines and bronchodilators may be required as well. Anyone with an anaphylactic reaction should be observed in a hospital setting for 12–24 hours, as the symptoms can recur. Persons with known anaphylactic reactions should be prescribed epinephrine injector kits to carry with them for immediate access at all times when they could be exposed. Desensitization therapy can also be offered to those with known anaphylaxis, as their risk of future severe reactions can be reduced by up to 50%.

Animal Bites

Nearly 5 million animal bites occur in the United States each year. The most common animals involved are dogs, cats, and humans.

The initial management should focus, as always, on the ABCs and on protection of the current injury (splinting of fractures, protection of cervical spine, etc.), as well as control of bleeding and assessment of the injuries incurred. History should be gathered on the type of animal involved in the bite, the situation regarding the bite (whether provoked or unprovoked), and the vaccination status of the animal, particularly to document rabies vaccination status.

Local cleaning of the wound(s) with soap and water, irrigation with saline, and debridement of devitalized tissue should take place as soon as possible. Often, for minor wounds, these treatments are all that is needed.

The risk of infection is dependent on numerous factors. Larger and deeper wounds are more likely to become infected than smaller, superficial wounds. Hand wounds also tend to have an increased risk of infection. Host factors, such as the presence of chronic illnesses or immune suppression, also play a role. The animal involved in the bite is important. Approximately 20% of dog-bite wounds become infected, whereas cat and human bites have a higher occurrence of infection.

Many different bacteria can be involved in bite wound infections. Both cats and dogs can carry staphylococci, streptococci, anaerobic species, and *Pasteurella* species. Humans carry staphylococci, streptococci, *Haemophilus* species, *Eikenella* species, and anaerobes.

The treatment of bite wounds starts with local care—cleaning, irrigation, and debridement. The primary closure of bite wounds is controversial, but obviously infected wounds should not be primarily closed. Tetanus vaccination should be updated in those patients at need. Animal control authorities should be contacted for guidance regarding rabies vaccination.

Patients with moderate to severe wounds from dog, cat, or human bites, who are seen early after the injury and without signs of active infection, should receive antibiotic prophylaxis for 3–5 days. Amoxicillin-clavulanate (Augmentin) given orally is an appropriate prophylaxis for most bite wounds. When cellulitis is present, longer courses of antibiotic, usually 7–14 days, are required. Hospitalization and surgical intervention may be required for more severe infections, osteomyelitis, joint infections, and in patients with complicating medical conditions.

Comprehension Questions

[43.1] Which of the following therapeutic options is common to the treatment of both bee stings and bite wounds?

    A. Antibiotic prophylaxis with amoxicillin-clavulanate
    B. Antihistamines for itching
    C. Tetanus vaccination
    D. Surgical wound debridement

[43.2] A 22-year-old woman develops a progressively enlarging red, hot area on her leg following a yellow jacket sting. She sees you in the office a day after the sting and says that the lesion is still enlarging. Which of the following statements is true?

A. This is an IgE-mediated reaction.
B. This is cellulitis that should be treated with antibiotic.
C. She should be prescribed an epinephrine kit to use if she gets stung again.
D. This type of reaction is unlikely to happen if she were to get stung again.

[43.3] You see a 7-year-old boy a day after he was bitten by his pet dog. According to the mother, the dog bit the child after he snuck up on the dog and grabbed its tail. The dog has had all its vaccinations, including rabies. The child has had no fever, has full movement of the injured limb, and has no sign of neurologic or vascular injury. The wound is on the child's forearm, is not deep, and is not bleeding, but has developed about 2 cm of erythema surrounding the site. Which of the following is the most appropriate treatment?

A. Hospitalization for IV antibiotic
B. Oral amoxicillin-clavulanate for 3–5 days
C. Oral amoxicillin-clavulanate for 7–14 days
D. Local care without any antibiotic

Answers

[43.1] **C.** Tetanus vaccination is common to the management of both bee stings and bite wounds. Bee stings rarely become infected and do not require antibiotic therapy.

[43.2] **A.** This patient is having a large, local reaction to her sting. This is an IgE-mediated reaction. It may respond to a course of oral steroid. There is at least a 50% chance that a similar reaction will occur if she were stung again, but she is unlikely to develop anaphylactic reactions in the future.

[43.3] **C.** This child is developing cellulitis from the bite wound. Based on his presentation, he does not appear to require hospitalization. He can be treated with oral antibiotics for 1–2 weeks.

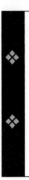

CLINICAL PEARLS

❖ Anyone with a history of anaphylactic reactions should be given a
   prescription for an epinephrine injector kit and instructed in the
   importance of keeping it at hand. These prescriptions need to be
   updated often, as the medication expires in 6–12 months.
❖ Human "bite" wounds are not always the result of a bite. A punch
   to the mouth can cause a serious inoculation and infection to the
   knuckles of the puncher.

REFERENCES

Golden DBK. Stinging insect allergy. Am Fam Physician 2003;67:2541–2546.
Goldstein EJC. Human and animal bites. In: Schlossberg D (ed). Current therapy of
   infectious disease. Philadelphia: WB Saunders, 2002:66–68.
Maguire JH, Pollack RJ, Spielman, A. Arthropod bites and stings. In: Kasper DL,
   Braunwald E, Fauci AS, et al. (eds). Harrison's principles of internal medicine.
   16th ed. New York: McGraw-Hill, 2005. Accessed on-line at: www.accessmed-
   icine.com/ resourceTOC.aspx?resourceID=4
Presutti RJ. Prevention and treatment of dog bites. Am Fam Physician 2001;63:
   1567–1574.

A 60-year-old male is brought to the emergency room by ambulance because of slurred speech and left-side weakness. His wife states the patient went to bed approximately at 11 P.M. the night before and was well. At 5 A.M., the time they usually get up, she noticed that he had some difficulties talking and moving his left arm and leg. They arrived at the emergency department at 6 A.M. He has history of long-standing hypertension (HTN), heart attack 10 years before, and high cholesterol. He is taking baby aspirin, an angiotensin-converting enzyme (ACE) inhibitor, and a statin on daily basis. He heavily consumed alcohol in the past, but stopped after the heart attack. He still smokes a half pack of cigarettes daily. His wife remembers that about 3 months ago he complained of mild bilateral leg pain during their morning walk and had to stop after 15 minutes. Also, she remembers that 1 month ago he had "slight right eye blackout" for 5 minutes. On presentation to the emergency department his blood pressure is 195/118 mm Hg, his pulse is 106 beats/min, his respiratory rate is 18 breaths/min, his temperature is 99.8°F, and his oxygen saturation is 97% on room air. Although his pupils are equal and reactive and the ocular movements are intact, he is unable to turn his eyes voluntarily toward the left side. The neck is supple, there is no jugular venous distension, and there are no bruits. The lungs are clear, the heart sounds regular without murmurs, and the abdomen is normal. The limbs are not well-perfused distally. The neurologic examination reveals that he is alert and oriented, although he does not recognize he is sick. He is right-handed. He shows loss of awareness and attention with respect to objects or stimuli on his left side. He has mild dysarthria but his speech is fluent and he understands and follows commands very well. There is mild weakness on the left side of the face and left-sided homonymous hemianopsia, but there is no nystagmus or ptosis, and no tongue or uvula deviation. He is not able to move his left arm and leg, has hyper-reflexia, and the left great toe is upgoing.

◆ **What is the most likely diagnosis?**

◆ **What is your next diagnostic step?**

◆ **What is your next step in therapy?**

ANSWERS TO CASE 44: Cerebrovascular Accident/Transient Ischemic Attack

Summary: The patient is a 60-year-old right-handed male with history of coronary artery disease, hypertension, and hypercholesterolemia, who presents to the emergency room complaining of slurred speech and an inability to move his left arm and leg. He had an episode of amaurosis fugax 1 month before admission. On physical examination, although he is alert and oriented, he has no awareness of his disability (anosognosia) and exhibits left-sided neglect. He has hypertension, dysarthria, and left hemiparesis. He also has left-sided homonymous hemianopsia, conjugate rightward gaze deviation, left hemifacial weakness, and left hyperreflexia.

◆ **Most likely diagnosis:** Cerebrovascular accident (CVA)

◆ **Next diagnostic step:** Obtain a brain computed tomography (CT) scan without contrast

◆ **Next step in therapy:** Determine advisability for acute treatment with thrombolytic agents

Analysis

Objectives

1. Recognize the significance of a correct diagnosis and evaluation of transient ischemic attacks (TIAs) and cerebrovascular accidents (CVAs).
2. Recognize the conditions that can mimic a stroke.
3. Understand that the clinical evaluation gives the most important clues about diagnosis of stroke.
4. Be familiar with the accepted approach for the early management of patients with ischemic stroke.
5. Be familiar with the current strategies for prevention of ischemic stroke and TIA.

Considerations

This 60-year-old patient has developed focal neurologic deficits, which is the usual presentation of patients with strokes. Considering that he has a history of hypertension, hypercholesterolemia, and vascular manifestations of atherosclerosis, such as coronary artery disease and peripheral vascular disease (lower-extremity claudication), ischemic stroke is the most probable diagnosis. Even more, he had a TIA (amaurosis fugax) 30 days before admission, which put him at risk for an ischemic stroke. His neurologic deficits are compatible with an ischemic stroke in the territory of the right middle cerebral artery, his non-dominant hemisphere, and the reason he is not aphasic.

Of immediate importance, the clinician should confirm that the neurologic impairments are secondary to ischemic stroke and not other conditions, especially intracranial hemorrhage. A brain CT without contrast should be obtained as soon as possible to exclude hemorrhage, tumor, and abscess. Blood sugar, serum electrolytes, renal function tests, and a drug screen also are important. A cardiac monitor should be attached and a 12-lead EKG obtained so as to exclude acute myocardial infarction or atrial fibrillation.

Because it probably has been more than 3 hours from the onset of symptoms (and as many as 7 hours), this patient is not a candidate for thrombolytic therapy. The initial ABC (Airway, Breathing, and Circulation) survey should guide treatment if the vital signs are compromised. Although his blood pressure is elevated, in the setting of an acute CVA, blood pressure management should be cautious. The patient should be admitted to the hospital for further evaluation and management. Deep venous thrombosis prophylaxis should be used. An evaluation of his swallowing function and early physiotherapy consultation should be obtained. Further imaging with a brain magnetic resonance imaging (MRI), magnetic resonance angiography, or CT angiography can help to clarify the etiology of the stroke and guide treatment.

Management of his chronic medical conditions, to try to reduce his risk of subsequent strokes, is critical. In this patient, these measures include tight control of his hypertension and hypercholesterolemia, along with smoking cessation. Because this patient had a stroke while taking aspirin, an alternative antiplatelet agent should be considered.

APPROACH TO CVA/TIA

There are 700,000 people that suffer from stroke in the United States each year, and the incidence of TIA is approximately 200,000–500,000 per year. Strokes remain the third-leading cause of death in North America. **TIA is defined as a focal neurologic deficit lasting less than 24 hours;** a stroke is diagnosed if the symptoms persist for more than 24 hours. However, with the development of new imaging techniques, a new definition of TIA has been proposed: a "brief episode of neurologic dysfunction caused by a focal disturbance of brain or retinal ischemia, with clinical symptoms typically lasting less than 1 hour, and without evidence of infarction."

Patients with a TIA are at increased risk of a subsequent stroke. The reported occurrence of a stroke after a TIA is as high as 5.3% within 2 days and 10.5% within 90 days. Patients with a TIA often require hospital admission, further evaluation, and the same long-term management as stroke patients.

Hypertension is the single most important risk factor for stroke, and the incidence of stroke in the United States has decreased as a result of better efforts to control hypertension in the past few decades. **Other risk factors are diabetes mellitus, age** (the older the patient, the greater the risk), **sex, race** (most frequent in females and in African-Americans), **heart disease** (atrial fibrillation, valvular heart disease, acute myocardial infarction, left ventricle thrombus, cardiomyopathy, etc.), **cigarette smoking** (a major independent risk factor), and **hyperlipidemia.**

Most strokes are cerebral infarctions, which can be classified as large-artery atherosclerotic infarction (intracranial or extracranial); embolism (usually from a cardiac source); small-vessel disease; other causes such as dissection, hypercoagulable states, and sickle cell disease; and infarcts of undetermined cause. Ninety-five percent of TIAs are a consequence of atherothromboembolism, cardiogenic embolism, and small-vessel disease.

Diagnosis and Evaluation

Sudden onset of focal neurologic deficit is the usual presentation of stroke patients, although some patients can have a gradual worsening of symptoms. Unless there is a hemispheric infarct, basilar artery occlusion, or cerebellar stroke with edema, nearly all of the patients are alert. If the middle cerebral artery territory is affected, the patient would experience aphasia (when dominant hemisphere is involved), contralateral hemiparesis, sensory loss, spatial neglect, and contralateral impaired conjugate gaze. When the territory of the anterior cerebral artery is affected, foot and leg deficits are more frequent than arm deficits. These patients often have associated cognitive and personality changes. Vertebrobasilar stroke symptoms and signs include motor or sensory loss in all four limbs, crossed signs, disconjugate gaze, nystagmus, dysarthria, dysphagia. There can be ipsilateral limb ataxia and gait ataxia if the cerebellum is affected.

Assessment of the vital signs is important in the initial examination. Severe high blood pressure can be suggestive of hypertensive encephalopathy or intracranial hemorrhage as causes of the symptoms. A fever may lead to consideration of an infectious cause. A rapid or irregularly irregular pulse may imply atrial fibrillation as a potential cause of the stroke. A timely general physical examination and comprehensive neurologic examination should follow.

The differential diagnosis of acute neurologic symptoms and signs is broad. Along with CVAs, these symptoms can be caused by seizures, acute confusional states, syncope, metabolic and toxic encephalopathy (hypoglycemia), brain tumors, CNS infections, and subdural hematoma. When it is determined that a stroke is the cause of the presentation, **it is crucial to differentiate between ischemic and hemorrhagic stroke because of the implications on further treatment.**

The initial assessment should establish if the patient is eligible for thrombolytic treatment. Establishing the time of symptom onset is the most important factor. The onset of symptoms is assumed to be the time that the patient was last known to be free of symptoms.

Brain Imaging

A CT scan of the brain without contrast is the initial imaging test of choice. CT of the brain can exclude most cases of intracranial hemorrhage, tumors, or abscesses. It is more available and takes less time than MRI. CT can also be used to detect a hemorrhagic transformation of an infarct in a patient with an ischemic stroke whose symptoms deteriorate.

Further imaging studies may be indicated to clarify the etiology of the stroke and to detect intracranial or extracranial arterial occlusions, which may affect treatment decisions. Evaluation of the cerebrovascular system can be accomplished with magnetic resonance angiography (MRA), CT angiography, catheter angiography, or transcranial Doppler ultrasonography.

Other Tests

A 12-lead EKG should be done in all stroke patients in order to detect acute myocardial infarctions, which can both cause strokes or be the result of a stroke. An EKG will also aid in the diagnosis of atrial fibrillation. Echocardiography may also be necessary to adequately assess the heart. Transesophageal echocardiography is particularly useful in detecting cardiac sources of embolism, such as thrombus caused by myocardial infarction, endocarditis, rheumatic heart disease, valvular prostheses, and atrial septal defects.

Blood glucose, electrolytes, renal function tests, and drug screening are important to exclude hypoglycemia and metabolic and toxic encephalopathy. If the patient is on anticoagulant therapy, the prothrombin time, partial thromboplastin time, and platelet count should be measured and are required before considering thrombolytic therapy. Lumbar puncture is indicated if subarachnoid hemorrhage is considered and the CT is not diagnostic or if a CNS infection is possible.

Treatment

As in every critical patient, **the initial survey should assess the ABCs.** If hypoxia is detected, supplemental oxygen should be administered to maintain oxygen saturation above 95% and the cause of the hypoxia investigated (partial airway obstruction, aspiration pneumonia, atelectasis). An endotracheal tube should be placed if the airway is threatened. **A cardiac monitor should be placed to detect atrial fibrillation or any other arrhythmias.**

Unless a hypertensive encephalopathy, aortic dissection, acute renal failure, or pulmonary edema is present, the **treatment of arterial hypertension should be cautious.** Antihypertensive medication is recommended when the systolic blood pressure is >220 mm Hg or the diastolic blood pressure is >120 mm Hg. If the patient is suitable for thrombolytic treatment, medication should be initiated to decrease the systolic blood pressure to <185 mm Hg and the diastolic blood pressure <110 mm Hg. The agents most frequently used are IV labetalol, nicardipine, and sodium nitroprusside.

The presence of a fever after stroke onset is associated with an increase in morbidity and mortality. If a patient is febrile, the pateint should receive antipyretic medications while the source of the fever is investigated.

Except when thrombolytic therapy is given, **most patients with a nonhem-orrhagic stroke should receive aspirin within the first 48 hours**. Urgent anticoagulation is not recommended.

Judiciously selected patients can benefit from intravenous administration of recombinant tissue-type plasminogen activator (rtPA) if they can be treated within 3 hours of the onset of ischemic stroke. The risk of hemorrhage associated with rtPA treatment is approximately 5% and there are numerous contraindications to the use of thrombolytic therapy, including recent surgery, trauma, myocardial infarction, use of anticoagulant medications, and uncontrolled hypertension.

Early posttreatment care includes mobilization once the patient is stable and evaluations of the patient's ability to swallow and nutritional status. The presence of a fever should prompt a work-up for common causes, such as pneumonia (both community acquired and aspiration) and urinary tract infections. When thrombolytic therapy is not used, deep vein thrombosis prophylaxis should be provided. Family support and treatment of depression should be also initiated when appropriate.

Prevention of Stroke in Patients with Previous Ischemic Stroke or TIA

A history of a previous TIA or CVA confers a high risk for future events. Aggressive risk factor control should be undertaken in these patients. All patients should be counseled to quit smoking and to reduce alcohol intake. Hypertensive patients should be treated per JNC-7 (Joint National Committee on Prevention, Detection, Evaluation and Treatment of High Blood Pressure, 7th report) guidelines (see Case 30). High cholesterol should be treated with a goal low-density lipoprotein (LDL) of <100 mg/dL. Tight diabetic control should be sought. Antiplatelet agents such as aspirin (50–325 mg/d), the combination of aspirin and extended-release dipyridamole, or clopidogrel should be started in patients with a history of noncardioembolic ischemic stroke or TIA.

Carotid endarterectomy (CEA) can reduce the risk of stroke in someone with a history of previous TIA/CVA and carotid artery stenosis. It is indicated for symptomatic patients with carotid stenosis >70% when it can be performed by an experienced surgeon with a low rate of perioperative complications. CEA can be considered for symptomatic patients with a 50–70% stenosis, but is not indicated when there is <50% stenosis.

Anticoagulation with warfarin reduces the risk of stroke in certain circumstances. It is indicated to reduce the risk of embolic strokes for patients with persistent or paroxysmal atrial fibrillation. It is also useful for patients with an ischemic stroke caused by an myocardial infarction and existence of left ventricular thrombus. Warfarin is indicated patients with cardiomyopathy, rheumatic mitral valve disease, and prosthetic heart valves.

Comprehension Questions

[44.1] Which of the following statements is true regarding TIA?

A. The neurologic dysfunction typically lasts less than 1 hour.

B. The risk of a subsequent stroke after a TIA is less than 1% within 90 days.

C. A previous TIA is an indication for warfarin therapy.

D. Infarction can usually be seen on CT or MRI of the brain.

[44.2] Which of the following statements is true considering the initial work up in a stroke patient?

A. Lumbar puncture is indicated if a subarachnoid hemorrhage is considered and the brain CT is negative.

B. Chest x-ray should be obtained as soon as possible.

C. Brain CT with contrast is useful to rule out intracranial hemorrhage.

D. MRI of the brain is the initial diagnostic imaging study of choice.

[44.3] Which statement is true regarding treatment of stroke patients?

A. Fever is a defense mechanism and should not be treated unless >102°F.

B. Blood pressure should be aggressively lowered in the acute setting.

C. Thrombolytic therapy is safe and effective for use in most stroke patients.

D. Early mobilization should be routine.

[44.4] Which statement is true regarding prevention of stroke in patients with ischemic stroke or TIA?

A. Patients with noncardioembolic stroke benefit from oral anticoagulation.

B. After a stroke, patients with carotid stenosis >25% benefit from carotid endarterectomy.

C. For patients with noncardioembolic stroke, aspirin is an acceptable option for initial therapy.

D. LDL cholesterol should be treated with a goal of <130 mg/dL.

Answers

[44.1] **A.** A TIA is a brief neurologic episode, typically less than 1 hour in duration, that does not cause infarction. The occurrence of stroke after TIA is as high as 5.3% within 2 days and 10.5% within 90 days. Warfarin is indicated in specific circumstances, such as the presence of atrial fibrillation, but is not routinely used following a TIA.

[44.2] **A.** Routine chest x-rays affect the clinical management in few patients with stroke, and are not recommended as routine initial work up. CT of the brain *without* contrast can exclude most cases of intracranial hemorrhage, tumors, or abscesses, and is the initial test of choice in most situations. When a subarachnoid hemorrhage is suspected but not seen on CT, a lumbar puncture is indicated for diagnosis.

[44.3] **D.** Mobilization of stroke patients should be started when they are considered medically stable. In the setting of an acute stroke, management of high blood pressure should be cautious. Thrombolytic therapy can be beneficial in selected patients, but carries significant risks and has numerous contraindications. Fever should be treated and a work-up performed to determine its etiology, as it carries an increased risk of morbidity and mortality.

[44.4] **C.** Patients with stroke but no detected sources of embolism benefit from antiplatelet agents, not anticoagulants. Aspirin, clopidogrel, or a combination of aspirin and dipyridamole are acceptable regimens. For patients with recent TIA or ischemic stroke and ipsilateral severe (>70%) carotid artery stenosis, carotid endarterectomy is recommended. When the degree of stenosis is <50%, there is no indication for CEA. Patients with a history of symptomatic cerebrovascular disease should be treated to an LDL goal of <100 mg/dL.

CLINICAL PEARLS

❖ Hypertension is the single most important risk factor for stroke.
❖ Although most strokes are cerebral infarcts, it is crucial to differentiate between ischemic and hemorrhagic stroke because of the implications on further treatment.
❖ CT of the brain without contrast is the initial imaging test of choice in most suspected strokes.
❖ Unless a hypertensive encephalopathy, aortic dissection, acute renal failure, or pulmonary edema is present, the treatment of arterial hypertension should be cautious.

REFERENCES

Adams HP, Adams RJ, Brott T, et al. Guidelines for the early management of patients with ischemic stroke: a scientific statement from the Stroke Council of the American Stroke Association. Stroke 2003;34:1056–1083.

Adams H, Adams R, Del Zoppo G, Goldstein LB. Guidelines for the early management of patients with ischemic stroke: 2005 guidelines update. A scientific statement from the Stroke Council of the American Heart Association/American Stroke Association. Stroke 2005;36:916–923.

Goldstein LB, Larry B, Simel DL. Is this patient having a stroke? JAMA 2005;293:2391–2402.

Sacco RL, Adams R, Albers, G, et al. Guidelines for prevention of stroke in patients with ischemic stroke or transient ischemic attack. Circulation 2006;113:e409–e449.

Shah KH, Edlow JA. Transient ischemic attack: review for the emergency physician. Ann Emerg Med 2004;43:592–604.

A 39-year-old homeless man presents to the emergency department for cough and fever. He says that his illness has been worsening over the past 2 weeks. He initially felt short of breath and now is short of breath at rest. On questioning, he tells you that he lives in a homeless shelter when he can, but he frequently sleeps on the streets. He has used IV drugs (primarily heroin) "on and off" for many years. He denies medical history but the only time he gets medical attention is when he comes to the emergency department for an illness or injury. On review of systems, he complains of fatigue, weight loss, and diarrhea. On examination, he is a thin, disheveled man appearing much older than his stated age. His temperature is 100.5°F, his blood pressure is 100/50 mm Hg, his pulse is 105 beats/min, and his respiratory rate is 24 breaths/min. His initial oxygen saturation is 89% on room air, which comes up to 94% on 4 L of oxygen by nasal cannula. Significant findings on examination include dry mucous membranes, a tachycardic but regular cardiac rhythm, a benign abdomen, and generally wasted-appearing extremities. His pulmonary examination is significant for tachypnea and fine crackles bilaterally, but no visible signs of cyanosis. His chest x-ray is read by the radiologist as having diffuse, bilateral, interstitial infiltrates that look like "ground glass."

◆ **What is the most likely cause of this patient's current pulmonary complaints?**

◆ **What underlying illness does this patient most likely have?**

◆ **What testing and treatment should be started now?**

ANSWERS TO CASE 45: HIV and AIDS

Summary: A 45-year-old, homeless, IV drug abuser is seen with fever, cough, dyspnea, and fatigue. He is found to be tachypneic, febrile, and hypoxemic. His chest x-ray reveals bilateral interstitial infiltrates.

◆ **Most likely cause of current illness:** *Pneumocystis jiroveci* (formerly known as *Pneumocystis carinii*) pneumonia

◆ **Most probable underlying illness:** AIDS

◆ **Recommended current testing and treatment:** Complete blood count (CBC), electrolytes, arterial blood gas; HIV enzyme-linked immunosorbent assay with confirmatory Western blot; CD4 cell count; sputum for *P. jiroveci*; start treatment with trimethoprim-sulfamethoxazole (TMP-SMX).

Analysis

Objectives

1. Know the common risks and modes of transmission of HIV/AIDS.
2. Be aware of common presentations of persons infected with HIV.
3. Learn the role of antiretroviral therapy and other adjunctive treatments in the chronic management of HIV and AIDS.
4. Be able to identify common complications and opportunistic infections associated with HIV/AIDS.

Considerations

Pneumocystis jiroveci (formerly known as *Pneumocystis carinii*) pneumonia is an AIDS-defining illness in someone infected with HIV. *P. jiroveci* is a fungus that may colonize many people, but typically causes disease only in those with profound immune deficiencies, such as AIDS infections or cancers treated with chemotherapy. *P. jiroveci* pneumonia usually presents with nonproductive cough, fever, and dyspnea that worsens over a few days to a few weeks. Patients usually are found to be febrile, tachypneic, and hypoxic, although their lung examination may be unremarkable (other than tachypnea). The presence of a bilateral interstitial infiltrate on chest x-ray, often described as having a ground-glass appearance, is classic for *P. jiroveci* pneumonia. The identification of the organism in sputum, either spontaneously produced or induced, is diagnostic, but treatment is usually started prior to definitive diagnosis in those with a classic clinical picture.

As *P. jiroveci* pneumonia occurs after the CD4 count has markedly reduced, patients often will have symptoms and signs of other AIDS-related complications as well. It is common to see oral or esophageal candidiasis, diarrhea, Kaposi sarcoma, wasting syndrome, and other complications in a patient presenting with

P. jiroveci pneumonia. Although it presents in the setting of advanced disease, *P. jiroveci* pneumonia remains a common presenting illness in those who did not know that they were infected with HIV and is a frequent initial opportunistic infection in those with known HIV disease. The incidence of *P. jiroveci* pneumonia is decreasing in the United States with more widespread awareness of HIV disease, broader usage of antiretroviral therapy, and prophylactic use of TMP-SMX in patients with CD4 counts of <200 cells/μL.

APPROACH TO HIV AND AIDS

Epidemiology

HIV infection is a chronic infection with a variable course. The HIV pandemic has spread to every country in the world and has infected 59 million persons worldwide. It is estimated that more than **20 million people have died from AIDS and its complications.** HIV disease is caused by the human retroviruses, HIV-1 and HIV-2. HIV-1 is more common worldwide, whereas HIV-2 has been reported in western Africa, Europe, South America, and Canada.

In the United States, more than 1 million people are estimated to be infected with HIV, with **approximately 25% unaware of their infection.** The highest prevalence of HIV occurs in men who have sex with other men and in IV drug users, although the occurrence in heterosexual sexual contact is increasing. African-Americans are disproportionately affected with infection, both in total numbers of cases and in development of new infections.

Transmission

HIV is transmitted from person to person through contact with infected blood and body fluids. Sexual contact is the most common mechanism of transmission, with receptive anal intercourse or the presence of genital lesions (ulcerations, mucosal disruptions) conferring increased risk of infection. Infection can be passed during vaginal, anal, and oral intercourse. The risk of transmission can be reduced by the proper and consistent use of latex condoms (either male or female condoms). Because HIV can pass through lambskin condoms, these are not recommended.

Sharing needles by IV drug users is the second most common source of transmission of HIV. Vertical transmission from an infected woman to her baby has been found to occur during pregnancy, during the process of delivery of a baby, and from breast-feeding. Blood and blood-product transfusions have been linked to infection, although the routine screening of donor blood for HIV now makes this an extremely rare event.

Healthcare workers have been infected with HIV through accidental punctures with needles used on HIV-infected patients. There is also a risk of infection by infected blood entering through open skin wounds or mucous membranes. The risk of transmission to healthcare workers is low and is related to the viral load of the patient, the amount of blood to which the worker is exposed, and the depth of the inoculum. Postexposure risk of developing HIV infection can be reduced by immediate and careful cleaning of the exposure/puncture site along with postexposure prophylactic treatment with antiretroviral therapy.

HIV has been measured in small amounts in saliva and tears of HIV-infected patients, but no cases of transmission based on exposure to these have been documented. Transmission has been reported to occur in bite wounds from infected individuals, but only when significant tissue damage and bleeding has occurred. Measurable amounts of HIV have not been found in sweat. No case of HIV has been documented to have occurred via an insect vector.

Primary Infection

Following initial exposure to HIV, some patients will complain of nonspecific symptoms, such as low-grade fever, fatigue, or myalgias. This illness typically occurs 6–8 weeks following the infection and is self-limited. The primary infection is also known as acute seroconversion syndrome, as the symptoms are thought to be related to the development of antibodies to the virus.

Following the resolution of the primary infection symptoms (if any occur), there is a period of clinical latency. During this time, most infected persons are asymptomatic, although some may have lymphadenopathy. This period usually extends for 6–9 months following the transmission of the virus.

Clinical Categorization of HIV/AIDS Infections

The Centers for Disease Control and Prevention defines three clinical categories and three laboratory categories (based on CD4 cell counts) of HIV infection. The clinical categories are A, B, and C; the laboratory categories are 1, 2, and 3. **For classification purposes, HIV-infected patients can be defined with both a clinical and laboratory category** (e.g., A3, B2, etc.).

The laboratory categories are as follows:

1. CD4 cell count ≥500 cells/μL
2. CD4 cell count 200–499 cells/μL
3. CD4 cell count <200 cells/μL

Clinical **category A** includes asymptomatic HIV infection, primary HIV infection (above), and persistent generalized lymphadenopathy. Persistent generalized lymphadenopathy is defined as enlarged lymph nodes involving at least two noncontiguous sites other than inguinal nodes.

Category B infections are symptomatic conditions in an HIV-infected person that are either indicative of a defect in cell-mediated immunity or that have a course or management complicated by HIV infections. These are not AIDS-defining illnesses and were previously known as AIDS-related complex. Table 45–1 lists some of these infections, which are not AIDS-defining illnesses. Table 45–2 lists some of the **category C** conditions, which are

Table 45–1

SOME EXAMPLES OF HIV CLINICAL CATEGORY B CONDITIONS

Bacillary angiomatosis	Idiopathic thrombocytopenic purpura
Oropharyngeal candidiasis	Listeriosis
Persistent, recurrent, or difficult to treat vaginal candidiasis	Pelvic inflammatory disease (especially if complicated by tuboovarian abscess)
Cervical dysplasia or carcinoma in situ	Peripheral neuropathy
Oral hairy leukoplakia	Herpes zoster, 2 or more episodes involving more than 1 dermatome

Information from Centers for Disease Control and Prevention. 1993 Revised classification system for HIV infection and expanded surveillance case definition for AIDS among adolescents and adults. MMWR 1992;41 (RR-17).

Table 45–2

HIV CLINICAL CATEGORY C CONDITIONS

Candidiasis of bronchi, trachea or lungs	Esophageal candidiasis	Invasive cervical Cancer
Coccidioidomycosis (disseminated or extrapulmonary)	Extrapulmonary *Cryptococcus*	Intestinal cryptosporidiosis (>1 month's duration)
Cytomegalovirus disease	HIV-related encephalopathy	Herpes simplex: chronic ulcer, bronchitis, pneumonitis, or esophagitis
Disseminated or extrapulmonary histoplasmosis	Intestinal isosporiasis (>1 month's duration)	Kaposi sarcoma
Burkitt lymphoma	Immunoblastic lymphoma	Primary brain lymphoma
Mycobacterium avium complex (disseminated or extrapulmonary)	*Mycobacterium tuberculosis* (any site)	*P. jiroveci* pneumonia
Pneumonia, recurrent	Progressive multifocal leukoencephalopathy	Recurrent *Salmonella* septicemia
Toxoplasmosis of brain	Wasting syndrome caused by HIV	

Information from Centers Disease Control and Prevention. 1993 Revised classification system for HIV infection and expanded surveillance case definition for AIDS among adolescents and adults. MMWR, 1992;41 (RR-17).

AIDS-defining illnesses. The presence of a CD4 cell count <200 cells/μL, with or without symptoms, is also considered diagnostic of AIDS.

For classification purposes, a patient's **HIV is defined by the highest clinical category in which the patient has ever qualified.** For example, someone with oral candidiasis (category B) who is treated and now asymptomatic remains in clinical category B. Similarly, once a category C condition has occurred, the person will remain in category C.

Diagnostic Evaluation

The standard screening test for HIV infection is the detection of HIV antibodies using the enzyme-linked immunosorbent assay (ELISA). **Samples that are repeatedly positive on ELISA testing are must be confirmed by Western blot testing.** The Western blot test is an electrophoresis that detects antibodies to HIV antigens of specific molecular weights.

When HIV is diagnosed, a complete history and physical examination should be performed. Emphasis should be placed on identifying comorbid conditions, determining the presence of any category B or C conditions, reducing risky behaviors, and assisting with coping strategies. **HIV is reportable to local health authorities, but partner notification laws vary by state,** so it is important to know the local regulations.

Before instituting therapy, laboratory testing should include HIV genotype testing to identify strains that may be resistant to therapy. HIV RNA levels can help to assess disease activity. CD4 lymphocyte counts should be measured at baseline and, generally, every 3–6 months thereafter to monitor for disease staging, progression, and the risk of complications. A complete blood count (CBC), comprehensive metabolic panel, and urinalysis should be performed at baseline and periodically thereafter to monitor for complications of HIV and of the medications that are used in treatment.

Screening for other sexually transmitted diseases (syphilis, hepatitis B and C, gonorrhea, chlamydia) **should be performed** initially and repeated, if needed, because of any ongoing risks identified. Hepatitis B and A vaccination should be offered to those who lack immunity. A purified protein derivative (PPD) test should be done, and if initially negative, repeated annually. Women should have regular Papanicolaou (Pap) smears to evaluate for cervical dysplasia or cancer.

Treatment

Because of the complexity of treatment regimens and frequently changing treatment guidelines, **patients with HIV/AIDS should be referred, in almost all cases, to a physician with expertise in treating these conditions.** In general, antiretroviral therapy is used in patients who have AIDS (by laboratory or clinical criteria), who have symptoms of disease, or who are pregnant (to reduce the risk of vertical transmission).

Prophylactic treatments to reduce the risk of infection are also important in immunosuppressed patients. HIV patients should receive annual influenza vaccination and should be offered pneumococcal vaccination (preferable before the CD4 counts fall below 200 cells/µL). Live virus vaccines are contraindicated in both HIV patients and their close (household) contacts. Prophylaxis against *P. jiroveci* pneumonia should be instituted using TMP-SMX when the CD4 count falls below 200 cells/µL and *Mycobacterium avium-intracellulare* complex prophylaxis, using azithromycin or clarithromycin, is recommended if the CD4 count falls below 50 cells/µL.

Comprehension Questions

[45.1] A 42-year-old woman has AIDS, with a CD4 count of 125 cells/µL. She is on antiretroviral therapy. Which of the following treatments is recommended at this time?

   A. Discontinue retroviral treatment
   B. Varicella vaccination to reduce the risk of herpes zoster
   C. TMP-SMX for *P. jiroveci* pneumonia prophylaxis
   D. Clarithromycin for *Mycobacterium avium-intracellulare* complex prophylaxis

[45.2] Which of the following is an AIDS-defining condition?

   A. Oral thrush
   B. Cervical carcinoma in situ
   C. Listeriosis
   D. Kaposi sarcoma

[45.3] Which of the following is ineffective in preventing the transmission of HIV?

   A. Female condom
   B. Male latex condom
   C. Male lambskin condom
   D. Antiretroviral therapy in pregnancy to reduce vertical transmission

Answers

[45.1] **C.** With this level of cell count, the patient should continue antiretroviral therapy and start *P. jiroveci* pneumonia prophylaxis. The level is not yet low enough to recommend *Mycobacterium avium-intracellulare* complex prophylaxis. Varicella is a live virus vaccine and is contraindicated in HIV>

[45.2] **D.** Kaposi sarcoma is a category C, AIDS-defining condition. All of the other conditions listed are category B.

[45.3] **C.** Lambskin condoms are ineffective in reducing the transmission of HIV. All of the other listed options can reduce the risk of infection.

CLINICAL PEARLS

❖ Because of the complexity of the drug regimens and the ever-changing guidelines, persons with HIV should be comanaged with an infectious disease specialist or other physician with expertise in treating HIV.

❖ The use of antiretroviral therapy during pregnancy can reduce the risk of vertical transmission of HIV. Women with high HIV viral titers at term should be offered elective cesarean delivery, as this further reduces the risk of vertical transmission.

❖ The risk of transmission of HIV to healthcare workers by accidental needle sticks from HIV-infected patients is very low. It is important to report these injuries promptly, as early prophylactic treatment can significantly lower the risk of developing HIV disease.

REFERENCES

AIDS Education and Training Centers. Clinical manual for management of the HIV-infected adult, 2005 edition. Available at: www.aidsetc.org/aetc/aetc?page= cm-00–00.

Centers for Disease Control and Prevention. 1993 Revised classification system for HIV infection and expanded surveillance case definition for AIDS among adolescents and adults. MMWR 1992; 41(RR-17).

Khalsa AM. Preventive counseling, screening, and therapy for the patient with newly diagnosed HIV infection. Am Fam Physician 2006;73(2):271–280.

A 33-year-old African-American male presents to the office for an acute visit with nausea and diarrhea that he has had for the past week. Along with these symptoms, he has had a low-grade fever, some right upper quadrant abdominal pain, and has noticed that his eyes seem yellow. He has no significant medical history and takes no medications regularly. He denies alcohol, tobacco, or IV drug use. He works as a pastor in a local church that went on a mission to build a medical clinic in a rural area of Central America about 5 weeks ago. He had a mild case of traveler's diarrhea while there, but otherwise has felt well. On examination, he is a well-developed man who appears to be moderately ill. His temperature is 99.8°F, his blood pressure is 110/80 mm Hg, his pulse is 90 beats/min, and his respiratory rate is 14 breaths/min. He has a prominent yellow color to his sclera and under his tongue. His mucous membranes are moist. Lung and cardiac examinations are normal. His abdomen has normal bowel sounds and tenderness in the right upper quadrant. His liver edge is palpable just below the costal margin. There are no other masses felt, no rebound, and no guarding. On rectal examination, he has clay-colored soft stool that is Hemoccult negative.

◆ **What is the most likely diagnosis?**

◆ **When and how did he most probably contract this illness?**

◆ **How can you confirm the diagnosis?**

◆ **What is the treatment at this point?**

ANSWERS TO CASE 46: Jaundice

Summary: A 33-year-old male with no significant medical history develops diarrhea, abdominal pain, and jaundice about a month after traveling to Central America. He is noted to have yellow eyes and tender hepatomegaly.

◆ **Most likely diagnosis:** Acute infection with hepatitis A.

◆ **Most probable timing and source of infection:** Ingestion of contaminated food or water while on his mission to Central America 5 weeks earlier.

◆ **Test to confirm the diagnosis:** Antihepatitis A immunoglobulin (Ig) M.

◆ **Treatment of acute hepatitis A:** Supportive care and symptomatic treatment for the patient; report infection to local health department; consider giving Ig prophylaxis to close household or sexual contacts.

Analysis

Objectives

1. Develop a differential diagnosis for adults with jaundice.
2. Know the symptoms, management, complications, and modes of transmission of hepatitis A, B, and C.
3. Be able to interpret the results of hepatitis viral serology tests.

Considerations

This presentation of diarrhea along with nonspecific, crampy abdominal pain is most often caused by viral gastroenteritis. However, this patient has several symptoms and signs that serve as clues to point to other potential diagnoses. Of particular importance, the complaint of yellow eyes should prompt an evaluation for jaundice.

Bilirubin is a breakdown product of red blood cells. During the breakdown of hemoglobin, bilirubin is formed and bound to albumin, which carries it to the liver. In the liver, a portion of the bilirubin is made water soluble by conjugation to a glucuronide. This "conjugated bilirubin" is excreted in the bile and then largely excreted in the stool. Bilirubin that is not conjugated ("unconjugated bilirubin") in the liver remains bound to albumin.

Most cases of **jaundice can be characterized as having prehepatic, hepatic, or posthepatic causes.** Prehepatic jaundice is most often from hemolysis of red blood cells, which overwhelms the liver's ability to conjugate and clear the bilirubin through its normal pathways. This produces a hyperbilirubinemia that is primarily unconjugated.

Hepatic causes of jaundice can lead to either unconjugated or conjugated hyperbilirubinemia. Viruses, such as hepatitis, and alcohol reduce the liver's ability to transport bilirubin *after* it has been conjugated, resulting in a conjugated hyperbilirubinemia.

Posthepatic jaundice is usually caused by obstruction to the flow of bile through the bile ducts. This can be caused by bile duct stones, strictures, or tumors that narrow or block the ducts. Posthepatic jaundice is, therefore, a conjugated hyperbilirubinemia.

APPROACH TO JAUNDICE

History and Examination

The most important information in the diagnostic evaluation usually comes from the history. In patients presenting with jaundice, the history should be thorough and should include questions focused on identifying the common causes of jaundice. Specific information should include when the jaundice commenced and whether it is of acute or gradual onset. The presence of gastrointestinal symptoms, such as abdominal pain, nausea, vomiting, diarrhea, or changes in stool color can be significant. Itching is common in jaundice and this symptom may, in fact, precede the onset of the yellow color.

Associated symptoms, such as unintended weight loss or the development of adenopathy may lead to the consideration of certain diagnoses, including malignancies. Bruising or bleeding disorders may suggest severe hepatic dysfunction that is interfering with the production of clotting factors. Increasing abdominal girth may be caused by ascites and peripheral edema by obstruction of venous return from the lower extremities or hypoalbuminemia.

A complete review of the past medical history is necessary. **Any medications, whether prescription, nonprescription, or herbal supplements, should be reviewed.** Acetaminophen is a widely used over-the-counter agent that, in toxic amounts, can cause hepatocellular damage. Numerous herbal agents have been associated with liver damage as well.

The **social history is of critical importance in a patient with jaundice.** The abuse of alcohol is the most common cause of cirrhosis. IV drug use or unsafe sexual practices can lead to infection with hepatitis B or C. Hepatitis is also associated with getting tattoos if unsterilized equipment is used. Travel history, especially the location and timing of any international travel, can lead to the consideration of hepatitis A.

A comprehensive physical examination is also important in the work-up of someone with jaundice. Along with a general physical examination, certain areas should be emphasized. Jaundice may first be noticed as a yellowing of the sclera, especially in persons with darker skin types. Yellow discoloration can also commonly be seen under the tongue.

Examination of the skin should document the jaundice and also look for clues to its cause. The stigmata of alcohol abuse (e.g., caput medusa, spider veins) or IV drug use (needle track marks) should be noted. Large hematomas, by themselves, could be a cause of jaundice as the blood resorbs. Signs of bruising or bleeding should also be documented.

Abdominal examination must include, among other things, evaluation of the general contour of the abdomen, the presence of any ascites, the presence of organomegaly, and any tenderness. Hepatomegaly may or may not occur as a part of liver disease. Right upper quadrant tenderness can be associated with acute hepatitis but also with gallstone disease. Splenomegaly could suggest portal hypertension from cirrhosis or could be caused by malignancy.

Laboratory Testing

The most important initial laboratory evaluation of jaundice is the bilirubin level, which is usually reported as both a total bilirubin and direct bilirubin. **The reported direct bilirubin is a measurement of the conjugated bilirubin level.** Unconjugated bilirubin can be determined by subtracting the directed bilirubin from the total bilirubin.

The relative relationship of conjugated and unconjugated bilirubin in a jaundiced person can be indirectly evaluated by performing a urinalysis. **Conjugated bilirubin is excreted in the urine, whereas unconjugated bilirubin is not.** A urinalysis on a jaundice patient who has a high level of bilirubin suggests that the patient has a conjugated hyperbilirubinemia; absence of bilirubin on the urinalysis suggests that it is an unconjugated hyperbilirubinemia.

Unconjugated Hyperbilirubinemia

A mild unconjugated hyperbilirubinemia, usually identified as an incidental finding when liver enzymes are tested for some other reason, is often caused by **Gilbert syndrome.** Gilbert syndrome is a congenital reduction of conjugation of bilirubin in the liver. It occurs in approximately 5% of the population and is of no health significance. Occasionally, the bilirubin level will increase during times of illness and then recover to its baseline, slightly elevated level, after the illness resolves. In a patient with mildly elevated unconjugated bilirubinemia, otherwise normal liver enzymes and complete blood count (CBC), and who is otherwise well, no further work-up is indicated.

Hemolysis can cause an unconjugated hyperbilirubinemia in proportion to the amount of hemolysis that occurs. It is most often diagnosed by identification of anemia along with the presence of red cell fragments or abnormalities (spherocytosis, thalassemias, Sickle cell disease). The management is to treat the cause of the hemolysis.

Conjugated Hyperbilirubinemia

Hepatitis A is a viral infection of the liver primarily transmitted via fecal–oral contamination. Contaminated food and water are the primary sources of infection, although risks also include drug use (both injection and noninjection) and male–male sexual contact. Hepatitis A infection is widespread in Africa, Asia, and Central and South America. Travelers to these areas are at risk for infection.

Hepatitis A causes a self-limited illness characterized by jaundice, fever, malaise, and abdominal discomfort. The incubation period is 2–8 weeks, with an average of 4 weeks. While the symptoms can be mild, even asymptomatic in younger patients, there is an approximately 2% fatality rate in those older than age 50 years. The illness tends to last for 4–6 weeks, although some people have an illness that will last up to 6 months. There is no specific treatment for hepatitis A. Supportive care and symptomatic treatments are indicated.

Hepatitis A is diagnosed based on the presence of a conjugated hyperbilirubinemia, elevated hepatic transaminases, and serology. An acute infection causes an elevation of antihepatitis A virus (HAV) IgM. An elevated anti-HAV IgG but negative IgM indicates a history of a previous hepatitis A infection but not acute illness.

Hepatitis A vaccination is available and recommended for those at high risk, including travelers to endemic areas, persons with chronic liver disease, men who have sex with men or children who live in areas with high rates of the illness. Household or sexual contacts of persons infected with hepatitis A can be offered prophylaxis with injections of immunoglobulin.

Hepatitis B virus infection is transmitted via contact with contaminated blood or body fluids. Sexual contact and needle sharing are common mechanisms of infection. Hepatitis B may also be vertically transmitted from mother to baby. The incubation period from exposure to clinical symptoms is 6 weeks to 6 months. Only 50% of infections with hepatitis B are symptomatic. Approximately 1% of infections result in hepatic failure and death. Along with the acute symptoms, which are similar to hepatitis A, hepatitis B can cause a chronic infection. **Chronic hepatitis B is highly related to the age of the patient**—90% of infected infants and 60% of children younger than age 5 years develop chronic hepatitis B, which can lead to cirrhosis and hepatocellular carcinoma.

Serologic studies, using several markers, are necessary to determine the presence and type of hepatitis B infection that is present. Hepatitis B surface antigen (HBsAg) is present in both acute and chronic infections. Its presence is associated with contagiousness to others. Patients with the e antigen (HBeAg) are 100 times more infectious than those lacking the HBeAg. **Antibody to the surface antigen (anti-HBs) is seen in resolved infections and is the serologic marker produced after hepatitis B vaccination.** An IgM antibody to the hepatitis B core antigen (anti-HBcAg IgM) is diagnostic of an acute infection. A measurable level of HBsAg with a negative anti-HBcAg IgM is diagnostic of chronic hepatitis B. Figures 46–1 and 46–2 show the serologic studies associated with acute hepatitis B infection and chronic hepatitis B infection.

Acute hepatitis B infection is treated supportively. Persons with chronic hepatitis B may be candidates for antiviral therapy. They should be referred to

Acute hepatitis B with recovery

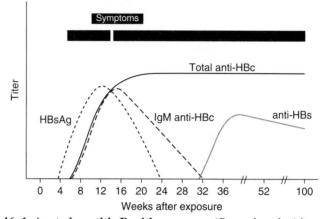

Figure 46–1. Acute hepatitis B with recovery. (*Reproduced with permission from Briscoe, DB. Lange Q&A: USMLE Step 3. 4th ed. New York: McGraw-Hill, 2005:48.*)

a specialist both to evaluate the appropriateness of therapy and to monitor for the development of hepatocellular carcinoma or cirrhosis.

Hepatitis B vaccination is universally recommended for children. Vaccination is also recommended for adults at high risk of disease, including healthcare and public safety workers, IV drug users, persons with chronic liver disease, and dialysis patients.

Chronic hepatitis B infection

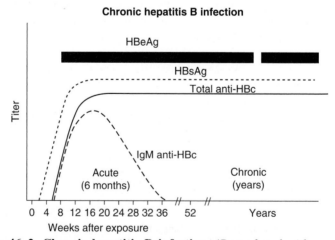

Figure 46–2. Chronic hepatitis B infection. (*Reproduced with permission from Briscoe, DB. Lange Q&A: USMLE Step 3. 4th ed. New York: McGraw-Hill, 2005:48.*)

Hepatitis C, formerly known as non-A, non-B hepatitis, is the most common cause of chronic liver disease in the United States, with more than 4 million infected persons. Transmission occurs via exposure to infected blood or body fluids via sexual contact, needle sharing, or accidental exposure of healthcare workers, and by vertical transmission. Blood or blood-product transfusion was a common source of exposure prior to 1992.

The virus can be detected in the blood within 1–3 weeks of exposure, with liver cell injury detectable in 4–12 weeks. Most infections are asymptomatic, but hepatitis C can cause an acute illness with jaundice, malaise, and anorexia. **Of those infected with hepatitis C, 60–85% will develop a chronic infection,** with measurable levels of hepatitis C virus RNA (HCV RNA) for more than 6 months.

Chronic hepatitis C can lead to cirrhosis and hepatocellular carcinoma. Disease activity can be monitored by serial measurements of HCV RNA along with transaminases levels. Chronic hepatitis C can be treated with antiviral therapy, using ribavirin and/or interferon, but results are variable and there is no cure. There is currently no vaccination available for hepatitis C.

Alcohol abuse can cause an acute, severe hepatitis, or chronic fatty liver, hepatitis, and cirrhosis. Alcohol leads to a conjugated hyperbilirubinemia by impairing bile acid secretion and uptake. **Transaminase levels from alcohol abuse typically show the aspartate aminotransferase (AST) being elevated out of proportion to the alanine aminotransferase (ALT);** viral hepatitis usually causes greater elevations of the ALT (see Case 41 for a more thorough discussion of alcohol abuse).

Physical obstructions of bile drainage can also cause conjugated hyper-bilirubinemia. Common etiologies include gallstones that become impacted in the bile ducts, postoperative biliary strictures or extrinsic compression of the bile ducts by tumors, such as pancreatic cancer. Imaging of the bile system with ultrasound, computed tomography (CT) scan, or magnetic resonance imaging (MRI) is usually diagnostic. Endoscopic retrograde cholangiopancre-atography (ERCP) can be diagnostic and, in some cases, therapeutic.

Comprehension Questions

[46.1] A 32-year-old male with no significant medical history comes in for evaluation of an elevated bilirubin level that was detected on blood work required for a preemployment physical. The bilirubin level was 1.5 mg/dL (normal up to 1.0 mg/dL) with an elevated unconjugated component. He feels fine, takes no medications, occasionally drinks a beer, and is married and monogamous. His liver enzymes, chemistries, and complete blood count (CBC) are normal. What is the next step in his evaluation?

    A. Reassurance
    B. Counsel on alcohol reduction
    C. Abdominal ultrasound
    D. Hepatitis serologies

[46.2] Six months after diagnosis with an acute infection with hepatitis B, a patient has the following serologic studies: HBsAg negative; anti-HBsAg positive; HBeAg negative; anti-HBcAg positive. What is your interpretation of these results?

A. Chronic active hepatitis B
B. Resolved acute infection
C. Resolved acute infection but contagious to sexual contacts
D. Resolved infection but at risk for reinfection in the future

[46.3] Which of the following is most likely to cause an unconjugated hyper-bilirubinemia?

A. Hepatitis A
B. Gallstone in the common bile duct
C. Chronic alcohol use
D. Spherocytosis

Answers

[46.1] **A.** This is a classic case of Gilbert disease, a benign mild elevation of unconjugated bilirubin. In the face of otherwise normal history, examination, and liver enzymes, no further work-up is indicated.

[46.2] **B.** These serologies are consistent with resolved hepatitis B infection and ongoing immunity. This patient has both negative surface and e antigens, so is not a risk to spread the disease to others.

[46.3] **D.** Hemolytic anemia from spherocytosis or other causes is likely to cause an unconjugated hyperbilirubinemia. All of the other listed options cause a primarily conjugated hyperbilirubinemia.

CLINICAL PEARLS

❖ The acute onset of painless jaundice in a patient older than age 50 years should prompt an examination for pancreatic cancer (malignancy in the head of the pancreas causing compression of the bile ducts).

❖ All pregnant women should be screened for the presence of HBsAg. If positive, treating the newborns with hepatitis B immunoglobulin (HBIg) and vaccination can reduce the risk of vertical transmission.

❖ One of the greatest risks for the development of cirrhosis in those with chronic hepatitis C is alcohol use. Anyone with chronic hepatitis C should be counseled to avoid all alcohol intake.

REFERENCES

Centers for Disease Control and Prevention. Diagnosis and management of food-borne illnesses. MMWR 2004;53(RR04):1–33.

National Institutes of Health. Management of hepatitis C: 2002. Consensus statement. Available at: http://consensus.nih.gov/2002/2002hepatitisC2002116html.htm.

Roche SP, Kobos R. Jaundice in the adult patient. Am Fam Physician 2004;69: 299–304.

Workowski KA, Levine WC. Sexually transmitted diseases treatment guidelines, 2002. MMWR 2002;51(RR06):1–80.

A 52-year-old man presents to the office with approximately 2 weeks of upper abdominal pain. His symptoms are difficult for him to describe, but include some "discomfort" in the epigastric region that comes and goes. He has had some "heartburn" and nausea, but no vomiting or diarrhea. He has noticed that his stool looks darker than it used to, but he has not seen any blood. He feels full quickly after eating. He tried taking some over-the-counter antacid, which helps a little, but not much. His only other medication is an over-the-counter nonsteroidal antiinflammatory drug (NSAID) that he takes "once or twice" a day because of arthritis in his knees. He does not smoke cigarettes or drink alcohol. On examination, he is pale appearing, but in no acute discomfort. He is afebrile, his blood pressure is 120/80 mm Hg, his pulse is 95 beats/min, and his respiratory rate is 14 breaths/min. Head, ears, eyes, nose, and throat (HEENT) examination is notable only for pale conjunctiva. Cardiac and pulmonary examinations are normal. His abdomen has normoactive bowel sounds and tenderness in the epigastrium. There is no mass, rebound, or guarding. Rectal examination reveals normal tone, no masses, and dark black stool that is strongly heme positive. The remainder of his examination is unremarkable.

◆ **What is the most likely diagnosis?**

◆ **What evaluation and treatment is indicated at this point?**

◆ **What can be done to reduce the risk of recurrence of this problem?**

ANSWERS TO CASE 47: Peptic Ulcer Disease

Summary: A 52-year-old male presents with vague upper abdominal discomfort, nausea and early satiety. He is a daily NSAID user. He appears pale on examination, suggesting that he may be anemic. He has mild abdominal tenderness and melanotic stool on examination.

◆ **Most likely diagnosis:** Bleeding peptic ulcer

◆ **Evaluation and treatment at this point:** A stat complete blood count (CBC), discontinuation of his NSAID, upper GI endoscopy, and testing for *Helicobacter pylori*. He should be treated with a proton pump inhibitor (PPI) and antibiotics for *H. pylori*, if tests confirm its presence. He may need a blood transfusion (dependent on the result of his CBC). He will also require evaluation with a colonoscopy.

◆ **Reduce risk of recurrence by:** Discontinuation and avoidance of NSAID or, if unable to completely discontinue, use of PPI with the NSAID; eradication of *H. pylori.*

Analysis

Objectives

1. Learn the risk factors for the development of peptic ulcer disease (PUD).
2. Know how to diagnose and treat peptic ulcers.
3. Understand the role of *H. pylori* in PUD, including methods for testing for and treatment of PUD.
4. Know the "alarm symptoms" for which endoscopy is indicated.

Considerations

Dyspepsia is defined as chronic or recurrent upper abdominal pain or discomfort. Approximately 10% of dyspepsia is caused by peptic ulcer disease. Other common causes include gastroesophageal reflux disease (GERD) and functional dyspepsia. The diagnostic work-up and treatment of patients with dyspepsia varies and is dependent on the age of the patient, the presenting symptoms and signs, and the response to the initial management offered.

Early diagnostic **endoscopy should be considered for patients with new-onset dyspepsia who are older than age 55 years or who have symptoms that may be associated with upper GI malignancy** (Table 47–1). For those younger than age 55 years and without alarm symptoms, testing for *H. pylori,* either by urea breath test or stool antigen testing, is recommended. For those who test positive, treating the *H. pylori* followed by acid-suppression therapy is indicated. For persons who test negative, empiric therapy with a PPI for 4–8 weeks

Table 47–1

"ALARM" SYMPTOMS FOR WHICH EARLY UPPER GI ENDOSCOPY
IS RECOMMENDED

- Weight loss
- Progressive dysphagia
- Recurrent vomiting
- Gastrointestinal bleeding
- Family history of cancer

is a cost-effective intervention. Endoscopy or reconsideration of the diagnosis should be considered for those who continue to be symptomatic following these interventions.

APPROACH TO PEPTIC ULCER DISEASE

PUD is a term used to encompass both duodenal and gastric ulcers. **Duodenal ulcers are more prevalent overall, whereas gastric ulcers are more common in NSAID users.** Risk factors for the development of PUD include *H. pylori* infection, the use of an NSAID, cigarette smoking, and personal or family history of PUD. Black and Hispanic populations have a higher likelihood of developing PUD as well. The lifetime risk of developing PUD in the United States is approximately 10%.

History and Examination

Dyspepsia symptoms are common and there is significant overlap between the symptoms of PUD, GERD, and functional dyspepsia. Patients with symptoms primarily of heartburn or acid regurgitation are more likely to have GERD. **Classic symptoms associated with PUD include epigastric abdominal pain that is improved with the ingestion of food, or pain that develops a few hours after eating.** Nocturnal symptoms are also common with PUD. The symptoms are often gradual in onset and present for weeks or months. Patients often self-medicate with over-the-counter antacid medications, which usually provide some relief, prior to presenting to the physician.

The examination should both attempt to confirm your suspicion of PUD and rule out other diagnoses that may present with abdominal pain. PUD often will only have the examination finding of epigastric tenderness. The presence of GI bleeding may be documented by stool occult blood testing; however, the bleeding from PUD may be episodic and a negative single office occult blood test does not completely rule out bleeding. Signs of anemia (pale conjunctiva or skin, tachycardia, hypotension, orthostasis) should be evaluated and managed as needed.

Many potential diagnoses must be considered in your differential. Finding right upper quadrant tenderness may suggest gallbladder or biliary disease.

Appendicitis, while classically causing right lower quadrant pain, may present with only vague abdominal symptoms (especially with a retrocecal appendix). Epigastric pain radiating to the back and associated with nausea and vomiting may be pancreatitis. Pelvic infections, pelvic pathology, and even ectopic pregnancy must be considered as possibilities in women. Myocardial ischemia should be considered in those at risk.

Helicobacter pylori

H. pylori is a corkscrew-shaped Gram-negative bacillus that is the causative agent of most non–NSAID-related ulcers. *H. pylori* is also associated with the development of gastric cancer. The **presence of the organism is associated with a 5–7 times increased risk of the development of PUD.** How *H. pylori* is transmitted is not entirely understood.

Several tests are available to diagnose infections with *H. pylori*. **Serologic testing for anti-*H. pylori* antibodies** is widely available, inexpensive, and noninvasive. It is highly sensitive for the presence of a history of infection but cannot distinguish an active infection from a treated infection.

Active infection can be confirmed by **urea breath testing.** This test is performed by having the patient ingest a carbon-labeled urea compound, which is then metabolized by urease from the *H. pylori* organism. The labeled CO_2 released by this process is measured in exhaled breath. This test is highly sensitive and specific, but is limited by availability and expense.

During endoscopy, *H. pylori* testing can occur on a **biopsy specimen.** The bacterium can either be visualized microscopically using a variety of staining methods, cultured, or detected by rapid testing of the specimen. Endoscopy also allows for direct visualization of ulcers and evaluation for the presence of malignancy or other pathology in the esophagus, stomach, or duodenum. Endoscopy is invasive and expensive, limiting its utility to certain clinical situations.

Management of Suspected PUD

After the initial history and physical examination, focused testing appropriate to evaluate the suspected clinical syndromes should be ordered. A CBC should be drawn to evaluate for anemia, even when stool studies are negative for occult blood. A patient who has been vomiting or not eating should have basic chemistry studies performed. Liver enzymes, amylase, and lipase tests may be ordered when biliary or pancreatic disease is suspected. An EKG can be done if cardiac disease is a consideration, and an upright chest x-ray is the test of choice for possible abdominal organ perforation. Abdominal ultrasonography is indicated when gallstones are suspected. A pregnancy test should be ordered on reproductive-age women, and cervical cultures performed if infection is suspected.

Patients with significant anemia, hemodynamic instability (hypotension, tachycardia, orthostasis) or suspected acute abdomen should be hospitalized. IV rehydration and blood transfusion should be performed when necessary. Urgent surgical evaluation should be obtained if an acute abdomen is present.

Dyspepsia in patients younger than age 55 years with no alarm symptoms can be managed with a noninvasive *H. pylori* "test-and-treat" protocol. A **test for an active *H. pylori* infection (urea breath test, presence of *H. pylori* antigens in stool) should be performed.** If positive, treatment to eradicate the infection, along with a PPI to suppress acid production, should be prescribed (Table 47–2 lists *H. pylori* treatment regimens). Those with no evidence of active infection can be treated with acid suppression alone for 4–6 weeks. If symptoms resolve, no further testing is indicated. Along with treatment, offending agents, such as NSAIDs and tobacco, should be discontinued.

Patients older than age 55 years or with alarm symptoms should be referred for upper GI endoscopy to exclude the possibility of malignancy. Endoscopy is preferred over radiologic procedures because of better visualization and because of the ability to perform biopsy. Endoscopy also can be therapeutic, if a source of bleeding can be identified and cauterized. **A patient who is older than age 50 years and who has blood in the stool should also undergo a colonoscopy regardless of the upper endoscopic findings,** to ensure that there is not a colon cancer also contributing to the GI blood loss.

Table 47–2

FOOD AND DRUG ADMINISTRATION-APPROVED TREATMENT REGIMENS FOR *H. PYLORI* INFECTION

Omeprazole 40 mg QD and clarithromycin 500 mg TID for 2 weeks, then omeprazole 20 mg daily for 2 weeks
Ranitidine bismuth citrate (RBC) 400 mg BID and clarithromycin 500 mg TID for 2 weeks, then RBC 400 mg BID for 2 weeks
Bismuth subsalicylate 525 mg QID and metronidazole 250 mg QID and tetracycline 500 mg QID for 2 weeks and H_2-receptor blocker as directed for 4 weeks
Lansoprazole 30 mg BID and amoxicillin 1 g BID and clarithromycin 500 mg TID for 10 days
Lansoprazole 30 mg TID and amoxicillin 1 g TID for 2 weeks (only use if allergic to clarithromycin or if infection known resistant to clarithromycin)
RBC 400 mg BID and clarithromycin 500 mg BID for 2 weeks, then RBC 400 mg BID for 2 weeks
Omeprazole 20 mg BID and clarithromycin 500 mg BID and amoxicillin 1 g BID for 10 days
Lansoprazole 30 mg BID and clarithromycin 500 mg BID and amoxicillin 1 g BID for 10 days

Information from Centers for Disease Control and Prevention, available at: www.cdc.gov/ulcer/md.htm#fda.

Surgical intervention should be considered for peptic ulcers that are intractable, for hemorrhage that cannot be controlled, for perforation, and for obstruction.

Comprehension Questions

[47.1] A 30-year-old asymptomatic woman comes to you for advice. She attended a health fair where she tested positive for *H. pylori* on a blood test. What can you tell her about the result of this test?

  A. She may or may not have an *H. pylori* infection.
  B. She probably has a peptic ulcer.
  C. She has an *H. pylori* infection but may or may not have an ulcer.
  D. She should be treated immediately for *H. pylori*.

[47.2] A 62-year-old man is found to be anemic and has a gastric ulcer, which was diagnosed on upper GI endoscopy. A biopsy and testing confirm an *H. pylori* infection. What further testing is indicated at this time?

  A. Upper GI radiographic series with small bowel follow through
  B. Abdominal ultrasound
  C. Colonoscopy
  D. Urea breath test

[47.3] A 41-year-old male presents for evaluation of upper GI discomfort that he's had for about 2 months. He has had no blood in his stool, no vomiting, and no dysphagia. He has lost about 10 lb. Which of the following is most appropriate?

  A. *H. pylori* "test and treat"
  B. Empiric therapy for *H. pylori*
  C. Admission to the hospital
  D. Referral for endoscopy

Answers

[47.1] **A.** *H. pylori* blood tests are testing for anti-*H. pylori* antibodies. They cannot distinguish active infections from old infections nor can they diagnose the presence of ulcers. Treating a positive serum test in an asymptomatic person is not indicated.

[47.2] **C.** The presence of blood in the stool or anemia in a patient older than age 50 years, even when an ulcer is found, is an indication for colonoscopy, as this may also represent a presentation of a concomitant colon cancer. An urea breath test may be beneficial after completion of treatment to confirm eradication of the infection.

[47.3] **D.** This patient presents with the alarm symptom of weight loss. He should be referred for early endoscopy.

CLINICAL PEARLS

❖ Persons who require long-term NSAID therapy may benefit from testing for active *H. pylori* infection, followed by eradication, if positive, as this may lower their risk of developing an ulcer. PPI therapy, along with the NSAID, can also lower the risk.

❖ Commonly held beliefs, such as ulcers being caused by stress or spicy foods, are incorrect. The vast majority of ulcers are caused by *H. pylori* and NSAIDs.

REFERENCES

Graham DY, Rakel RE, Fendrick AM, et al. Symposium on peptic ulcer disease. Postgrad Med 1999;105(3);93–137.

Talley NJ. American Gastroenterological Association medical position statement: evaluation of dyspepsia. Gastroenterology 2005;129(5):1753–1755.

Townsend CM, Beachamp RD, Evers BM, et al. Sabiston textbook of surgery. 17th ed. Philadelphia: WB Saunders, 2004:1289.

An 18-month-old girl is brought to the office by her mother for an acute visit because of a rash. She had a fever for the past 3 days, along with some mild respiratory symptoms. She was given acetaminophen for the fever but no other medication. The fever has gone down in the past day, but today she developed a rash. The rash came up suddenly, starting on the trunk, and spreading to the extremities. The child has no significant medical history and no known ill contacts, although she attends daycare 3 days a week. On examination, she is mildly fussy but easily consolable in her mother's lap. She has a noticeable erythematous rash of small macules and papules that blanch on palpation. The remainder of her examination is normal.

◆ **What is the most likely diagnosis?**

◆ **What is the most likely cause of this illness?**

◆ **What is the appropriate treatment?**

ANSWERS TO CASE 48: Fever and Rash

Summary: An 18-month-old girl is brought in for evaluation of a rapidly spreading rash that started after 3 days of fever. She has diffuse, blanching, erythematous macules, and papules but otherwise appears well.

◆ **Most likely diagnosis:** Roseola

◆ **Most likely cause of the illness:** Human herpes virus 6

◆ **Treatment:** Supportive only, as the rash is likely to resolve in 24–48 hours

Analysis

Objectives

1. Be able to identify common rashes associated with viral infections in children.
2. Know the appropriate management of febrile illness associated with rashes in children.

Considerations

Febrile illness and rashes are extremely common presentations in family medicine and pediatric offices. Most of the time these presentations represent mild, self-limited illness that requires no specific therapy. However, some of these presentations will represent serious, or even life-threatening, infections that need urgent interventions.

Rashes associated with fever may be caused by viruses, bacteria, spirochetes, or undetermined causes. History should attempt to identify any exposures that may cause these syndromes. Specific information that may be helpful include the duration of the illness, other associated symptoms, contact with any other ill person, history of recent travel, use of medications or exposure to animals and insects (e.g., ticks). A review of immunization status is critical, as many vaccine preventable diseases can cause fever and rash. **Immunization does not guarantee immunity** but may result in a less-severe presentation of the disease.

Physical examination should include thorough general and skin examinations. Examination findings can both lead to a specific diagnosis and identify complications of the causative agent. For example, the presence of exudative pharyngitis along with fever and rash may suggest scarlet fever caused by a group A streptococcus infection while an abnormal lung examination in a patient with crops of vesicles of different ages may lead to a diagnosis of varicella (chicken pox) complicated by pneumonitis.

The ability to accurately describe skin lesions is necessary for documentation purposes. It is also important when you are not certain what the diagnosis is. Knowing the definitions of macules, papules, pustules, and the like, will make it much easier and more accurate to look for information in a textbook or journal or when you discuss a case with a colleague or consultant. The better the information that you can provide, the more likely you are to get correct information in return. See Case 13 for definitions of many of the terms used to describe common skin lesions.

APPROACH TO FEVER AND RASH

Definitions

Enanthem: An eruption on a mucous membrane as a symptom of a disease.
Exanthem: An eruption on the skin as a symptom of a disease.

Common Viral Infections

Roseola

Human herpes virus 6 is a ubiquitous virus that infects most children before the age of 3 years, although most infections are asymptomatic. The virus has an incubation period of 1–2 weeks and causes an illness associated with fever and mild respiratory symptoms, which tends to last for no longer than 5 days. **Following defervescence, a characteristic rash appears suddenly.** It is an erythematous maculopapular eruption that starts on the trunk and spreads rapidly to the extremities, with sparing of the face. The rash tends to disappear in 1–2 days. The diagnosis is primarily clinical, based on the history and examination. Because of the short-lived nature of the disease, no treatment is usually required other than reassurance.

Varicella

The varicella zoster virus is a highly contagious virus that causes two clinical syndromes. **Chickenpox** is the more common childhood infection. A typical case of chickenpox includes a fever and a rash, which tends to develop in clusters. The initial exanthem is often papules or **vesicles on an erythematous base,** described as "dewdrops on a rose petal." The vesicles then progress to shallow, crusted erosions. Patients may also develop enanthems, with lesions on the oral, nasal, or gastrointestinal mucosa. In rare cases, serious complications may develop, which include encephalitis, meningitis, and pneumonitis. The diagnosis is usually clinical, but may be confirmed with Tzanck smear or identification of the virus on DNA probe testing. Antiviral therapy using acyclovir, valacyclovir, or famciclovir may shorten the course of the illness if started within 72 hours of onset. Varicella vaccination is now universally recommended at age 12–18 months and has significantly reduced the incidence of childhood chickenpox.

   Shingles is a reactivation of the varicella virus, which can remain dormant in a dorsal root ganglion following the initial infection. The reactivated virus causes a vesicular eruption, usually along a single dermatome and not crossing the midline. The reaction can occur at any age, but is more common in the elderly or immunosuppressed. The rash can be extremely painful and can result in a neuralgia that lasts long after resolution of the rash. Antiviral therapy started within 72 hours of the rash may reduce the incidence of the postherpetic neuralgia.

Erythema Infectiosum

Parvovirus B19 causes a characteristic syndrome known as erythema infectiosum or **fifth disease.** This virus tends to infect children younger than 10 years of age and occurs most commonly in the winter or spring. The rash usually starts as confluent erythematous macules on the face, which usually spares the nose and periorbital regions. This gives the classic **"slapped cheek" appearance** that is commonly diagnostic of the infection. The facial rash lasts for 2–4 days, followed by lacy, pruritic exanthem on the trunk and extremities that usually lasts for 1–2 weeks, but can have a relapsing course for several months. Parvovirus B19 tends to cause a more severe illness, with rheumatic complaints such as arthritis. The virus can be transmitted from mother to fetus during pregnancy, resulting in fetal hydrops and pregnancy loss.

Common Bacterial Infections

Group A β-Hemolytic Streptococcus

Group A β-hemolytic *Streptococcus* (GAS) is associated with numerous diseases, particularly in children. It is the causative agent of streptococcal pharyngitis and its complications, which include rheumatic fever and glomerulonephritis. It can also cause a cellulitis of the skin.

The rash of **scarlet fever** usually starts about 2 days after the onset of sore throat. The rash consists of punctate, raised, erythematous eruptions that can become confluent and feel like sandpaper. The rash tends to start on the upper trunk and spreads to the rest of the trunk and the extremities. The exanthem can also be associated with an enanthem, causing the appearance of a "strawberry tongue." The rash fades and desquamation occurs 4–5 days after the first appearance of the rash.

GAS infections can be confirmed by rapid antigen testing or culture from a throat swab. The first-line treatment for GAS infections is penicillin, with cephalosporins or macrolides as alternatives in the penicillin allergic.

Neisseria Meningitidis

The **meningococcus causes an acute, life-threatening infection,** often associated with a rash. Meningococcemia can cause a severe illness with high fevers, hypotension, and altered mental status. Most people with meningococcemia progress to develop frank meningitis, with its associated signs of meningeal irritation. The **rash**

of meningococcemia often starts as an erythematous maculopapular eruption that progresses to form petechiae.

Someone with suspected meningococcemia should be immediately hospitalized, usually in the intensive care unit. The ABCs (Airway, Breathing, and Circulation) should be urgently evaluated, blood and cerebrospinal fluid cultures collected, and empiric antibiotic therapy instituted. A common regimen includes vancomycin and ceftriaxone, with adjustments based on culture results. A meningococcal vaccine is now recommended for routine childhood immunization and also should be offered to patients at risk for the disease (asplenic, those living in dormitories or military barracks). Close contacts of someone with meningococcal infection should be offered prophylaxis with rifampin.

Tick-borne Diseases

Rocky Mountain Spotted Fever

Rocky Mountain spotted fever (RMSF) is an acute, life-threatening infection caused by the organism *Rickettsia rickettsii*, which is transmitted via a tick bite. The infection occurs more often in the summer months, when people are more likely to be outdoors. The illness causes acute fever, headache, myalgia, and fatigue. The **classic exanthem is a macular, papular, or petechial eruption that starts on the wrists and ankles.** Laboratory tests often show a low white blood cell count, low platelet count, and elevated liver enzymes. The diagnosis is confirmed with serology, but this is not helpful in the acute setting. Suspected RMSF should be treated empirically with doxycycline.

Lyme Disease

Lyme disease is endemic in many areas of the United States, including New England and the Mid-Atlantic regions. The causative spirochete, *Borrelia burgdorferi,* is transmitted via bite of the *Ixodes* tick. Because the tick is very small, infected persons are often unaware of a history of a tick bite. The characteristic rash, **erythema migrans,** develops 3–30 days following infection. The exanthema is typically an expanding erythematous macule with central clearing, often described as appearing like a "bull's-eye." In this stage of disease, treatment with oral doxycycline can prevent progression to the more serious complications of Lyme disease, including arthritis, carditis, and complete heart block. The diagnosis can be confirmed with serologic studies.

Comprehension Questions

[48.1] A 6-year-old is brought to your office with a fever and upper respiratory symptoms. On examination, he is noted to have a low-grade fever, a normal general examination, and an erythematous macular eruption on his cheeks. Which of the following is the most likely causative organism?

    A. Varicella zoster virus
    B. Parvovirus B19
    C. Human herpes virus 6
    D. Rubella virus

[48.2] A 10-year-old is found to have an exudative pharyngitis and a fine, sandpapery eruption on his trunk. He is allergic to no medications. Which of the following is the most appropriate first-line treatment?

    A. Doxycycline
    B. Vancomycin and ceftriaxone
    C. Erythromycin
    D. Penicillin

[48.3] You are called to see a 16-year-old in the emergency department. His parents say that he acutely developed fever, chills, and rash. He has been confused and not answering their questions. On examination he is toxically ill appearing, and is febrile, tachycardic, and hypotensive. He is noted to have a diffuse petechial rash. What is the most likely diagnosis?

    A. Meningococcemia
    B. Rocky Mountain spotted fever
    C. Scarlet fever
    D. Lyme disease

Answers

[48.1] **B.** Erythema infectiosum, fifth disease, characteristically causes the "slapped cheek" appearance described in this question. It is caused by parvovirus B19.

[48.2] **D.** Scarlet fever, caused by GAS infection, should be treated with penicillin in those who are not allergic to it. A macrolide, like erythromycin, is an alternative for use by the penicillin-allergic patient.

[48.3] **A.** This acute, severe illness is consistent with meningococcemia. This adolescent should be admitted to the ICU, his hypotension aggressively managed, and antibiotics started. His family should receive prophylactic therapy with rifampin.

CLINICAL PEARLS

❖   Shingles that approaches the eye, because of a reactivation involving
the trigeminal nerve, should be evaluated by an ophthalmologist.
A clue that the eye may become involved is seeing characteristic
lesions approaching the tip of the nose.

❖   Many vaccine-preventable illnesses, including measles, rubella, and
varicella, have characteristic rashes associated with them. Always
get a vaccination history on children presenting with fever and rash.
Also, consider the possibility that immigrants from other countries
may not be vaccinated if they present with similar symptoms.

REFERENCES

McKinnon HD, Howard T. Evaluating the febrile patient with a rash. Am Fam
    Physician 2000;62:804–816.
Scott LA, Stone MS. Viral exanthems. Dermatol Online 2003;9(3):4.

A 32-year-old woman presents for evaluation of a lump that she noticed in her right breast on a routine self-examination. She says that she doesn't examine herself often, but that she thinks that this lump is new. She has not had any nipple discharge and has no breast pain, although the lump is a bit tender. She has never noticed any masses before and has never had a mammogram. She has no history of breast diseases and has never had a biopsy. There is no history of breast cancer in the family. She takes oral contraceptive pills regularly, but no other medications. She does not smoke cigarettes or drink alcohol. She has never been pregnant. On examination, she is a well-appearing, but somewhat anxious, thin female. Her vital signs are within normal limits. Her general physical examination is normal. Examination of her breasts reveals no skin dimpling or retraction and no nipple discharge. In the lower outer quadrant of the right breast there is a 2-cm, firm, well-circumscribed, movable mass that is mildly tender. No other masses are felt, but the breast tissue is noted to be firm and glandular throughout. No axillary, supraclavicular, or cervical lymphadenopathy is appreciated.

 What is the most likely diagnosis of this breast lesion?

 What is the next step in evaluation?

 What is the recommended follow-up for this patient?

ANSWERS TO CASE 49: Breast Diseases

Summary: A 32-year-old woman presents for evaluation of a lump in her right breast that she found on a breast self-examination (BSE). The lump is found to be 2 cm in size, firm, and mobile. No adenopathy is noted.

◆ **Most likely diagnosis:** Breast cyst

◆ **Next step in evaluation:** Needle aspiration of cyst

◆ **Follow-up:** If aspiration of the cyst results in complete resolution of the mass, and if the fluid is clear/yellow, follow-up clinical examination in 1–2 months to ensure no recurrence; if aspiration does not make the mass disappear, if the fluid is bloody, or if the lesion recurs, further evaluation with biopsy of the lesion is indicated.

Analysis

Objectives

1. Learn how to work-up a breast mass.
2. Know the risk factors for breast cancer.
3. Know how to manage benign breast diseases.

Considerations

A palpable breast mass is a potentially frightening finding for a woman. The media has widely disseminated the statistic that 1 in 8 women will have breast cancer in their lifetime. Consequently, the evaluation of the breast mass is designed to answer the one question that is on the patient's mind, whether she says it or not: Is this lump breast cancer? Fortunately, most palpable breast masses are not cancerous. Unfortunately, a definitive determination of whether a lesion is benign or malignant cannot be made by history and physical examination findings only.

Certain factors have been identified as increasing a woman's risk of breast cancer. A family history of breast cancer in a first-degree relative (parent, sibling), especially if the cancer occurred in a premenopausal woman and was bilateral, is associated with an increased risk. Early age at menarche (<12 years), late age of menopause (>55 years), and nulliparity or first live birth after the age of 30 years are also associated with higher risks. The use of hormones, either estrogen alone or combined with progesterone, are considered to confer higher risks, although recent studies raise some questions and further information is needed. Lifestyle considerations, including obesity, physical inactivity, and alcohol use (>3 drinks per day), also are identified risk factors. Finally, a history of previous breast disease, especially biopsies showing atypical hyperplasia, carcinoma in situ, or prior breast cancer, are associated with increased risks.

In the case presented, there are several pieces of information presented that lead toward a likelihood of a benign process. Breast cancer can occur at any age, but approximately 70% of breast cancers occur in women older than age 50 years. You can never overlook the possibility of malignancy in a woman who is in her 30s, but the possibility of cancer is lower in her than in an older woman. The characteristics of the lesion are also more consistent with a benign, probably cystic, process. It is described as well-circumscribed, firm, mobile, tender, and with no overlying skin changes. Lesions that are hard, fixed in place, nontender, have indistinct borders, or have overlying skin dimpling/retraction are more suggestive of cancer. Nevertheless, no individual characteristic on examination is diagnostic and an appropriate evaluation is necessary.

APPROACH TO DISEASES OF THE BREAST

Palpable Breast Mass

Following a complete history, with an emphasis on factors that may confer an increased risk of cancer, a careful examination of both breasts should be performed. The breast examination should include a visual inspection for skin changes, dimpling, retraction, and asymmetry, and should note the presence and quality of any nipple discharge (color, presence of blood, etc.).

Palpatory examination should be performed in a systematic manner to include all quadrants of the breast, as well as the superficial, intermediate, and deep breast tissue. Specific characteristics of any palpable lumps, including size, location, tenderness, mobility, firmness, and distinction of the mass from the surrounding tissue, should be noted, both to assist in developing a diagnosis and to allow for serial examinations to determine if the mass is changing. The breast examination should also include palpation of the axilla and supraclavicular regions to identify the presence of enlarged lymph nodes.

Whenever possible, the identification of a new breast mass should prompt an immediate **fine-needle aspiration** (FNA). FNA can be both diagnostic and therapeutic. An FNA that identifies fluid that is clear, yellow, or green-tinged and that results in complete resolution of the mass is diagnostic of a benign cyst. In this setting, the fluid can be discarded and no further work-up is necessary. The patient should be seen in follow-up in 4–6 weeks for reexamination to evaluate for recurrence of the lesion.

If the mass does not completely resolve, if the fluid withdrawn is bloody, if no fluid is aspirated, or if the lesion is found to recur on follow-up, further evaluation is indicated. **Diagnostic mammography** is generally the next test to be performed. Along with routine mammographic views, compression and magnification views of the area of the palpable mass are performed so as to better characterize the lesion. **Ultrasonography** can be used as an adjunct to mammography in an effort to determine if the lesion is solid or fluid filled.

Lesions determined to be cystic should be aspirated. Ultrasound guidance assist in this procedure. As above, if clear fluid is removed and the cyst completely resolves, clinical follow-up is all that is needed. **Masses found to be solid or complex (containing both cystic and solid components) should be biopsied.**

Several biopsy techniques are used in practice. FNA can be performed on solid lesions. It is the least invasive and simplest procedure, but also has the highest risk of false-negative or nondiagnostic results. **Core-needle** biopsy and **mammotome** biopsy use larger cutting needles to obtain larger tissue samples. These are usually performed using ultrasound or mammographic guidance by a radiologist or surgeon. These procedures have a higher chance of providing a diagnostic sample but are more invasive and costlier than FNA. Although **surgical excision** is the most invasive and expensive diagnostic method, it is also therapeutic by removing the lesion in question. It is usually reserved for those at high risk or high suspicion for malignancy.

Breast Pain

Breast pain (mastalgia) is the most frequent breast-related complaint for which women present for evaluation. As with the presentation of a breast lump, the patient's primary fear, whether spoken or unspoken, is whether the pain is a manifestation of breast cancer. As such, the evaluation should include a history to evaluate for high breast cancer risk status, a careful breast examination, and a screening mammography in women for whom it is routinely indicated. Any abnormalities found in the primary evaluation should be worked-up as appropriate. **Breast pain is not a common presentation of breast cancer,** particularly when it is bilateral breast pain.

Most breast pain may be categorized as cyclic mastalgia, noncyclic mastalgia, or nonmammary pain. **Cyclic mastalgia** is usually diffuse, bilateral, and related to the woman's menstrual cycle. In some cases, it can be unilateral. **Noncyclic mastalgia** may be continuous or intermittent, but is not associated with the menstrual cycle. It is more commonly unilateral and more prevalent in postmenopausal women. **Nonmammary pain** is breast pain secondary to another etiology. This is often chest wall pain but, sometimes, the underlying cause may be difficult to determine.

Laboratory testing is usually unnecessary in the evaluation of mastalgia, although a pregnancy test should be performed in reproductive-age women. Hormonal contraceptives or hormone replacement therapy may be causes of breast pain and consideration should be given to discontinuation or reduction of estrogen dosages. An appropriately fitted supportive bra and lifestyle changes, such as tobacco cessation, caffeine elimination, and stress reduction techniques, are often successful in alleviating symptoms. **Evening primrose oil** is available over the counter, is well tolerated, and often provides relief. For women with unrelenting pain in spite of the above modifications, **danazol,** an antigonadotropin, is Food and Drug Administration (FDA) approved for the treatment of breast pain, but is relatively expensive and has numerous side effects (hair loss, acne, weight gain, irregular menses).

Nipple Discharge

Nipple discharge is usually caused by a benign process. Nipple discharge that occurs only with nipple stimulation, that is clear, yellow, or green, and that appears from multiple ducts is usually physiologic. This discharge often goes away if efforts are made to reduce nipple stimulation (including ceasing efforts to check to see if the discharge will still occur).

Discharge that is spontaneous, persistent, bloody, from a single duct, and associated with a mass is more likely to represent a pathologic process. In this setting, the most common causes are intraductal papillomas, duct ectasia, cancers, and infections. If the discharge is not obviously bloody, a Hemoccult card can be used to test for occult blood.

Following the initial history and physical examination, mammography should be performed in all women with a spontaneous or bloody discharge, and in any woman in whom routine mammographic evaluation is indicated. Palpable breast masses should be appropriately evaluated. The **treatment of most unilateral, spontaneous, or bloody nipple discharges is surgical excision of the terminal duct** involved. This both resolves the problem and allows for pathologic diagnosis of the problem.

Galactorrhea

Galactorrhea is an inappropriate discharge of breast milk or milky fluid. It is not associated with breast cancer. Galactorrhea may be associated with hypothyroidism, hyperprolactinemia, or the use of certain medications (contraceptives, phenothiazines, others). Offending medications should be discontinued, if possible. Prolactin and thyroid-stimulating hormone levels should be drawn to evaluate for endocrine abnormalities. Imaging of the pituitary with a head computed tomography (CT) scan or magnetic resonance imaging (MRI) is indicated if the prolactin level is elevated, to evaluate for a pituitary adenoma.

Comprehension Questions

[49.1] A 34-year-old woman notes that she has had breast nipple discharge for 2 months. The physician makes an assessment that the circumstances and characteristics are likely associated with a pathologic process. Which of the following characteristics is most concerning?

A. Yellow
B. Bilateral
C. Bloody
D. Present with nipple stimulation

[49.2] Which of the following tests is most appropriate for determination of whether a breast mass is solid or fluid filled?

    A. Palpation of the lesion
    B. Screening mammogram
    C. Diagnostic mammogram
    D. Ultrasound

[49.3] A 52-year-old woman has a palpable breast lump. An attempt at FNA does not result in aspiration of fluid. A mammogram is read as normal. What is the appropriate next step?

    A. Repeat clinical exam in 4–6 weeks
    B. Repeat mammogram routinely in 1 year
    C. Referral for biopsy
    D. Discontinuation of her hormone replacement therapy

Answers

[49.1] **C.** Nipple discharges that are spontaneous, unilateral, persistent, bloody, and associated with a mass are more likely to represent pathologic processes. Most of these are still benign (papilloma, duct ectasia), but evaluation and surgical intervention is usually required.

[49.2] **D.** Ultrasonography is much more sensitive at determining whether a lesion is cystic or solid than the other tests listed.

[49.3] **C.** A biopsy is the next appropriate step in this setting. A negative mammogram is not diagnostic of a benign process and does not rule out the possibility of having a breast cancer. A tissue diagnosis is needed in this setting.

CLINICAL PEARLS

❖ Approximately 1% of breast cancer occurs in men. A new palpable mass in a man's breast should prompt a diagnostic evaluation.

❖ Remember that the question in the mind of just about every woman presenting with a breast-related complaint is, "Do I have breast cancer?" The job of the physician is to both manage the presenting complaint and to answer this question.

REFERENCES

Institute for Clinical Systems Improvement. Diagnosis of breast disease. Bloomington, MN: Institute for Clinical Systems Improvement, 2005:1–51.

Klein S. Evaluation of palpable breast masses. Am Fam Physician 2005;71: 1731–1738.

Morrow M. The evaluation of common breast problems. Am Fam Physician 2000;61: 2371–2378, 2385.

Newman LA, Sabel M. Advances in breast cancer detection and management. Med Clin North Am 2003;87:997–1028.

A 28-year-old nulliparous woman presents for evaluation of irregular menstrual cycles for the past year. Her periods will come only every 2 or 3 months and she has gone as long as 4 months without a period. Currently, she gives a last menstrual period of 11 weeks ago. She says she had menarche at age 13 years and that her cycles have been "mostly" regular, usually occurring every 30 days, but she would miss one here and there. She has never been on hormonal contraception. She does not smoke, does not drink alcohol, and does not exercise. She is sexually active with a single partner and uses condoms for contraception. On review of systems, she reports a 30-lb weight gain in the past 18 months, but otherwise has felt fine. On examination, she is noted to be obese, with a body mass index of 30. Her vitals signs are otherwise normal. She has fine hair growth on her face and a velvety thickening of the skin on her neck. Her general physical examination is normal. A pelvic examination reveals normal external genitalia, no vaginal or cervical discharge, no cervical motion tenderness, and no uterine or adnexal masses.

◆ **What is the most likely diagnosis?**

◆ **What is the first laboratory test that should be performed?**

◆ **What treatment option can be used to regularize her menstrual cycle and prevent unintended pregnancy?**

ANSWERS TO CASE 50: Menstrual Cycle Irregularity

Summary: A 28-year-old woman presents for evaluation of irregular menstrual cycles for the past year. She is obese and noted to have gained 30 lb. She is found to be hirsute and to have acanthosis nigricans. Her pelvic examination is normal.

◆ **Most likely diagnosis:** Anovulatory menstrual cycles secondary to polycystic ovarian syndrome (PCOS)

◆ **Initial laboratory test:** Pregnancy test

◆ **Treatment to normalize cycles and prevent pregnancy:** Oral contraceptive pills

Analysis

Objectives

1. Learn some of the common causes of irregular menstrual cycles.
2. Develop an understanding of a rational work-up of menstrual cycle abnormalities.
3. Learn the management of common menstrual cycle disorders.

Considerations

Menstrual cycles are considered normal if they occur at regular intervals of 21–35 days in length. During their reproductive years, most women will, at some point, have late or missed menstrual cycles. When this occurs on a rare occasion and pregnancy is ruled out, watchful waiting is usually indicated, with resumption of normal menstrual cycles almost always occurring.

The differential diagnosis of persistent menstrual cycle irregularities is broad. In all cases, the initial diagnosis that must be considered in the case of a menstrual cycle change is pregnancy. After pregnancy is excluded, numerous neuroendocrine and genitourinary conditions must be considered.

In a normal (highly simplified) menstrual cycle, estrogen, which is produced by the ovary with regulation by the hypothalamus and pituitary, causes a build up of the endometrial lining of the uterus. After ovulation, the corpus luteum produces progesterone, which compacts the endometrium. If conception of pregnancy does not occur, the production of progesterone abruptly decreases, resulting in sloughing of the endometrium and a menstrual bleed.

In the case presented of an obese, hirsute woman with ongoing weight gain and irregular menses, PCOS should be the initial consideration (after pregnancy). PCOS is a syndrome of insulin resistance and androgen excess. **Anovulation is the menstrual cycle irregularity associated with PCOS.** Without ovulation, there is a failure of luteal production of progesterone, resulting in an absence of normal menstruation. Women with PCOS can have induced menstrual bleeds by providing periodic supplemental progesterone or by using oral contraceptive pills. Lifestyle modification—diet, exercise, weight loss—is necessary to address the underlying insulin resistance. Pharmacotherapy to reduce insulin resistance, including metformin and thiazolidinediones, has been tried in PCOS with varying degrees of success. Infertility associated with PCOS sometimes responds to the use of clomiphene citrate to promote ovulation.

APPROACH TO MENSTRUAL CYCLE IRREGULARITIES

Definitions

Amenorrhea: Absence of menstrual bleeding for 6 or more months when a woman is not pregnant.

Menometrorrhagia: Heavy menstrual flow or prolonged duration of flow occurring at irregular intervals.

Menorrhagia: Excessive menstrual flow, or prolonged duration of flow (>7 days), occurring at regular intervals.

Metrorrhagia: Bleeding occurring at irregular intervals.

Clinical Approach

A thorough history is the initial component of the evaluation of menstrual irregularities. The history of presenting complaint should examine both the specific abnormality that is occurring and when it was first noted. A menstrual calendar can be very valuable in this setting. Associated symptoms, including weight gain or loss, galactorrhea, heat or cold intolerance, and other forms of bleeding should be documented. A complete general health history is necessary. A complete reproductive health history, including age at menarche, history of any previous menstrual cycle abnormalities, medications, contraception, infections, surgeries, and sexual practices along with pregnancies and their outcomes is required. A social history focusing on stressors, substance use, exercise habits, and sexual activity can provide important information.

The general physical examination should attempt to identify medical conditions that can cause menstrual abnormalities. Extremes of body mass index—both overweight and underweight—can affect menstruation. Hirsutism or acne suggests androgen excess. The thyroid should be examined for size, consistency, and the presence of nodules. Skin and hair changes may also occur with thyroid conditions. Breasts should be examined for galactorrhea. Unexplained bruising or easy bleeding may occur with coagulopathies.

The pelvic examination is a critical component. In women having excessive or unusual bleeding, initial efforts should be made to determine whether the blood is coming from the uterus or another anatomic site. Urethral, rectal, vaginal wall, or cervical bleeding can easily be mistaken for menstrual abnormality. Signs of infection should be noted and cultures collected, as cervicitis may predispose to cervical bleeding. A Papanicolaou (Pap) smear should be performed. Bimanual examination should note the size and consistency of the uterus, the presence of any masses or tenderness. The adnexa should also be carefully examined for abnormality.

Abnormal Bleeding Associated with Regular Menstrual Cycles

Menorrhagia with regular intervals between bleeding is suggestive that regular ovulation is occurring. This implies that the endocrine pathways are functioning normally and that the problem may be anatomic within the genital system. **Leiomyomata** (fibroids), especially those that are submucosal in the uterus, are a common cause of this problem. They create an increased endometrial surface area with a resultant increase in menstrual bleeding. **Endometrial polyps** may cause menorrhagia by a similar mechanism. **Coagulopathy,** whether inherited, as a complication of another medical condition (e.g., liver disease) or from medications, is another common cause.

Reduced volume of menstrual bleeding associated with regular ovulation is a less common occurrence. **Asherman syndrome** is a scarring within the uterine cavity caused by trauma from uterine curettage. It can result in reduction in the size of the uterus as the walls become scarred to each other. This may cause minimal or even absent menstruation in the face of normal hormonal function. A scarred and obstructed cervical os can cause a similar picture.

Abnormal Bleeding Associated with Irregular Menstrual Cycles

Bleeding that is unpredictable in terms of timing and flow is known as dysfunctional uterine bleeding (DUB) and implies an abnormality within the hypothalamic–pituitary–ovarian axis. This pattern is common shortly after menarche and as a woman approaches menopause. At other times, it signals anovulation. In this setting, the endometrium is continuously stimulated by estrogen and sloughs off irregularly.

Continuous estrogen stimulation can also lead to endometrial hyperplasia and endometrial carcinoma. Risk factors for endometrial carcinoma include a history of anovulatory menstrual cycles, obesity, nulliparity, older than age 35 years, the use of tamoxifen, or of unopposed exogenous estrogen.

The **evaluation of a woman with DUB is dependent on age and risk factors.** In the period after menarche, watchful waiting is usually indicated, with correction of the problem usually occurring within 1–2 years. In women younger than the age of 35 years who are not at increased risk of endometrial cancer, treatment may be offered without work-up beyond the history and physical examination.

Further evaluation is indicated for women older than age 35 years, women of any age who have identified risk factors for endometrial cancer, women younger than age 35 years with continued symptoms in spite of treatment, and postmenopausal women with uterine bleeding. The work-up involved typically includes imaging of the pelvic organs with an ultrasound and sampling of the endometrial tissue. **Transvaginal pelvic ultrasound** provides information on uterine size and masses, and can assess the thickness of the endometrium, which correlates with the risk of hyperplasia. An **endometrial biopsy** can be performed quickly and easily in the office setting, using a thin, disposable, sampling device. The combination of sonographic measurement of endometrial thickness and endometrial biopsy is highly sensitive for the diagnosis of endometrial cancer. **Hysteroscopy** (endoscopic evaluation of the uterine cavity) can directly visualize endometrial masses, polyps, or other abnormalities, and can lead to directed biopsy. It is often performed with **dilation and curettage** (D&C), which sharply removes almost the entire endometrial lining for diagnostic and therapeutic purposes.

When the work-up does not reveal malignancy, **anovulatory bleeding is usually responsive to treatment with either combined estrogen and progestin oral contraceptives (OCPs) or progestin alone.** A progestin can be given for 7–10 days with a subsequent withdrawal bleed expected to occur within a week following the completion of the course. Both of these regimens reduce the risk of developing endometrial hyperplasia and carcinoma. When medical treatments fail, or when symptoms are severe, surgical options may be required. Hysterectomy provides definitive treatment and is necessary in the case of a malignancy. Endometrial ablative procedures are also available and widely used.

Comprehension Questions

[50.1] A 42-year-old woman presents for evaluation of irregular menstrual bleeding for a year. She has had painless vaginal bleeding in various amounts at various times of the month. She is on no medications and has no significant medical history. Her examination reveals her uterus to be slightly enlarged, but without masses or tenderness. The remainder of her examination is normal. A pregnancy test is negative. What is the most appropriate next diagnostic step?

A. D&C
B. Endometrial biopsy in the office
C. Empiric therapy with oral contraceptive pills
D. Hysteroscopy

[50.2] A 28-year-old woman has not had a period since she had a D&C for a missed abortion 8 months ago. Which of the following is the most likely reason for this?

A. Scarring from the D&C
B. Undiagnosed uterine perforation from the D&C
C. Premature menopause
D. Use of hormonal contraceptives following the D&C

[50.3] A 40-year-old woman complains of increased bleeding and cramping with her menstrual cycles that has become worse over the course of the past year. Her cycles remain regular. On examination, her uterus is enlarged, but no focal masses or tenderness is felt. What is the most likely diagnosis?

    A. Uterine leiomyoma
    B. Endometrial carcinoma
    C. Anovulatory bleeding
    D. Bleeding dyscrasia

Answers

[50.1] **B.** An endometrial biopsy can be performed in the office at the time of the visit, once pregnancy is excluded. The procedure is quick, safe, and relatively simple. This should be followed by a transvaginal ultrasound. D&C, hysteroscopy, and treatment with contraceptive pills may be indicated later in the process of evaluation and management.

[50.2] **A.** This patient likely has Asherman syndrome, that is, scarring that is resulting in an ablation of the uterine cavity and preventing the endometrial lining from developing. Treatment of this problem is surgical.

[50.3] **A.** Uterine leiomyomata (fibroids) is the most likely, and most common, cause of menorrhagia in this setting. The regularity of her cycles suggests that she is having ovulatory cycles. Although bleeding dyscrasia is possible, it is much less common than fibroids and would not account for the large, firm uterus on examination.

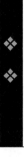

CLINICAL PEARLS

❖ The first test performed on a woman with menstrual cycle irregularities should be a pregnancy test.

❖ A history of anovulatory cycles does not confer absolute protection against pregnancy. Ovulation may occur intermittently and irregularly. If the woman does not want to become pregnant, she should be counseled on contraceptive options.

REFERENCES

Albers JR, Hull SK, Wesley RM. Abnormal uterine bleeding. Am Fam Physician 2004;69:1915–1926, 1931–1932.

Carr BR, Bradshaw KD. Disorders of the ovary and female reproductive tract. In: Kasper DL, Braunwald E, Fauci AS, et al (eds). Harrison's principles of internal medicine. 16th ed. New York: McGraw-Hill, 2005. Accessed online at: www.accessmedicine.com/resourceTOC.aspx?resourceID=4

A 30-year-old woman presents to your office with the chief complaint of a "yeast infection that I can't seem to shake." She also has noticed that she has been urinating more frequently, but thinks that it is related to her yeast infection. Over the last several years she has noticed that she has gained more than 40 lb. She has tried numerous diets, most recently a low-carbohydrate, high-fat diet. The patient's only other pertinent history is that she was told to watch her diet during pregnancy because of excessive weight gain. Her baby had to be delivered by cesarean because he weighed more than 9 lb. Her family history is not known, as she was adopted. On physical examination, her blood pressure is 138/88 mm Hg, her pulse is 72 beats/min, and her respiratory rate is 16 breaths/min. Her height is 65 inches and her weight is 190 lb (body mass index [BMI] = 31.6). Her physical examination reveals darkened skin that appears to be thickened on the back of her neck and moist, reddened skin beneath her breasts. Her pelvic examination reveals a thick, white, vaginal discharge. A wet preparation from the vaginal discharge reveals branching hyphae consistent with *Candida*. A urine dipstick is performed that is negative for leukocyte esterase, nitrites, protein, and glucose.

◆ **What is the most likely primary diagnosis for this patient?**

◆ **What physical findings does she have that are suggestive of the diagnosis and have implications for management?**

◆ **What diagnostic studies should be ordered at this time?**

ANSWERS TO CASE 51: Diabetes Mellitus

Summary: A 30-year-old obese woman presents with a difficult-to-treat yeast infection and polyuria. She has gained 40 lb in spite of her effort to lose weight. She has a history of significant weight gain and having been told to "watch her diet" during a pregnancy. On examination she is found to have a BMI of 31.6, acanthosis nigricans, candidal vaginitis ,but a negative urine dip.

◆ **Most likely diagnosis:** Type 2 diabetes mellitus

◆ **Significant physical findings:** Obesity, acanthosis nigricans, blood pressure that is elevated for a diabetic (goal is <135/85 mm Hg), candidal vaginitis, and possibly candidal skin infection under her breasts

◆ **Diagnostic studies:** Blood glucose measurement (random sugar can be checked in the office with a fingerstick sample); follow-up testing should include electrolytes, blood urea nitrogen (BUN), creatinine, fasting lipids, urine microalbumin:creatinine ratio, and hemoglobin A_{1c}.

Analysis

Objectives

1. Know the diagnostic criteria for diabetes mellitus, including, signs and symptoms, physical findings, and diagnostic studies.
2. Know the pathophysiologic and epidemiologic differences between type 1 and type 2 diabetes mellitus.
3. Learn the treatment options for diabetic patients.
4. Be aware of the acute emergencies that can occur to diabetics and how to manage them.

Considerations

Diabetes mellitus is one of the most common medical problems encountered in medical practice. There are an estimated 17 million diabetics in the United States and the number is increasing both in the United States and worldwide. Diabetes affects all ethnic groups, but there is a disproportionate burden of disease in African-Americans, Native Americans, and Hispanics. The global epidemic of obesity has led to a dramatic increase in the number of type 2 diabetics presenting with disease in their teens and 20s.

The complications of diabetes are myriad. Diabetics are 6–10 times more likely than nondiabetics to be hospitalized for cardiovascular disease and 15 times more likely to be hospitalized for peripheral vascular diseases. It is the leading cause of blindness in working-age adults in the United States, most of which is preventable. It is also the leading cause for end-stage renal disease and non-traumatic amputations. In 1997, the direct and indirect cost related to diabetes mellitus was estimated to be $98 billion dollars.

Other complications that may be less well known to patients but that are attributable to diabetes include neuropathic, gastrointestinal, and immunologic changes. Peripheral neuropathy, leading to reduced sensation or pain, can lead to the development of ulcerations, infections, or injuries of the extremities. Gastroparesis can be a difficult-to-manage problem that makes diabetes more difficult to manage by impairing the patient's ability to eat properly. Immunologic changes make diabetics more prone to opportunistic infections, such as fungal skin or genitourinary infections.

Impaired glucose tolerance or frank diabetes may be present for years prior to the diagnosis of type 2 diabetes. In the case presented, the history of excessive weight gain during pregnancy with a large baby and cautions on watching her diet may be a sign of a history of gestational diabetes. Women with gestational diabetes have an increased risk of developing nongestational diabetes.

As in the case presented, difficult-to-treat or recurrent fungal infections may be the initial presentation that leads to the diagnosis of diabetes. This patient has both vaginal and skin infections. Although, in this case, the diagnosis is diabetes, other immune deficiency states must be considered when recurrent fungal infections are found. In the appropriate setting, HIV or other immunosuppressive conditions must be considered.

The symptom of polyuria should also lead to an increased suspicion for diabetes. High serum glucose levels function as an osmotic diuretic, resulting in frequent urination. This is often associated with polydipsia, a state of extreme thirst. Patients with type 1 diabetes also may present with polyphagia. Their lack of insulin prevents their food intake from being appropriately metabolized, resulting in a state of hunger for which they will frequently eat but not feel sated.

The absence of glucose in the urine dipstick does not exclude the diagnosis and should not delay a blood glucose measurement. Glucosuria occurs when the blood glucose level is greater than a renal "threshold" level, above which the glucose will spill into the urine. The lack of glucosuria only shows that the blood sugar level is not above this threshold level. Overt signs of insulin resistance (acanthosis nigricans, elevated blood pressure, obesity) also make the diagnosis of type 2 diabetes more likely.

APPROACH TO DIABETES MELLITUS

Definitions

DCCT: Diabetes Control and Complications Trial, a large, prospective, randomized controlled study of the advantages and disadvantages of "tight" versus "loose" diabetic control in type 1 diabetes.

UKPDS: United Kingdom Prospective Diabetes Study, a large, prospective, randomized controlled study of interventions and outcomes in type 2 diabetes.

Clinical Approach

Diabetes mellitus is a general term for several different diseases that result in high blood sugar levels and that eventually lead to microvascular and macrovascular complications. The major classifications of diabetes mellitus are type 1 diabetes, type 2 diabetes, and gestational diabetes.

Type 1 diabetes (previously called juvenile diabetes, juvenile-onset diabetes mellitus [JODM] or insulin-dependent diabetes mellitus [IDDM]) results from destruction of insulin-producing pancreatic β cells. This destruction was previous thought to be viral related and to occur acutely. Recent studies indicate that there may be islet-cell antibodies present for years prior to the development of overt type 1 diabetes. Following the initial presentation, there may be a "honeymoon" period where there are still some functioning β cells that produce insulin. Eventually, there is a total loss of the production of insulin. This type of diabetes has a point mutation at HLA-DQ with increased DR3- and DR4-positive karyotypes. These individuals tend to manifest before their fourth decade.

Because of the lack of insulin, which is required for the metabolism of glucose, type 1 diabetics are prone to metabolize fats, with the resultant production of ketones. An extreme result of this process is **diabetic ketoacidosis,** a syndrome characterized by hyperglycemia, high levels of serum acetone, and an anion gap metabolic acidosis. This often occurs during times of physical stress, such as an infection or myocardial infarction, or when the patient does not use his or her insulin. Diabetic ketoacidosis is a medical emergency, requiring hospitalization, careful insulin management, correction of acidosis and electrolyte disturbances, and evaluation for the underlying cause of the condition.

Type 2 diabetes (previously called adult onset diabetes mellitus [AODM], non–insulin-dependent diabetes mellitus [NIDDM]) patients, in contrast to type 1 diabetics, in whom there is a lack of insulin, are typically hyperinsulinemic. Their disease results primarily from insulin resistance in the peripheral tissue and this resistance is often related to obesity. Type 2 diabetics often manifest signs of insulin resistance for many years prior to the diagnosis of overt diabetes. This type accounts for at least 90% of the diagnosed cases, and virtually all undiagnosed diabetes, in the United States.

Type 2 diabetes has a stronger familial predisposition than type 1. Type 2 diabetics often have a family history of the disease. The genetic factors are multifactorial and have not been identified. It is strongly associated with obesity and its complications: metabolic syndrome, hyperinsulinemia, hypertension, dyslipidemia, hyperglycemia, and central obesity.

Uncontrolled type 2 diabetics can achieve extremely high blood sugars without developing ketosis and acidosis. This type is more prone to hyperosmolar states because of the high blood sugar levels. **Nonketotic hyperosmolar syndrome** occurs when blood sugar levels become highly elevated, often approaching 1000 mg/dL. This may be the presenting symptom of type 2 diabetes, or may result from an intercurrent illness or failure to take medications. The serum osmolarity is elevated and the patient has a large fluid deficit. In severe cases, coma or death can occur. This can be managed with hospitalization, rehydration, treatment of underlying illnesses, and, sometimes, the judicious use of insulin to overcome the acute glucose toxicity.

Gestational diabetes occurs in 3–10% of all pregnancies. Typically, women have 50% more insulin in their third trimester. Gestational diabetes is triggered by increased insulin resistance caused by elevated chorionic somatomammotropin, progesterone, and estrogens. Women with gestational diabetes are more prone to develop non–pregnancy-related type 2 diabetes and should be screened with a glucose tolerance test postpartum.

Risk factors for gestational diabetes include age older than 25 years, member of a high-incidence racial group (Native American, African-American, Hispanic American, South or East Asian, Pacific Islander), body mass index ≥25, history of glucose intolerance, previous history of gestational diabetes, and history of diabetes in a first-degree family member. The American College of Obstetricians and Gynecologists recommends screening all women for gestational diabetes at 24–28 weeks' gestation, except for women who have no risk factors. Gestational diabetes is treated with careful diet management and, when necessary, insulin.

Diagnosis

The diagnostic criteria for diabetes are:

1. A random glucose ≥200 mg/dL along with classic symptoms that include polydipsia, polyuria, polyphagia, frequent infections and weight loss;
2. A fasting glucose >125 mg/dL on at least 2 occasions; and
3. A 2-hour plasma glucose ≥200 mg/dL after a 75-g glucose load.

Glycosylated hemoglobin or hemoglobin A_{1c} (HGA_{1c}) is not recommended for diagnosis. This test is used to estimate the average glucose over the past 3 months in those who are diagnosed with diabetes. Measurement of C-peptide and insulin levels can be used to distinguish type 2 from type 1 diabetes when the history, physical examination, and other tests, such as serum ketones and osmolality, are not enough. Other tests recommended by the American Diabetes Association are fasting lipid profiles (at the time of diagnosis and, at least, annually thereafter), serum creatinine, urinalysis, urine microalbumin:creatinine ratios (at time of diagnosis in type 2 diabetics and annually thereafter; in type 1 diabetics who have had disease for 5 years and annually thereafter), annual dilated eye examinations, regular foot examinations, EKG (in adults), and, in type 1 diabetics, thyroid disease screening with a thyroid-stimulating hormone (TSH).

Management

The treatment for type 1 diabetes involves the use of insulin. In most cases, combination therapy using a short-acting insulin prior to meals and an intermediate- or long-acting basal insulin is used. Insulin pump therapy, which provides a continuous subcutaneous infusion of short-acting insulin, is an alternative.

Insulin management requires careful and frequent self-monitoring of glucose, often with adjustment of insulin dosage based on the glucose levels, amount of physical activity, and caloric/carbohydrate intake (Table 51–1 summarizes some of the available insulin products).

Type 2 diabetics should be educated on the importance of diet and exercise as key components of their management. In some cases, that will be all that is needed to achieve appropriate control. An initial goal that is achievable by many is a 10% weight loss. When lifestyle changes alone do not result in adequate control, numerous oral agents are available.

Biguanides (metformin) act on the liver to **decrease glucose output during gluconeogenesis.** Secondary actions include improved insulin sensitivity in the liver and muscle and a hypothesized decrease in intestinal absorption of glucose. Metformin can lower the HGA_{1c} by 1.5–2%. The UKPDS showed a significant reduction in cardiovascular events, diabetes-related deaths, and all causes of mortality in those who used metformin. Other advantages include no potential hypoglycemia, reduced insulin levels, a potential weight loss, and a reduction in triglycerides and low-density lipoprotein (LDL) cholesterol. The efficacy, safety, and improved outcomes make it a popular first-line agent in type 2 diabetes.

The most common side effects are gastrointestinal, such as nausea and diarrhea. These side effects are reduced by starting with lower doses and giving the medication with meals. The more dangerous side effect is the development of lactic acidosis. The risk of this potentially fatal side effect is increased by renal insufficiency. Metformin use is contraindicated in those with a creatinine >1.5 mg/dL, hepatic insufficiency, or congestive heart failure. It is Category B

Table 51–1
INSULIN PREPARATIONS

TYPE OF INSULIN	ONSET OF ACTION	PEAK OF ACTION	DURATION OF ACTION
Rapid acting (lispro or aspart insulin)	15 minutes	30–90 minutes	3–5 hours
Short acting (regular insulin)	30–60 minutes	60–120 minutes	5–8 hours
Intermediate acting (neural protamine hagedorn [NPH] insulin)	1–3 hours	7–15 hours	18–24 hours
Long acting (glargine insulin)	1 hour	None	24 hours

Source: Information from U.S. Food and Drug Administration. Available at: www.fda.gov/fdac/features/2002/chrt_insulin.html

in pregnancy and contraindicated in nursing mothers. It is the oral agent of choice in type 2 diabetes in children older than age 10 years.

Sulfonylureas were the first oral agents available for type 2 diabetes. Their principal action is to function as **insulin secretagogues** that stimulate β cells in the pancreas to secrete insulin. Advantages include a potential 2% reduction in HGA$_{1c}$, once- or twice-a-day dosing, and relatively low cost. Disadvantages are poor response in 20% of patients, a tendency of the users to gain weight, and a tendency for the medications to lose effectiveness over time. As insulin secretagogues, sulfonylureas carry a risk of causing hypoglycemia.

The principal action of **thiazolidinediones** (TZDs) is **improving insulin sensitivity in muscle and adipose tissue.** Secondary actions are decreased hepatic gluconeogenesis and increased peripheral glucose utilization. Among their advantages is a decrease in triglyceride and increase in high-density lipoprotein (HDL) cholesterol levels. Because they are metabolized in the liver, they can be used in patients with renal impairment. They also do not, when used by themselves, cause hypoglycemia. Disadvantages include a slight increase in LDL cholesterol, weight gain, and a slow onset of action. These agents may take up to 12 weeks to fully become effective. They cause water retention, which is of concern with renal compromise and congestive heart failure. TZDs may be used by themselves, but are often used as adjuncts with sulfonylureas or insulin.

Meglitinides are **short-acting secretagogues** that increase insulin secretion from the pancreas. These medications are taken no more than 1 hour before meals because of the rapid onset and short duration of action. They are useful in patients whose blood sugars vary at mealtime but who have controlled fasting glucose levels. They reduce HGA$_{1c}$ levels from 0.5–2%. The disadvantages include a risk of hypoglycemia (especially if the medication is taken but no meal is then eaten) and expense. They should not be used in patients with hepatic dysfunction.

α-Glucosidase inhibitors delay carbohydrate absorption by inhibiting α-glucosidase in the small intestine, which decreases postprandial hyperglycemia. They reduce HGA$_{1c}$ levels by 0.7–1.0%. This class of medication may offer benefits to patients with erratic eating habits, as hypoglycemia will not occur if meals are skipped. The principal side effects are GI, including flatulence. These medications are contraindicated in ketoacidosis and in hepatic disorders.

The goal of diabetic management is to safely lower the blood sugar so as to reduce the risk of macrovascular and microvascular complications. Both the UKPDS and DCCT showed lower rates of complications in controlled diabetes. The goal of treatment is to achieve a HGA$_{1c}$ of less than 7%, although some authorities are now advocating 6.5% as a goal. Goal fasting blood sugar is <120 mg/dL and 2-hour postprandial sugar is <140 mg/dL.

Other treatments are equally important to tight glucose control in the effort to reduce adverse events, such as heart attacks and strokes. The UKPDS clearly showed that tight blood pressure control is effective in reducing cardiovascular events. The blood pressure goal in diabetes is <135/85 mm Hg. Diabetes is considered a coronary heart disease risk equivalent for decisions regarding lipid management. The goal LDL cholesterol level is <100 mg/dL. All diabetics should be advised to be immunized with the pneumococcal vaccine and to get annual influenza vaccination.

Management of Hypoglycemia

Hypoglycemia can cause the symptoms of sweating, tachycardia, nausea, headache, confusion, and even coma. When hypoglycemia is suspected and the patient is conscious and cooperative, juice, soda, candy, or some other sugar-containing product can rapidly alleviate the symptoms. If the person is not able to take something by mouth, rapid administration of IM glucagon can be effective. In a hospital setting, or when IV access is available, an injection of 50% dextrose (D_{50}) rapidly corrects the problem. Following any of these therapies, the patient should be closely watched, as the hypoglycemia may recur (especially if the patient uses a long-acting insulin or oral hypoglycemic agent).

Comprehension Questions

[51.1] Which of the following test results is diagnostic of diabetes mellitus?

  A. Single fasting glucose of 150 mg/dL
  B. A 2-hour oral glucose tolerance test greater than 200 mg/dL with a 100-g glucose load
  C. A random glucose greater than 200 mg/dL with symptoms such as polydipsia or polyuria
  D. A HGA_{1c} greater than 7.5%

[51.2] A 7-year-old is brought to the office with symptoms of polydipsia, polyphagia, polyuria, and weight loss. For the past 24 hours he has had abdominal pain and vomiting. Urinalysis done in the office shows the presence of glucose and ketones. A fingerstick blood glucose is >500 mg/dL. Which of the following is the most appropriate management?

  A. Prescription for oral metformin and referral to a nutritionist
  B. Hospitalization with institution of insulin and IV fluids
  C. Prescription for insulin to be started at home, with follow-up in 24 hours
  D. Treatment for acute gastroenteritis and referral to an endocrinologist

[51.3] Which of the following classes of medications has the lowest incidence of causing hypoglycemia when given as single-agent therapy?

  A. Biguanide
  B. Insulin
  C. Sulfonylurea
  D. Meglitinide

Answers

[51.1] **C.** Diabetes mellitus can be defined by two separate measurements of a fasting glucose >125 mg/dL; a random glucose ≥200 mg/dL with classic symptoms or a 2-hour glucose tolerance test of ≥200 mg/dL after a 75-g glucose load. HGA_{1c} should not be used in diagnosing diabetes.

[51.2] **B.** This is a typical presentation of diabetic ketoacidosis, a medical emergency. This is a not uncommon initial presentation of type 1 diabetes. This child requires immediate hospitalization, IV fluids, and insulin.

[51.3] **A.** Biguanides (metformin) are effective medications for the treatment of type 2 diabetes; they do not cause hypoglycemia when given as monotherapy. Insulin and insulin secretagogues carry a significant risk of hypoglycemia as a complication of therapy.

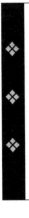

CLINICAL PEARLS

❖ Diabetes is one of the most common diseases in clinical practice. The criteria for diagnosis have been lowered to decrease complications, including death.

❖ Type 2 diabetes accounts for more than 90% all diabetes in the United States. The increasing presence of obesity is, unfortunately, driving the incidence of type 2 diabetes even higher.

❖ Biguanides are gaining favor in the treatment of type 2 diabetes because of their potency and demonstrated reduction in morbidity and mortality.

REFERENCES

American Diabetes Association. Standards of medical care for patients with diabetes mellitus. Diabetes Care 2002;25(Suppl 1):S33–S49.

Accessed online at: www. accessmedicine.com/resourceTOC. aspx?resourceID=4.

Isley WL, Oki J. Diabetes mellitus, type 2. 2005. Available at: http://www.emedicine.com /med/topic547.htm.

Knowler WC, Barret-Connor E, Fowler SE, et al. Reduction in the incident of type 2 diabetes with lifestyle intervention or metformin. N Engl J Med 2002;346: 393–403.

Kumar V, Fausto N, Abbas A. Robbins and Cotran pathologic basis of disease. 7th ed. Philadelphia: WB Saunders, 2004:1189–1205.

Lavis V, Hays L. Guidelines for treatment with insulin in the hospital. UT-Houston Endocrinology Dept. Insulin Administration Guide 2006. Available at: http/www.uth.tmc.edu/school/med/imed/endo/Insulin.

Powers A. Diabetes mellitus. In: Kasper DL, Braunwald E, Fauci AS, et al. (eds). Harrison's principles of internal medicine. 16th ed. New York: McGraw-Hill, 2005.

Schneider AS, Szanto PA. Pathology: board review series. 2nd ed. Baltimore: Lippincott Williams & Wilkins, 2001:352–355.

Tallia AF, Cardone DA, Ibsen KH, et al. Swanson's family practice review. 5th ed. St. Louis: CV Mosby, 2004:126–135, 700–702.

A 74-year-old African-American female enters your office with the complaint that she has been developing bruises all over her extremities for the last several days. She also has noticed that her stool seems to be a lot darker. She describes it looking almost like coffee grounds. She relocated to your area to live with her daughter after her home in New Orleans was destroyed several months ago. This is her initial visit to your office, as she had refills available for all of her medications and previously felt fine. Her past medical history is notable for being hypertensive, postmenopausal, having an irregular heartbeat that she doesn't remember the exact name for, and having a touch of diabetes and arthritis. Her prescribed medications are hydrochlorothiazide and warfarin. Her over-the-counter medications include aspirin which she started taking since moving to your city, a multivitamin, acetaminophen for her arthritis and ibuprofen for when her knees really bother her. She also admits to regularly drinking herbal teas.

◆ **What is the differential diagnosis for this patient's presentation?**

◆ **What diagnostic studies are indicated?**

◆ **Why are the elderly at increased risk for the development of adverse drug reactions?**

ANSWERS TO CASE 52: Adverse Drug Reactions and Interactions

Summary: A 74-year-old woman presents with easy bruising and dark stools for several days. She is new to your practice, but is on an antihypertensive medication and a blood thinner. She is also taking numerous over-the-counter medications.

◆ **Differential diagnosis:** Includes an adverse drug interaction involving her warfarin and the aspirin, nonsteroidal antiinflammatory drugs (NSAIDs) and acetaminophen that she is currently taking. Other (much less likely) possibilities include bleeding from a gastrointestinal malignancy, liver disease, or hematologic abnormality (acute leukemia).

◆ **Necessary diagnostic studies:** This patient should have a test for stool occult blood in the office, a stat complete blood count (CBC), a prothrombin time (PT) with international normalized ratio (INR), a metabolic panel, and an EKG. It would be appropriate to consider this patient for observation status in the hospital while her studies are pending.

◆ **Reasons for increased risk of drug reactions in the elderly:** Numerous issues, including polypharmacy, changes in renal and hepatic function, and pharmacodynamic considerations (change in body composition and volume of distribution) that develop with aging.

Analysis

Objectives

1. Understand the scope and risk of the problem of drug interactions and adverse effects.
2. Learn some mechanisms to reduce these risks.
3. Know why the elderly are particularly vulnerable to potential complications.

Considerations

The extensive use of medications—including prescribed, over-the-counter, herbal, and homeopathic products—makes adverse drug reactions and interactions a significant public health concern. A Harvard study revealed that **6.5% of hospital inpatients experienced a documented injury secondary to medications.** Because of physiologic changes and the use of multiple medications for multiple medical conditions, the elderly are at increased risk. **An estimated 3–11% of hospital admissions in the elderly are related to adverse drug reactions.**

The patient presented has numerous risks for the development of serious problems related to her medications. As noted before, her age alone is a risk.

The use of warfarin is another, as its use should be closely monitored. Having been on this medication while not under the care of a physician, after leaving New Orleans and prior to establishing care, is a danger in itself. Warfarin also has numerous drug–drug interactions, among them are an increased risk of bleeding with the concomitant use of aspirin, NSAIDs, or acetaminophen.

Because of her age, the presence of bruising (suggesting an increased PT from her medications), and the possibility of rectal bleeding, she should have a Hemoccult test done and she should be screened for anemia with a CBC. She should also have a PT with INR to evaluate her degree of anticoagulation and risk for ongoing hemorrhage. Because of her age and comorbid conditions, she should also have a metabolic panel to evaluate her glucose, electrolytes, and renal and liver functions, and an EKG to evaluate for signs of ischemia. With the possibility of significant abnormalities on these tests that may require urgent management, it would be reasonable to place her in observation status in the hospital for monitoring and treatment. Eventually, although probably not necessary in the acute setting, she would require a colonoscopy to ensure that there is not an underlying colorectal cancer contributing to her bleeding.

If she is found to have a prolonged PT, several therapeutic options are available, depending on the clinical situation and the magnitude of the abnormality. For mildly over-anticoagulated patients with no evidence of bleeding, temporary discontinuation of warfarin or dose reduction is often all that is needed. For more prolonged prothrombin times, vitamin K—given IM, IV, or PO along with stopping the warfarin—can correct most abnormalities within a few days. When the PT is very high, or if there is evidence of bleeding, replacement of coagulation factors with a transfusion of fresh-frozen plasma will rapidly reverse the coagulopathy.

APPROACH TO ADVERSE DRUG REACTIONS AND INTERACTIONS

Definition

Cytochrome P450 (CYP): A hepatic enzyme system that is composed of more than 20 isoenzymes, and which is responsible for the metabolism of numerous medications. The **CYP isoenzymes can be induced,** resulting in increased drug metabolism and reduced therapeutic benefit of a medication, **or blocked,** resulting in decreased drug metabolism and potential for drug toxicity.

Clinical Approach

Etiologies of Adverse Drug Effects

Side effects are defined as effects from drugs that are beyond their intended therapeutic scope. These effects may be either adverse or beneficial. Adverse side effects can range from minor nuisances, such as nausea or diarrhea, to severe or life-threatening, such as cardiac arrhythmias precipitated by antiar-rhythmic or stimulant medications. Other side effects have been found that are beneficial. For example, peripheral α-adrenergic blockers, initially used as antihypertensives, were found to alleviate obstructive symptoms from prostatic hyperplasia and are now widely used for this purpose. Another example is minoxidil, also an antihypertensive agent, which was found by some users to result in hair growth, so it is now marketed as an antibaldness treatment.

Drug interactions account for 5–10% of adverse reactions. Drug interactions may be caused by pharmacokinetic effects, resulting in a change in either the drug's concentration or the drug's effect. Some of these interactions may be predictable, as a consequence of chemical effects secondary to enzymatic effects, protein binding, renal and hepatic interactions, and pharmacodynamic interactions. Warfarin may interact with several other medications and dietary factors to increase the active form of this drug to toxic levels, resulting in over-anticoagulation with resultant bruising and hemorrhage.

Drugs also may have additive effects caused by using two or more agents designed to produce a similar outcome working synergistically. An example of this is using a β-adrenergic blocking agent with certain calcium channel blockers (diltiazem, verapamil). Both medications can decrease heart rate but by different mechanisms of action. Combining the two may result in profound bradycardia and hypotension.

Other **interactions may be more directly related to the chemical characteristics** of the medications or the solutions in which they are delivered. For example, mixing glargine insulin with other insulin types in the same syringe may result in precipitation of the insulin product, rendering them ineffective. Similarly, some IV medications must be administered individually while others can be combined.

Drug Metabolism

Many drugs are metabolized in the liver. **Medications with a high first-pass hepatic clearance may be particularly susceptible to adverse events caused by alterations in hepatic metabolism.** Diseases that change the effective circulatory volume, such as congestive heart failure, may also alter the rate of drug or metabolite elimination because of the effects on hepatic and renal blood flow.

The CYP system plays a significant role in many real or potential adverse drug events. Although more than 20 CYP isoenzymes have been identified, 6 of these isoenzymes have been found to account for most of the clinically significant interactions.

CYP1A2 is induced by tobacco. Drugs that depend on the 1A2 isoenzyme include theophylline and imipramine. Consequently, smokers who use these medications may have increased metabolism and decreased clinical effect. Similarly, drugs that decrease this enzyme form, such as ciprofloxacin, will decrease drug metabolism and result in higher effective drug levels.

CYP2C9, CYP2D6, and CYP2C19 have evidence of genetic polymorphism. This can result in different individuals having different rates of metabolism. As an example, certain individual users of warfarin may have higher effective plasma levels of the drug and a longer period to achieve steady states because of an increased half-life for this drug as a result of decreased metabolism by CY2C9.

Alcohol has effects on the 2E1 isoenzyme. This isoenzyme can produce a hepatotoxic metabolite of acetaminophen. Because of this, the use of alcohol and acetaminophen is dangerous and an acetaminophen overdose, which is already potentially toxic to the liver, is made worse if mixed with alcohol.

Drugs that have a significant first-pass effect may have an effect on metabolism in the liver or absorption in the intestine. For example, increased levels of the 3A isoenzyme may result in alterations in the level, and therefore therapeutic effect, of cyclosporine.

Competition for enzyme binding also may result in an effect on the metabolism of certain medications. Warfarin competes with antifungal medication fluconazole for metabolism by the CYP system. This may result in reduced warfarin metabolism and may result in over-anticoagulation.

Many drugs are albumin bound. When multiple agents are competing for the same albumin binding sites, there is a potential to have greater amounts of unbound medication, resulting in higher circulating free drug levels. This causes particular concern for drugs that have a smaller volume of distribution, rapid onset of action or narrow therapeutic index.

Renal considerations are related to interaction of drugs at renal sites and decreased renal function. Renal interactions are often a result of alterations in the elimination of water-soluble drugs because of competition for the renal tubular system. These effects may be either positive or negative. An example of the beneficial effect of this is the concomitant administration of probenecid with penicillin. Probenecid decreases renal excretion of penicillin, resulting in an increased level and therapeutic effect of the antibiotic.

Other renal considerations include decreased kidney function secondary to either disease processes, such as hypertension or diabetes, or from the natural decline in renal function that occurs with aging. Many medications have recommendations for alteration in dosing amount or interval based upon the patient's creatinine clearance. Creatinine is a product of muscle and the elderly may have falsely elevated calculated creatinine clearance rates because they have decreased muscle mass. Creatinine clearance can be estimated using the following equation:

Creatinine clearance

$$= \frac{[(140 - \text{age}) \times (\text{ideal body weight in kg})] (\times 0.85 \text{ for women})}{72 \times \text{serum creatinine (mg/dL)}}$$

Interventions to Reduce the Risk of Adverse Drug Events

There are many possible interventions to reduce the risk of adverse drug events or interactions, especially in the older population, including the following:

- Only prescribe those medications that are clearly indicated. However, do not avoid a necessary medication.
- Obtain a history of adverse events related to medications on all patients.

- Maintain a list of all medications that a patient is taking, including pre-scribed, over-the-counter, herbal, and homeopathic. Update this list at every visit.
- Instruct your patients to bring in **all** of their medications regularly to make sure your medication list is accurate.
- Routinely perform drug interaction surveys on patients taking multiple medications. There are computerized tools available to perform these sur-veys, including several personal digital assistant (PDA)-based products.
- Have knowledge of renal, hepatic, and circulatory issues that affect your patients.
- Consider issues related to individual patients, such as unique genetic or racial factors.
- Document and report suspected adverse drug effects.

Comprehension Questions

[52.1] A 62-year-old man is prescribed a new medication. He is warned not to drink alcohol because this medication may result in the production of a hepatotoxic metabolite. Which of the following is the most likely agent?

A. Warfarin
B. Aspirin
C. Acetaminophen
D. Carafate

[52.2] Which of the following factors is most likely to increase the risk of adverse drug reactions in the elderly?

A. Increased glomerular filtration rate
B. Polypharmacy
C. Inability to open medicine containers
D. Increased hepatic blood flow

[52.3] A 63-year-old female patient has been reading on the Internet about the dangers of medicine interactions and adverse side effects. In your coun-seling of the patient, which of the following statements is most accurate?

A. All drug interactions are inherently dangerous.
B. All medication side effects are, by definition, adverse.
C. The primary goal of medication therapy is to eliminate all side effects.
D. Some medication side effects can be beneficial to patients.

Answers

[52.1] **C.** Alcohol induces a specific CYP isoenzyme that results in the production of a hepatotoxic metabolite of acetaminophen.

[52.2] **B.** A multitude of factors result in the elderly being particularly vulnerable to adverse drug events. Included among these are polypharmacy, decreased renal and hepatic function, and pharmacokinetic and pharmacodynamic considerations.

[52.3] **D.** Some medication side effects have turned out to be beneficial to patients, such as increased hair growth with minoxidil or relief of obstructive symptoms in patients with prostatic hypertrophy who use α-adrenergic blocking agents. The goal of medication therapy should be to maximize therapeutic benefit and minimize adverse effects or risks as safely as possible.

CLINICAL PEARLS

❖ Along with the biochemical changes that occur with aging, several physical conditions may also affect medication compliance. Arthritic patients may have difficulty opening prescription caps (especially childproof caps). Reduced vision may interfere with the ability to properly use a medication. Memory difficulties may cause trouble adhering to regimens involving multiple medications. All of these factors, and many others, need to be considered when prescribing medications to the elderly.

REFERENCES

Brunton LL (ed). Goodman and Gillman's the pharmacological basis of therapeutics. 11th ed. New York: McGraw-Hill, 2006.
Taylor RB (ed). Fundamentals of family medicine: the family medicine clerkship textbook. 3rd ed. New York: Springer-Verlag, 2003.

SECTION III

Listing of Cases

Listing by Case Number

Listing by Disorder (Alphabetical)

LISTING BY CASE NUMBER

LISTING BY DISORDER (ALPHABETICAL)

❖ INDEX

Note: Page numbers followed by *f* or *t* indicate figures or tables, respectively.